Here is an essential interdisciplinary reference book that brings together the most significant current research in problems of development and aging from a variety of fields. Distinguished investigators including immunologists, pathologists, cell biologists, and workers in related areas report their most recent theories and findings. Their explorations demonstrate the intimate interconnections among the processes of development, differentiation, and aging.

Comprehensive in scope, the work dynamically investigates the molecular, genetic, and cellular levels as well as organ systems and homeostasis. Particular emphasis is focused on:

- ontogeny of the immune response
- differentiation of immunologically committed cells
- aging of immune response

An important discussion of some of the sociological implications of aging is included. This volume answers the need for a thorough, up-to-date resource for the many students and professionals whose work brings them into contact with the aging process.

BIOLOGY OF AGING AND DEVELOPMENT

FASEB MONOGRAPHS

General Editor: KARL F. HEUMANN

A Continuation Order Plan is available for this series. A continuation order will bring delivery of each new volume immediately upon publication. Volumes are billed only upon actual shipment. For further information please contact the publisher.

BIOLOGY OF AGING AND DEVELOPMENT

Edited by
G. Jeanette Thorbecke
New York University School of Medicine

FASEB, Bethesda
PLENUM PRESS, New York and London

Library of Congress Cataloging in Publication Data

Main entry under title:

Biology of aging and development.

(FASEB monographs; v. 3)
Originally published in Federation proceedings, v. 34, no. 1-2, 1975.
Includes bibliographies and index.
1. Aging—Congresses. 2. Developmental biology—Congresses. I. Thorbecke,
G. Jeanette. II. Series: II. Federation of American Societies for Experimental
Biology. FASEB monographs; v. 3. [DNLM: 1. Aging—Congresses. W1 F202/
WT104 B615 1974]

QP86.B52   612.6'7   75-34295
ISBN 0-306-34503-X

The material in this book originally appeared in *Federation Proceedings*
Vol. 34, No. 1, January 1975 and No. 2, February 1975. First published in the
present form by Plenum Publishing Corporation in 1975.

Plenum Press, New York is a Division of Plenum Publishing Corporation
227 West 17th Street, New York, N.Y. 10011

United Kingdom edition published by Plenum Press, London
A Division of Plenum Publishing Company, Ltd.
Davis House (4th Floor), 8 Scrubs Lane, Harlesden, London, NW10 6SE, England

Printed in the United States of America

Contents

SESSION III
FINITE VERSUS INFINITE PROLIFERATIVE AND FUNCTIONAL CAPACITIES OF CELLS

SESSION IV
AGING OF HOMEOSTATIC CONTROL SYSTEMS

Contents

Introduction

One of the reasons for all the FASEB Societies to meet yearly is the possibility to interrelate recent progress in diverse areas of research. The FASEB Conferences have been organized to promote such interdisciplinary approaches. They center around a basic theme with the aim of discussing active research, including widely divergent approaches, towards a better understanding of a general biological phenomenon.

Because of the mounting interest in the subject of aging and development, this has been chosen as the theme for this year's symposia. We have necessarily been limited in the number of topics that could be covered. In our choice we have attempted to select those facets of the main subject which at this time are generating active research interest among our membership.

We have included invited speakers from abroad, such as Drs. Goldstein, Liew and Miller from Canada and Drs. Wolpert, Holliday and Williamson from England. I am sorry to say that the two speakers that we had invited from Russia, Dr. Frolkis, and from Czechoslovakia, Dr. Sterzl, were unable to attend.

The first symposium, to be chaired by Dr. Leslie Orgel, will highlight current theories in development and aging, as well as sociological aspects of aging. The second conference, for which Dr. Michael Potter is chairman, concerns some genetic aspects of development using various intriguing phenomena of the immune response as models. The mystery of the eternal life of certain cell lines is the topic of the third conference, which has been organized by Dr. Leonard Hayflick. Aging of homeostatic control systems will be considered in the next session, chaired by Dr. Paola Timiras, and in the fifth symposium we turn to the lymphoid tissue and its cell populations for development and aging at the organ level with Dr. William Paul as our chairman. In the final, sixth, conference Dr. Hamish Munro will preside over a program concerning development and aging at the molecular level.

G. J. THORBECKE, *Conference Chairman*
New York University Medical Center

1

Implications of aging research for society

BERNARD L. STREHLER

Neurophysiology Laboratory
Veterans Administration Hospital
Martinez, California 91553[1]

The success, until now, of the human species in controlling the resources of this planet for its own benefit is based on two features unique to man. The first of these is a brain capable of assimilating experience in memory, organizing such experience into abstract categories, making predictions based on regularities in nature, inventing structures (machines and societies) that have modified nature in man's interest, and finally the communication of subjective experience between members of the species symbolically through written and spoken languages. The second uniquely human feature is a sufficiently long life-span to make the above-mentioned qualities of the human brain useful. We are the longest lived of the highly evolved animals.

These two evolved properties go hand in hand, for there would be little evolutionary value to a brain capable of storing decades of experience and manipulating this data logically if there were insufficient longevity to use this mental ability; conversely, a relatively puny body unprotected by the brain's predictive and inventive powers would not survive even to reproductive maturity. Long-lived tortoises can hide within their armor; longevous birds (usually predators) can fly above their natural enemies, and ancient bristlecone pines tower over competing species for nourishment, resist insects with toxic oils and outlive fires with thick slow-burning bark. But man dominates through wit and inventiveness.

Not the least of man's inventions is the system of arriving at understanding of general rules of nature, science, whose application has made possible industrial societies and tentative probings of outer space and the inner mind. In view of the revolutionary events of the first three quarters of this century, it would not be surprising to witness, during the

[1] Sabbatical year address. Present address: Department of Biological Sciences, Univ. of Southern California, Los Angeles, CA 90007.

3

last quarter, the conquest of the two most perplexing puzzles: 1) the nature of the neural processes that give rise to the sense of self, and 2) the molecular-cellular bases of the slow decline that returns dust to dust. Unless the aging process differs in some mysterious and totally unforeseen way from other puzzles man has solved in the past, it is essentially inevitable that he will, before long, understand aging's sources, and with that understanding will come a considerable measure of control. The effects on the individual and society of that control will be even more pervasive than the revolutions that followed the invention of modern democracy, the steam and internal combustion engines, means to generate and distribute electricity, the transistor, nuclear reactors, digital computers, and the understanding of DNA—most of which were fathered in our country.

EFFECT DOMAINS OF GERONTOGENY

Societies are often not ready for scientific windfalls. What predictions, possibilities, and problems will societies encounter when the age-old puzzle yields? Some are easily foreseen; others can only be fantasized.

Gerontogeny is defined here as the development of means to achieve an enhanced healthy longevity. Its effects in various domains of life will depend on the degree of such life extension, which cannot be predicted on a sound basis until more is understood of the basic process itself.

The duration of life depends on the interaction of two variables; the effects of environment, and the intrinsic changes that occur during aging within a living system. Essentially all of the increase in life duration that has occured during the 20th century is due to an improved environment, particularly in the public health and pharmaceutical domains. Figure 1 shows the general trend in survivorship curves that has occurred in the last 100 years. It can generally be described as an asymptotic approach to the so-called "rectangular" survival curve. Assuming uniform genetic qualities a species will approach a rectangular survivorship curve as its environment improves. In the extreme case, for a genetically homogenous population living in a homogeneous environment, all individuals would die at precisely the same maximum age, like a myriad of "wonderful one-horse shays".

In heterogeneous populations, such as the human species, different maximum longevities are to be expected even in ideal environments, because different genetic endowments will lead to death from different inherent defects at different times. Figure 2 shows the compound rectangular survivorship that presently exists. The light lines represent different genetically limited rectangular curves, the heavy line the average curve produced by such heterogeneity. Figure 3 depicts the shape of survivorship curves if genetic defects could be compensated for through "heroic" measures such as the hoped for conquest of cardiovascular disease, cancer, and the like. It also shows what would occur if the intrinsic rate of aging were retarded to 90%, 75% and 50% of its present rate, the first two probably within reach in our lifetimes. In the remainder of this presentation the middle figure, a 25% reduction in the rate of aging, will be used as a basis for the anticipation of effects of aging research on society within the lifetimes of those now approaching adulthood.

Domain 1: Physical health

There is no way to increase longevity in an hospitable environment except

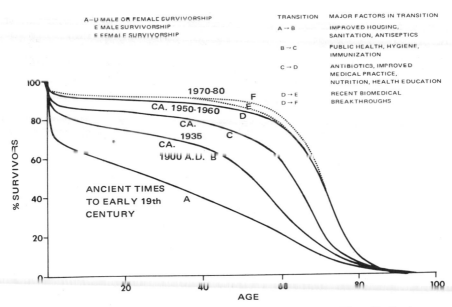

Figure 1. Human survivorship trends from ancient times to the present. These idealized curves illustrate the rapid approach to the limiting rectangular curve that has occurred during the last 150 years. The inset on the upper right lists major factors responsible for these transitions. Note that life expectancy for males has not changed since 1950 in the 50+ age group but that female survivorship has improved during this period, partially, at least, because of better treatment of reproductive system malignancies.

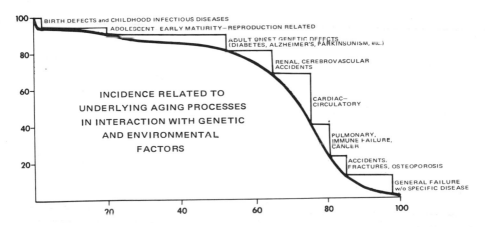

Figure 2. Composite origins of present rectangular survivorship curve in the U.S. Genetic predispositions to specific causes of death express themselves during different epochs of the total life span; the expression of these qualities appears to derive in considerable part from a general deterioration in a variety of structures and functions that has as its common denominator poorly understood "basic" aging processes. Among these the most important is a general decline in the rate at which reparative-homeostatic processes can proceed maximally. One common denominator may be the gradual loss of rDNA recently reported by Johnson et al. in post-mitotic cells.

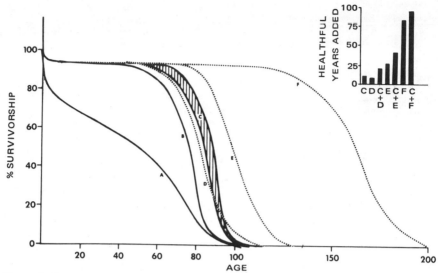

Figure 3. Past, present and potential human survivorship curves. *A*) ancient times to early 19th century. *B*) present survivorship curve. *C*) range of curves to be expected if the "major killers" were conquered (circulatory and neoplastic diseases). The basic reason that such conquest, the major direction of present biomedical research investment, would produce such a relatively minor change in survivorship derives from the fact that deaths due to "accidents," a measure of general homeostatic capacity, cause the same rate of death at about age 84 as do *all causes of death*, including the major killers, at age 68–72. Thus, a 15-year increment in longevity is the maximum to be expected from such research unless a retardation of aging is included in the therapeutic measures developed. *D*) survivorship that would derive from an 8–12% decrement in rate of aging, possibly derivable from pharmaceutical, dietary and immunological manipulations. *E*) hypothetical survivorship produced by a 20–30% decrease in rate of aging, potentially attainable through a 2–4 C decrease in body temperature. *F*) longer range hypothetical survivorship potentially derivable from a combination of factors in curves *D* and *E* plus means for reinstituting repressed gene functions and/or reinsertion of deleted portions of the genome. The basic conclusion to be derived from this graph is that an adequate investment in basic studies of the aging processes' origins, coupled with appropriate therapeutic measures should produce benefits in terms of added healthful and productive years far in excess of those to be expected from the major lines of biomedical research investment that exist today.

by improving the health state at all post-mature ages. Increased longevity, due to a retardation of the aging processes, will thus inevitably improve the health status of all age groups after age 21. (In the absence of aging the longevity of newly mature 21-year olds would exceed 2,000 years.)

Professional pessimists can take little comfort from their predictions of a society populated by ancient, wrinkled, toothless, decrepit, incontinent, mindless, Dorian Gray-like bodies, for such will not exist. It will take about as long to go through a terminal illness at age 150 as it does at 65 today. The real effect will be to increase the total number of years an individual spends in a healthful, and hopefully productive, state.

Domain 2: Mental health

Because we are the species most blessed (or cursed?) with the ability to predict the future, we are incapable of ignoring, in our innermost selves, the fact of our own impermanence. As a rule this awareness is suppressed or consciously ignored, like most unpleasant realities. But the ultimate reality is no less real than the April 15th income tax form. Although no one seems to have made a study of the effect of the individual's impermanence on this earth as a contributing factor to mental anguish and disease, one suspects that it is at least as important as many childhood hurts, insufficient self-esteem, marital incompatibility, impotence, frustrations in career fulfillments, and so on as a lingering source of mental disquietude and illness. It is accordingly more than likely that the postponement of aging's infirmities will decrease the incidence of mental disease and postpone the occurrence of age-related mental illness, e.g., depression.

Domain 3: Social effects

Biologists are not professionally schooled in such nebulous subjects as the intricacies of social forces. At best we are speculative spectators who are as confused by the premises, methods and predictions of social scientists as they themselves sometimes seem to be. Nevertheless, there are some rather obvious societal consequences of greatly increased life-spans. These range from poly-generational families to a decrease in intergenerational conflicts. It can be argued that much of the social upheaval of the last decade in the United States resulted from a disproportionate number of persons in the young adult category. Even today there is evidence of a changing emphasis as the postwar baby boom dies away. Enrollments in primary schools are decreasing; there is a surplus of teachers; in the next decade the population implosion will reach academia,

with uncertain results. The extension of the average life-span to 100 or 125 will make five-generation families a commonplace. Moreover, these concurrent generations will have much more in common than do the three-generation families that now exist. The average chronological age will be about 60, though the average physical state will be about 35–40.

The greatest benefit of such a social restructuring will be a greater sense of coherence and continuity in society, for the great preponderence of individuals will be in the productive, post-mature years, and the understandable conflicts that arise between the providers and the receivers in society should fade materially into the background. A potential danger than cannot be ignored is that the innovativeness of youth will be smothered by more established age groupings. It would be more than unfortunate if the blessing of increased healthful longevity were to be mixed with social inflexibility. On the other side of the ledger is the fact that a longer exposure to life permits a broader perspective among the more experienced — usually referred to as the "wisdom" that accompanies age.

Related to the above is the problem of tenure in positions of power. It would be disastrous to vest power to fashion social practice and policy in the limited hands and minds of those who acquired it at chronological age 45 – a fact all too well understood by younger faculty and reaching the proportions of ironic comedy if a Stalin, a Mao, or even some domestic statesmen were to hold political power for 10 decades!!!

Domain 4: Economic effects and poly-careers

The most extreme changes in society that will result from substantial life extension are in the economic area.

The existing patterns and trends toward early retirement versus productive employment will doubtless require rethinking. In today's industrial-technological societies, an individual contributes about half of his lifetime to the production of goods and services. For professionals about 25 years of dependence (childhood, education, and so on) are spent before the "loan" begins to be repaid to the community. Assuming retirement at 60–65 and 10 years of life beyond that, just about 35 years are spend in "production." It is improbable that retirement at 65 followed by 40 to 140 years of retirement-community living will be tolerated either by the "work force" or those who have retired with the energy implicit in a mind and body equivalent to today's 35- to 40-year-old. This means, in effect, that retirement will be postponed until well after 80 to 100 years of age, a grim prospect for those whose joys and creativity are at the level of the Archie Bunker prototype.

An obvious solution, which may well ensue, is the expansion of leisure time at all ages, accompanied by multiple and successive careers. Today's biological limitations make it difficult for all except the gifted, daring or foolish to give up the security of an established career to develop a new career interest. But if one had four successive 25-year periods in which to develop different skills and expertise, no such limitation would need to exist. Compulsory retirement might well be from one career to another.

Certain professions, particularly medicine, would benefit from extended periods of practices beyond what is now possible. For an excellent physician, extended experience is almost as important as excellent training, for one has to see many different kinds of illness in order to recognize subtle symptoms, and this kind of expertise can only be acquired over an appreciable period of time. In no professional area does an extended life-span offer such a beneficial side effect as in medicine. The wisdom that accompanies age would, in this case at least, be highly useful to us all. Another benefit would derive from the actual costs per year of life of medical care. If, as described earlier, the effect of extending life-span is to add to the "healthy middle years," and terminal illnesses cost about what they do now, the average expenditure per person/year of life will be correspondingly less than it presently is—a positive economic fallout.

The greatest problem posed by an extended life-span is how to supply the economic needs of persons, assuming retirement at some age. If one, as a rule of thumb, accepts 70% of the income level in the preretirement years as adequate for the postretirement years (fewer expenses), it is clear that an individual must accumulate a retirement investment from which he could derive the above at the then-existent interest rates, after inflation. Thus, a retirement income of $20,000 per annum would require an investment of about $400,000 at a return of 5%, over and above inflationary erosion, and this assumes also that there would be no use of the accumulated capital during the retirement years. This would require about $5,000 per annum to be accumulated (investment plus interest) over an average 40-year working lifetime or alternatively, with interest, about $1,500 per annum for a 70-year working lifespan.

Obviously, the more one accumulates per year, the earlier one can retire at the above-mentioned $20,000. Or, alternatively, if one chooses to work for a more extended period the decrement in usable resources during the working period would be correspondingly less. At any rate, while the above calculations are based on today's rate of return from investment and ignore the justifiable subsidies from the public treasury that social security benefit increases represent, as well as their magnitude in the future, it is more than obvious that both the business (particularly insurance) sector and the public bodies that are parts of the equation should begin now, if not yesterday, to make projections for the future. To base investment, governmental or private, on today's lifespan is to ignore rather clear handwriting on the palace wall, and the dislocations of a retirement income crisis could make the 1974 energy crisis look like an afternoon tea.

One of the factors that should reduce the economic load implicit in the above is the fact that most persons thrive on some kind of creative activity, whether it is called "work" or not. This is why new avenues to successive careers should be prepared for by individuals and society. In the absence of ready means to develop new outlets and interests, the result will be ennui for all except the very few. Who would want to be chairman of a study section, the department, the board or even the Supreme Soviet for 100 years?

While undoubtedly the preceding discussion can at best be only an improbable approximation to what life will be like 35 to 100 years from now, the greatest enemy in this writer's opinion will not be insecurity, poor mental or physical health, or even anonymity. It will be ennui, boredom, and the destructiveness that follow in their wake.

TO REACH THE GOLDEN ERA

Why are all these biological and human possibilities not being pursued with the vigor and inventiveness their potential promises? The answer is perhaps a kind of societal senescence. Could those who control policy and funding for the necessary fundamental research needed to bring the reality within reach of those of us now alive themselves be ensnared in time's net? Is the parochial promotion of professional status and career the moon behind which a sun of understanding lies? Are the available funds so necessary for the pursuit of today's ephemeral problems that we stand blindfolded before a lovely unfolding landscape?

As my late friend, Leo Szilard, who was as captured by this possibility as he previously was by the potential for nuclear fission, observed: "There are times when I would like to shout 'Help!' but all that comes out is 'Ha'!" Hungarians are like that!

REFERENCES

Because so little substantive work has gone into the anticipation of this problem, the relevant bibliography is minimal. It includes:

COMFORT, A. *The Biology of Senescence.* Boston, Mass: Routledge & Kegan Paul, 1964.
PALMORE, E. (editor) *Prediction of Life Span.* Lexington, Mass: Heath Lexington, 1971.
ROSENFELD, A. *The Second Genesis.* Englewood Cliffs, N. J.: Prentice Hall, 1969.
STREHLER, B. *Time, Cells, and Aging.* New York: Academic, 1962.
STREHLER, B. Myth and fact. *Center Mag.* III (4): 1970.
WHEELER, H. The rise of the elders. *Sat. Rev.* Dec. 5, 1970.

Current theories of biological aging[1],[2]

LEONARD HAYFLICK

Department of Medical Microbiology

Stanford University School of Medicine

Stanford, California 94305

ABSTRACT

Several lines of evidence have led to the notion that biological aging occurs as a result of changes in information-containing molecules either at the genetic or epigenetic level. The error theory, the redundant message theory, the codon restriction theory, and the transcriptional event theory represent the major current conceptualizations of biological aging as held by most gerontologists. The finding that cultured normal human and animal cells undergo a finite number of population doublings in vitro has provided new insights into age changes at the cellular level. The number of mitotic events that cultured normal animal cells can undergo appears to be inversely related to the age of the donor. A direct proportionality exists, however, between the mean maximum life-span of a species and the number of population doublings that their cultured embryonic cells will undergo. The several biochemical decrements known to occur prior to the cessation of mitotic activity in vitro are thought to herald those manifestations of senescence seen in the whole animal. Yet to be explained is how those cell classes such as the germ plasm and continuously propagable cancer cells escape from the inevitability of biological aging.— HAYFLICK, L. Current theories of biological aging. *Federation Proc.* 34: 9–13, 1975.

There is probably no other area of biological inquiry that is underpinned by so many theories as is the science of gerontology. This is due not only to the lack of sufficient fundamental data in the field, but also to the manifestations of biological changes that with time affect almost all biological systems from the molecular level to the whole organism. My purpose in this short exposition will be less to inform readers of all of the existing theories

[1] From Session I, *Theoretical Concepts of Developmental and Age Changes,* of the FASEB Conference on *Biology of Development and Aging,* presented at the 58th Annual Meeting of the Federation of American Societies for Experimental Biology, Atlantic City, N. J., April 9, 1974.

[2] Supported in part by grant HD04004 from the National Institute of Child Health and Human Development, National Institutes of Health, Bethesda, Maryland.

than to initiate small insurrections in the realm of their convictions in one selected area of hypotheses bearing on the science of aging.

The theories of aging to be considered are those that impinge on the finite lifetime of cultured normal cells in vitro and transplanted normal cells in vivo. In 1961 we observed that normal diploid human fibroblasts have a finite ability to replicate in vitro (25) and in 1965 we showed that the population-doubling potential of these cells is inversely related to the age of the donor (19). We interpreted these findings to be a manifestation of aging at the cellular level. In subsequent years these observations have been amply confirmed and extended in many other laboratories (8, 18, 20–23, 26, 31, 35). There is now some evidence supporting the notion that the numbers of population doublings of cultured embryonic fibroblasts are directly proportional to the mean life-span of the species (Table 1).

If normal human fibroblasts are preserved at the sub-zero temperatures of liquid nitrogen (−196 C), the population doubling potential of these cells remains unchanged. For example, in the case of normal human diploid embryonic fibroblasts that, unpreserved, undergo 50 ± 10 population doublings in vitro, the cumula-

tive number of population doublings after resurrection from the cold is always within this range regardless of the population-doubling level reached when the cells were first preserved. That is, the sum of population doublings undergone by normal fetal human fibroblasts both before and after preservation is always equal to 50 ± 10 (19). One such widely studied cell population, called WI-38, has been held in liquid nitrogen for 12 years and the total pre- and post-preservation population doublings of 50 ± 10 have remained unaffected by time. This is the longest period that normal human somatic cells have been preserved at sub-zero temperatures.

During the past decade it has also been learned that as cultured normal human cells approach the end of their in vitro lifetime (Phase III), a number of biochemical decrements occur which herald the approaching loss of division capacity (9, 24, 28). We do not interpret the loss of division capacity to necessarily produce age changes in vivo but would suggest that the biochemical decrements, which occur well before the cessation of mitotic capability, are the salient variables that produce those manifestations of biological aging that are familiar to all of us in the whole animal.

It has also been learned in the past decade that the in vivo transplantation of normal tissues to young donor animals, followed after these hosts age by transplantation again to young donors, also reveals a finite capacity for cell replication (10, 14, 15, 29, 38, 46). Thus in vitro and in vivo findings appear to be compatible with the notion that normal human and animal cells are capable of only a finite number of mitotic events. Based on such observations we have suggested that these findings may be associated with aging at the cellular level and that further ex-

TABLE 1. The finite lifetime of cultured normal embryonic human and animal fibroblasts[a]

Species	Range of population doublings for cultured normal embryo fibroblasts	Mean maximum life-span in years
Galapagos tortoise	90–125	175 (?)
Man	40–60	110
Mink[b]	30–34	10
Chicken	15–35	30
Mouse	14–28	3.5

[a] Data from ref 25.   [b] Dr. David Porter, personal communication. Data from 20 embryos.

ploration of this phenomenon might throw light on the fundamental mechanisms underlying the biology of aging (19–23, 25).

Since biological aging is thought to emanate from changes commencing at the molecular level and then up to the level of the whole animal, theories based on changes occurring at each increasingly greater level of complexity have been advanced. If the modern notions of biological development are rooted in signals originating from information-containing molecules, then it would seem reasonable to attribute fundamental causes of aging to similar molecular events. It would seem, therefore, that although many age changes, like developmental processes, occur at complexities greater than those at the genetic or epigenetic level, then the root causes of senescence should have a genetic basis also. Or at the least, they must be the result of fundamental changes that occur in information-containing molecules. If this supposition is to be believed then those classes of theories of biological aging which are based on observations made at the supramolecular level (for example, organelle, cell, tissue, and organ changes) are not likely to yield information on those fundamental molecular events which are presumed to be the essential variables leading to manifestations of aging at all higher organizational levels.

It is for this reason that I have chosen to restrict this presentation to those theories of aging that depend on molecular changes at the genetic or epigenetic level.

ERROR THEORIES

In 1963, Orgel proposed a model for biological aging that was based on a decrease in the fidelity of protein synthesis (34). This notion was first postulated by Medvedev (32).

Protein synthesis involves two steps in which discrimination between related molecules occurs. A unique amino acid must be selected by each activating enzyme and this must be attached to the appropriate tRNA. A codon of messenger RNA must then pair with the anticodon of an appropriate tRNA. These processes are probably prone to a small degree of error. The fidelity of protein synthesis could also be decreased by errors in RNA synthesis (34, 35). A repetition of events such as these, in which errors in proteins occur, could result in a convergence to a stable value of errors or it would diverge. If the former were the case, aging would not occur. In the latter case the error frequency would eventually become great enough to impair cell function (35). Although Orgel originally maintained the latter possibility, he has now abandoned this position because it is possible that a protein-synthesizing system containing a small number of errors might be capable of synthesizing a new protein-synthesizing system containing fewer errors. It is more plausible that this is the case in view of evidence for the existence of enzymes capable of scavenging error-containing proteins (17). There is one case in *Neurospora* where direct evidence exists for protein error frequencies increasing to the point where cell death ensues (36). This "error-catastrophe" hypothesis is also supported by evidence obtained by Lewis and Holliday (30) who have shown that the accuracy of protein synthesis in Leu-5 in *Neurospora* falls when the mutant is shifted from 25 C to 35 C and then remains virtually constant. After about 70 hours cell aging occurs rapidly with a simultaneous increase in the thermostability of glutamic dehydrogenase and a concomitant dramatic drop in the specific activity of this enzyme.

It has also been recently conjectured (27) that it may not be possible to distinguish between contributions to cellular aging caused by errors in protein synthesis from those due to an accumulation of somatic mutations. Inaccurate protein synthesis may be indistinguishable from inaccurate DNA synthesis, and in that sense they may be coupled phenomena (35). The accuracy of both processes may be completely dependent on the fidelity of the other. Orgel now subscribes to this more general notion in which positive feedback occurs where "the greater the number of errors that have accumulated in the macromolecular constituents of the cell, the faster the accumulation of further errors" (35). It is also envisioned that extracellular and intracellular mechanisms of aging are coupled since inaccurate protein synthesis must affect extracellular events.

REDUNDANT MESSAGE THEORY

Medvedev is the chief proponent of a notion that has considerable merit as a fundamental theory of biological aging. He proposes that the selective repetitions of some definite genes, cistrons, operons, and other linear structures on the DNA molecule, the bulk of which are repressed, behave as redundant messages to be called into action when active genome messages become faulty (33). He argues that the total genome of mammals is composed of not less than 10^5 structural genes or cistrons, but that in each cell hardly more than 0.2–0.4% of this number are expressed during biological development and maturity. If 1/500 of all genes are active and 499/500 are specifically repressed, and if mutagenic factors act equally on the repressed and active cistrons, the mutation rate of repressed genes must

yield more mutations than those occurring in active genes. Medvedev asserts that different species' life-spans may be a function of the degree of repeated sequences. Long-lived species should then have more redundant message than short-lived species. As errors accumulate in functioning genes, reserve sequences containing the same information take over until the redundancy in the system is exhausted resulting in biological age changes. The differences in species' life-spans is then thought to be a manifestation of the degree of gene repetition (33). The suggestion of gene repetition as a universal mechanism for phylogenetic evolution in eukaryotes has, of course, been made (2–4).

Thus the phenomenon of linear repetition of some genes can have not only evolutionary, but also gerontological, implications where there occurs a protective role of gene repetition against random molecular accidents. Conceptually this has merit not only as an explanation for the wide differences found in the life-span of species but also for the less variable life-span of individual members within a species. A repeated nucleotide sequence simply has a greater chance of preserving intact the final gene product during evolution or during a long life-span than does any unique sequence. It follows, therefore, that if an accumulation of errors occurs in unique genes then age changes may result from this kind of event. Certainly not all unique genes would be expected to have equal value for cell function or maintenance of cell life. The really vital unique sequences are likely to be restricted to some universally important genes of general metabolism. They may represent the essential group of genes whose failure ultimately results in manifestations of biological aging. Medvedev prefers the view that the derepression of unique genes during postembryonal or adult stages in development are the real initiators of age changes. This would be a manifestation of the deterioration with time of nonrepeated nucleotide sequences.

The theory that aging is due to the accumulation of gene mutations and chromosome anomalies has many supporters (5, 11–13, 43). Yet the failure of this theory to explain the quantitative aspects of normal and radiation-induced aging has been repeatedly observed (1, 6, 39).

CODON-RESTRICTION THEORY OF AGING AND DEVELOPMENT

Strehler has proposed a sophisticated mechanism of codon modulation that not only presents a theoretical framework for age changes but is offered as an explanation for ontogeny, development, immune tolerance, regeneration, and contact inhibition (41, 42). Briefly, he suggests that the kinds of proteins synthesized by cells are controlled by the set of code words that a cell can decode. Most theories accounting for biological aging can be divided into two concepts: one argues that age-dependent deterioration is the result of an active "self-destruct" program, and one that it is the result of passive "wearing out" processes. The former theories ascribe aging to a sequential program of events which, in turn, is ultimately specified by the order of DNA nucleotides in each species. Thus the operation of this program results in a predetermined series of events which cause aging and the eventual death of the individual (45). Strehler views the phenomenon of programmed cell death as observed during the embryogeny of limbs (37) and our observations of the finite lifetime of cultured cells (20, 25) as providing support for these theories. In the class of

theories based on a passive process, where accidental or stochastic events occur, there is a gradual accumulation of irreparable damage.

Strehler's codon restriction hypothesis is based on the following principles:

1) Although gene sequences are composed of about 61 usable triplets, only certain combinations of these are used in coding for any particular protein in differentiating systems.

2) The messages coding for the group of proteins synthesized by a cell are restricted to a codon array which is substantially less than the total complement of 61 that are potentially available.

3) The ensemble of codons a cell employs consists of those codons for which aminoacylated tRNA species are available in sufficient concentration. The two alternative loci at which regulation could occur would be in the production of usable tRNA species and the production of appropriate tRNA-synthetases. The latter alternative is emphasized by Strehler since messages for synthetases themselves must be translatable if they are to be produced. For this reason the mechanism allows for the sequential generation of different groups of synthetases as the language available to a cell is serially modified. The fact that the synthesis or repression of a particular group of synthetases occurs allows a new language set to become active at some future time as the cell progresses through its genetically determined developmental program.

4) A particular group of cell products therefore results from the prior activation of a limiting synthetase that then facilitates these new syntheses. Thus certain active language sets can decode messages both for new synthetases and for repressors of themselves or other syn-

thetases that had been expressed earlier in the cell's life cycle.

5) The repression of the use of certain code words simultaneously represses the production of all products specified in messages using these words. The ultimate results are manifestations of aging as the product previously manufactured deteriorates through stochastic events.

Strehler has discussed various experiments whose results bear on this model and although definitive evidence is not yet available, this model represents one of the most advanced theoretical designs bearing on the role of decrements in informational macromolecules and their possible role in biological senescence.

CONTROL OF AGE CHANGES BY TRANSCRIPTIONAL EVENTS

This thesis, championed by von Hahn (44), suggests that the control of cellular aging is functional at the level of the transcription of genetic information from DNA into the intermediary messenger RNA. This notion maintains that: 1) with increasing age, deleterious changes occur in the metabolism of differentiated post-mitotic cells; 2) the alterations are the result of primary events occurring within the nuclear chromatin; 3) there exists in the nuclear chromatin complex a control mechanism responsible for the appearance and the sequence of the primary aging events; and 4) this control mechanism involves the regulation of transcription although other regulated events may occur.

Von Hahn notes that there are several a priori assumptions involved in this hypothesis, the most important being that there exists a universal physiological aging process, deleterious to the cell, due to intrinsic causes, and progressively acting with increasing chronological age. These are the essential criteria characterizing biological aging that have been proposed by Strehler (40) and appear to be generally valid.

The central event of aging, at whatever level of biological complexity, seems to be the progressive diminution in adaptation to stress and in the capacity of the system to maintain the homeostatic equilibrium characteristic of the adult animal at the end of growth and full development (7).

Von Hahn suggests that two types of primary events, previously referred to here in another context, can interfere with transcription. One is genetically controlled and is based on a genetic program and the other is random involving stochastic processes similar to those discussed in the "error hypothesis."

Von Hahn offers data suggesting that there is an age-related increase in the stability of the DNA double helix which is dependent on the presence and degree of binding of certain proteins. In old nucleoprotein a particular protein fraction is bound to DNA in such a way as to increase the energy required for the separation of the two strands in the helix. Since strand separation is an essential step in transcription, blocking the process will block transcription leading to a loss of genetic information within the cell.

PROLIFERATING AND NONPROLIFERATING CELLS

Most gerontologists agree that there is probably no single cause of aging. A phenomenon which probably comes closer to a unifying theory relates to those concepts based on genetic instability as a cause of aging. It also seems that the genetic contribution to the aging process is foremost in the determination of a lifespan that is characteristic of each species. This is so because the range of variation in the maximum life-span among different species is obviously much greater than the range of individual life-spans within the species. One fundamental problem in relating genetic processes to aging is to attempt to separate the genetic basis of differentiation from a possible genetic basis for aging. I believe that a distinction should be drawn, at least operationally, between processes of development and of aging, or the concept of "first we ripen, and then we rot."

In metazoan aging, we are concerned essentially with three types of cell populations. The first are fixed postmitotics. These are represented by neurons and muscle cells that are essentially unable to divide. A second category includes slowly dividing cells, for example, those found in the liver. The third group would be inter-mitotic cells; cells that divide at a faster rate, that is, fibroblasts and blast cells generally.

There are essentially three types of proliferative cell populations that one can use to illustrate the processes by which these last two categories of dividing cells replicate. The first would be a population whose numbers increase with time; for example, embryonic tissue or tumor tissue, the latter case exemplifying antisocial behavior. The second type of proliferation would be a steady-state renewal system, where the rate of cell death equals the rate of cell birth; for example, the hair follicles in the skin. Finally, there is a population that is decreasing in numbers. This situation is perhaps programmed as a part of differentiation; for example, the massive destruction of cells during vertebrate embryogenesis (37) or in the thymus. A recent hypothesis bearing on causes of cycling cells becoming noncycling has been offered (16).

Genetic instability as a process can be further subdivided. One category is the progressive functional deterioration of these fixed postmitotic cells. The second is the progressive accumulation of faulty copying in dividing cells, or the accumulation of errors. These errors can be categorized as previously described. A third class consists of cross-linking effects in information-carrying molecules postulated by von Hahn (44), which is relevant not only in respect to DNA but to RNA as well. Cross-linkages occurring between proteins and DNA are known, and this concept of permanent gene repression may be responsible for the manifestations of aging, where repressors are irreversibly bound to structural genes.

The progressive accumulation of errors in function of either fixed postmitotics or actively dividing cells could act as a clock. This would initiate secondary types of mischief that would ultimately be manifest as biological aging as we know it. Thus aging could be a special case of morphogenesis. Cells may be programmed simply to run out of program.

FUNCTIONAL AND MITOTIC FAILURE

We may call the lapse of time during which these results become manifest as the "mean time to failure." The concept of mean time to failure has a precise relevance to the deterioration of mechanical as well as biological systems and it can be simply illustrated by considering the mean time to failure of, for example, automobiles. The mean time to failure may be 5 to 6 years, which may be extended or decreased by the competence of repair processes. Barring total replacement of all vital elements, deterioration is inevitable. Similarly, the progressive decrease in the adequacy of the cellular transcription mechanism may ultimately result in a catastrophe of errors in which cell function or cell division is impaired or wrongly directed.

By virtue of the concept that biological activities (and repair mechanisms) are imperfect, we are led to the conclusion that the ultimate death of a cell, or loss of or misdirected functionality, is a programmed event having a mean time to failure. Just as mechanical systems of different purpose have different mean times to failure it is proposed that such differences have their counterpart in informational molecules. Consequently the mean time to failure may be ultimately applicable to a single cell, clone, tissue, organ, or the intact animal itself. It is proposed that the genetic mechanism simply runs out of accurate program which results in a mean time to failure of all the dependent biological systems.

The existence of different average life-spans for each animal species and among the cells, tissues and organs of different animals may be the manifestation of the evolution of more perfect repair mechanisms in those biological systems of greater longevity.

In what way can we fit this concept to account for those biological systems that, seemingly, have escaped from the inevitability of aging? Specifically one must consider the continuity of the germ plasm and continuously propagable or transplantable tumor cell populations. Cancer cells can replicate indefinitely in vitro and in vivo. Is it possible that cancer cells, unlike normal cells, can exchange genetic information thereby insuring their apparent immortality? Gametes do not have an unlimited propensity to multiply unless they unite to form a zygote. Thus, the exchange of genetic material may serve to reprogram or to reset a more perfect biological clock. By this mechanism, species survival is guaranteed but the individual animal is ultimately programmed to failure.

CONCLUSION

A biological system will age if there is a progressive change in its structure and function causing the organism to deal less effectively with its environment. If repair processes corrected errors at the same rate as they were produced, then the steady state achieved would disallow the expression of senescence. Since senescence does occur in most living organisms it is supposed that the genetic program which orchestrates the development of an individual is incapable of maintaining it indefinitely. It is assumed that the accumulation of errors or instability in the genetic program may play the essential role in manifestations of aging phenomena.

REFERENCES

1. ALEXANDER, P. In: *Perspectives in Experimental Gerontology*, edited by N. W. Shock. Springfield, Ill.: Thomas, 1966.
2. BRITTEN, R. J., AND D. E. KOHNE. *Carnegie Inst. Washington, Yearbook* 66: 73, 1968.
3. BRITTEN, R. J., AND D. E. KOHNE. *Science* 161: 529, 1968.
4. BRITTEN, R. J., AND D. E. KOHNE. In: *Handbook of Molecular Cytology*, edited by A. Lima-de-Faria. Amsterdam: North-Holland, 1969, p. 21 and 38.
5. BURNET, M. J. *Brit. Med. J.* 1965: 337.
6. CLARK, A. M. *Advan. Gerontol. Res.* 1: 207, 1964.
7. COMFORT, A. *Gerontologia* 14: 224, 1968.
8. CRISTOFALO, V. J. In: *Advances in Gerontological Research 3*, edited by B. L. Strehler. New York: Academic, 1972.
9. CRISTOFALO, V. J., B. V. HOWARD AND D. KRITCHEVSKY. In: *Organic, Biological and Medicinal Chemistry 2*, edited by V. Gallo and L. Santomarra. Amsterdam: North-Holland, 1970.

10. CUDKOWICZ, G., A. C. UPTON, G. M.
SHEARER AND W. L. HUGHES. *Nature*
201: 165, 1964.
11. CURTIS, H. J. *Science* 141: 688, 1963.
12. CURTIS, H. J. *Federation Proc.* 23: 662,
1964.
13. CURTIS, H. J. In: *Perspectives in Experimental Gerontology*, edited by N. W.
Shock. Springfield, Ill.: Thomas, 1966.
14. DANIEL, C. W., K. B. DE OME, J. T.
YOUNG, P. B. BLAIR AND L. J. FAULKIN,
JR. *Proc. Natl. Acad. Sci. U.S.* 61: 53, 1968.
15. FORD, C. E., H. S. MICKLEM AND S. M.
GRAY. *Brit. J. Radiol.* 32: 280, 1959.
16. GELFANT, S., AND J. GRAHAM-SMITH, JR.
Science 178: 357, 1972.
17. GOLDBERG, A. L. *Proc. Natl. Acad. Sci.
U.S.* 69: 427, 1972.
18. GOLDSTEIN, S. *New Engl. J. Med.* 285:
1120, 1971.
19. HAYFLICK, L. *Exptl. Cell Res.* 37: 614,
1965.
20. HAYFLICK, L. *Exptl. Gerontol.* 5: 291, 1970.
21. HAYFLICK, L. In: *Aging and Development,
Band 4*, edited by H. Bredt and J. W.
Rohen. Stuttgart: F. K. Schattauer
Verlag, 1972.
22. HAYFLICK, L. *Am. J. Med. Sci.* 265: 433,
1973.
23. HAYFLICK, L. *Gerontologist* 14: 37, 1974.
24. HAYFLICK, L. In: *Theoretical Aspects of
Aging*, edited by M. Rockstein. New
York: Academic. In press.
25. HAYFLICK, L., AND P. S. MOORHEAD.
Exptl. Cell Res. 25: 585, 1961.
26. HOLECKOVÁ, E., AND V. J. CRISTOFALO
(editors). *Aging in Cell and Tissue Culture.*
New York: Plenum, 1970.
27. HOLLIDAY, R., AND G. M. TARRANT.
Nature 238: 26, 1972.
28. HOUCK, J. C., V. K. SHARMA AND L.
HAYFLICK. *Proc. Soc. Exptl. Biol. Med.*
137: 331, 1971.
29. KROHN, P. L. *Proc. Roy. Soc. London, Ser. B*
157: 128, 1962.
30. LEWIS, C. M., AND R. HOLLIDAY. *Nature*
228: 877, 1970.
31. MARTIN, G. M., C. A. SPRAGUE AND C. J.
EPSTEIN. *Lab. Invest.* 23: 86, 1970.
32. MEDVEDEV, ZH. A. *Usp. Sovrem. Biol.*
51: 299, 1961.
33. MEDVEDEV, ZH. A. *Exptl. Gerontol.* 7: 227,
1972.
34. ORGEL, L. E. *Proc. Natl. Acad. Sci. U.S.*
49: 517, 1963.
35. ORGEL, L. E. *Nature* 243: 441, 1973.
36. PRINTZ, D. B., AND S. R. GROSS. *Genetics*
55: 451, 1967.
37. SAUNDERS, J. W. In: *Topics in the Biology
of Aging*, edited by P. L. Krohn. New
York: Interscience, 1966, p. 159.
38. SIMINOVITCH, L., J. E. TILL AND E. A.
MCCULLOCH. *J. Cellular Comp. Physiol.*
64: 23, 1964.
39. STREHLER, B. L. *Quant. Rev. Biol.* 34:
117, 1959.
40. STREHLER, B. L. *Time, Cells and Aging.*
New York: Academic, 1962, p. 12.
41. STREHLER, B. L. *Proc. Intern. Congr.
Gerontol.* Vienna: Wein Medikalische
Academie, 1966, p. 177.
42. STREHLER, B., G. HIRSCH, D. GUSSECK,
R. JOHNSON AND M. BICK. *J. Theoret.
Biol.* 33: 429, 1971.
43. SZILARD, L. *Proc. Natl. Acad. Sci. U.S.*
45: 30, 1959.
44. VON HAHN, H. P. *Exptl. Gerontol.* 5: 323,
1970.
45. WILLIAMS, G. C. *Evolution* 11: 398, 1957.
46. WILLIAMSON, A. R., AND B. A. ASKONAS.
Nature 238: 337, 1972.

Towards a theory of development[1]

L. WOLPERT AND J. H. LEWIS

Department of Biology as Applied to Medicine

The Middlesex Hospital Medical School

London W1P 6DB, England

ABSTRACT

A theory of development would effectively enable one to compute the adult organism from the genetic information in the egg. The problem may be approached by viewing the egg as containing a program for development, and considering the logical nature of the program by treating cells as automata and ignoring the details of molecular mechanisms. It is suggested that development is essentially a simple process, the cells having a limited repertoire of overt activities and interacting with each other by means of simple signals, and that general principles may be discerned. The complexity lies in the specification of the internal state which may be described in terms of a gene-switching network. Pattern formation is a central feature in development; it is the process whereby states are assigned to the cells according to their positions, such that the appropriate type of cytodifferentiation is selected from the repertoire. The morphogenesis of the chick limb is briefly discussed. Genetic networks that account for such features as memory, competence and interpretation of positional information are given. The question of how these component parts are organized into a complete control system for development is posed as a problem for future study.—WOLPERT, L., AND J. H. LEWIS. Towards a theory of development. *Federation Proc.* 34: 14–20, 1975.

Development is the process relating genotype to phenotype. The central problem is to understand how the genetic information of the zygote becomes expressed in the multicellular pattern that we recognize as the adult organism. As Sydney Brenner once put it, is the adult computable from the egg? The egg must contain essentially all the information for making the adult, but in what form? Arguments that there cannot be enough information in the egg or that the information content mysteriously increases in development are not valid (1). For the egg need not contain a description of the adult, but only a program for making it; and a simple generative program can yield very complex patterns of behavior

[1] From Session I, *Theoretical Concepts of Developmental and Age Changes*, of the FASEB Conference on *Biology of Development and Aging*, presented at the 58th Annual Meeting of the Federation of American Societies for Experimental Biology, Atlantic City, N. J., April 9, 1974.

(14, 24). It is one of our main aims to show that in this sense, development, though it leads to a complex result, is essentially a simple process, and that general principles are involved. To understand the development of an embryo eventually in terms of molecular biology, we focus our attention on the cell. It is the meeting point of two investigations: molecular biology views it as a system to be broken down into smaller parts, while embryology views it as the basic unit from which a larger system is built up. We shall consider the cell as an automaton (or a finite state machine (24)), which receives cues from its environment, and displays a response through differentiation, metabolic activity, and so on. Our problem is to relate the internal logic of the automaton to the spatial organization of many similar automata as in tissues and organs.

Automata, in general, have a constant aspect—their constitution— and a variable aspect—their state. The constant aspect of the cell is its genome; the variable aspect is its content of other molecules. The way we specify the state of the cell depends on the type of change that we want to discuss. The changes of state that concern us in development are those with relaxation times of the order of hours; we are working on the epigenetic time scale, rather than the metabolic, which has relaxation times of the order of seconds (10). In these circumstances, we can largely specify the state of the cell in terms of its macromolecules alone. To simplify we pair up macromolecules with genes, and suppose that each gene can be characterized as 'off' or 'on' according as its active product (RNA or protein) is absent or present. Each gene is thus regarded as a two-way switch, and the states of all the gene-switches are taken jointly to define the state of the cell as a whole (see for example (19)). In the course of development, that state must change. Some genes may be turned on or off directly by cues from outside the cell, and other genes may follow suit through control connections between one gene and another. These control connections may, for example, depend on binding of proteins to chromosomes, or factors governing translation, or processing of messenger RNA or selective replication of mRNA itself, or even of such mechanisms as the production of heritable changes in DNA structure (3). But we do not want to speculate on the nuts and bolts of the genetic control network (reviewed (13,25)): our concern in this paper is with its logical organization: that is, which genes, by switching on or off, switch on or off which other genes? In choosing this level for our analysis, we avoid many problems of cell physiology. Cell division and movement, for example, are treated as basic elementary activities in the repertoire of our cell automata. We inquire only into the logic of the system that calls them up in response to external signals or internal changes in state.

One can distinguish three related processes in development: cytodifferentiation, pattern specification, and the molding of form. Cytodifferentiation consists in the production of specific sets of luxury macromolecules, such as hemoglobin, which effectively define the final differentiated states such as we see in red blood cells, muscle cells or nerve cells. Histologists recognize only about 200 such distinct cell types, in, for example, a vertebrate. Pattern specification is the process by which cells acquire different states according to their positions, and thereby select one or other from the basic repertoire of 200-odd possible courses of cytodifferentiation, so as to form a well-defined spatial pattern of cell types, such as the muscle, cartilage, dermis, etc., in the vertebrate limb. It is variety in the spatial pattern, and not in the basic cell repertoire of cytodifferentiated types, that accounts for the variety of vertebrates. The molding of form is a matter of cellular mechanics; the shape of an embryo changes because cells exert forces.

CHANGES IN FORM

The basic range of cellular activities responsible for the molding of form is very small and thus general principles are emerging. For example, our studies of early sea urchin development (14) showed how it was possible to account for a large variety of changes in form in terms of a very limited repertoire of cellular activities: localized cellular contractions and variations in adhesiveness between cells. There is now substantial evidence that localized contraction, associated with the actin-like microfilaments, is the dominant mechanism for bringing about the change of form in cell sheets in such varied systems as the gastrulating sea urchin (14, 35) and the developing salivary gland (29). From our point of view, such problems thus reduce to calling into operation a contractile subroutine or cytodifferentiation that exerts forces (such as matrix formation by cartilage (11)) at particular positions in the embryo. It is a general feature of such processes that there are complex mechanical consequences from the simple cellular activities that generate forces.

Cell movement falls under the same heading, and a great deal of effort has been devoted to the problem of the sorting-out of mixtures of cell types; type-specific differences in cell adhesiveness are usually invoked as the mechanism for organizing pattern in these systems (7, 30). However, we know of no histological patterns that arise in vivo by the sorting-out of random mixtures of cells in different states. On the contrary, when cells move, as, for instance, in the formation of retino-tectal connections (9) or of sea urchin mesenchyme (14), the motion is a response to position-dependent cues. The cells are first assigned states according to where they are, and these states govern their subsequent movement. The question of how the state assignments are linked to position, and then interpreted by the cell to determine its behavior, is a part of the problem of pattern specification.

PATTERN SPECIFICATION

We thus view the problem of pattern specification as central to any theory of development. The first requirement is that the state of a cell should be somehow related to the states and positions of its neighbors. There seem to be two main ways in which this is achieved. In the so-called mosaic eggs, it is brought about by cytoplasmic localization in the egg, the daughter cells being assigned states according to their cytoplasmic constitution when the egg is divided up (5, 6); in principle there need be no interaction between cells, though the absence of such interaction is not established (12, 15). The second way of linking state to position involves interactions between cells, and may be of much more widespread importance. In the simplest case, a signal is generated across a set of cells so that cells at opposite poles acquire different characters. In more general terms it has been suggested (38) that cells may have their positions specified with respect to certain boundary or reference regions as in a coordinate frame, and may then interpret this positional information by selecting an appropriate course of differentiation according to their genome and developmental history. One of the attractions of the positional information concept is that a universal mechanism for specification of position may be involved. There is already quite a lot of evidence that pattern mutants alter the response rather than the specification of position (31), that positional fields are small, say 50 cells long, so that signaling is always short range, and that there are common rules for pattern regulation and regeneration in very different systems (38).

A cellular character can of course be transmitted clonally, but where diversity among the progeny arises, it is determined by position. Of particular interest is the recent work of Garcia-Bellido et al. (8) who show that the cells during development of *Drosophila* form apparently discrete compartments, corresponding to discrete states of determination, which do not intermingle; the compartments of fields grow and become repeatedly subdivided. The behavior of a cell depends also, however, on its relative position within its compartment (22).

We would stress that the signals are usually of a rather unspecific character. The classical instance is that of neural plate induction in amphibians, which can be evoked by all sorts of different and unnatural substances (28). If specificity does not lie in the signal, it must lie in the system that responds. The same is probably true for positional information as clearly indicated by the autonomy of expression of different genotypes in the same positional field (31, 38). Indeed, at any stage of its development, a cell has only a very few alternative courses of behavior immediately open to it, and the choice between them can be guided by simple yes/no signals. The essential point is that the choice, once made, will control what options become available for the next decision. The cell has a

memory, and its behavior is determined by its history. Its highly specific state represents the record of a sequence of simple signals (like a message in Morse code). If there are 20 yes/no signals, there can be 2^{20}, i.e., a million, different messages, hence a million significantly different ways to assign the cell's final state. In general there are far more functionally distinct cell states than the mere 200-odd modes of cytodifferentiation: it is a commonplace in embryology that a cell can change its state of determination without changing its outward show of differentiation. Thus, the interpretation of positional information is the key process in pattern formation (37, 38).

All this we take as reinforcing the view that complexity and variety come from the mechanism inside the cell that records and interprets the morphogenetic signal, and not from the character of the signal itself. Our emphasis is very different from that of Turing (36), whose whole concern is with the generation of patterns of chemical activity by diffusion and cross-catalysis. He takes no account of the lasting effect on cells of the previous signals to which they have been exposed, nor of the capacity of cells to interpret present signals in a complex way according to that past history.

CHICK LIMB MORPHOGENESIS

It may be helpful to illustrate our approach with respect to the vertebrate limb, which shows features in common with many developmental systems. In the chick the limb starts as a very small bulge from the flank, and grows out as a tongue-shaped mass consisting of mesenchyme encased in ectoderm (Fig. 1). From the beginning of outgrowth, thanks to previous specifications, the mesenchyme has already a distinctive intrin-

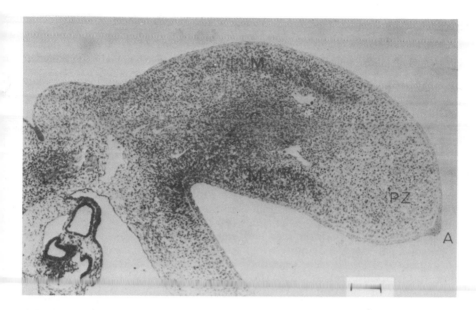

Figure 1. Section of a chick limb bud at the time when the presumptive hand is beginning to emerge from the progress zone. At the tip the thickened apical ectodermal ridge (A) can be seen. The progress zone (PZ) extends back in the undifferentiated mesenchyme about 300 μm. Further back cartilage (C) can be seen to be forming in the central region and muscle (M) is differentiating more laterally. (Bar is 100 μm.)

sic state appropriate to the limb and different for leg and wing (27); that is, it is determined as wing or leg mesenchyme. We have suggested that the overall shape of the limb bud may depend on the mechanics of the ectoderm and in particular on the mechanical role of the thickened apical ridge. The elements are formed from the mesenchyme and are laid down in a proximodistal sequence. With Summerbell we have proposed that the pattern of these elements is specified by a mechanism in which the cells first acquire positional values, i.e., records of their position along the proximodistal, anteroposterior, and dorsoventral axes. This positional information is then interpreted in terms of muscle, cartilage, loose connective tissue, and so on, according to rules that depend on the previous specification as leg or wing (33).

The positional value along the proximodistal axis is determined by the length of time the cells have spent in a special region at the tip—the progress zone—marked out by a signal from the apical ridge, which is a thickened part of the covering ectoderm. Possibly the cells count their divisions in the progress zone, thus linking growth to pattern formation. It seems that the length of each main cartilaginous rudiment corresponds initially to the length of tissue that emerges from the progress zone during the time equivalent to one cell cycle: this length amounts to about 20 cell-diameters and appears to be specified with a remarkable precision:

an error not greater than 5% (34). The later development of the cartilaginous elements is dependent on how much the cells divide and secrete matrix, and we suggest that this is governed by the positional value: the presumptive humerus grows much more than the presumptive wrist. There is remarkable autonomy and apparent absence of interaction along the proximodistal axis—for example, a young progress zone grafted to the tip of an older stage develops autonomously and gives rise to a limb with elements repeated in tandem (Fig. 2). Along the anteroposterior axis, by contrast, the positional value coordinate seems to be specified by a signal from a region at the posterior edge of the progress zone (26, 32). This may be analogous to the situation in other systems such as the insect epidermis (21, 23) and hydra (39) where positional information may be supplied by a gradient in a diffusible substance. Similarly, the progress zone model for the proximodistal axis may have wide applications especially where epimorphic growth and regulation are in-

volved (38). We do not yet know the biochemical basis of these mechanisms, but only how to recognize them when they are found.

A nice example of both determination and universality is provided by the experiment in which a piece of presumptive thigh from the chick leg bud is grafted into the progress zone of the wing bud, where it develops into a toe (27).

GENE CONTROL NETWORKS

We can thus view development as a process in which cells change their state both in response to external cues and autonomously, and use that state to call up the appropriate type of overt cellular activity or differentiation from the limited basic repertoire. Our task now is to work out how the set of states and transitions can be generated by an appropriate gene switching network inside the cell. This is a standard type of problem in the design of digital computers. The solution is arbitrary in several respects: there are many ways of constructing a given logical function out

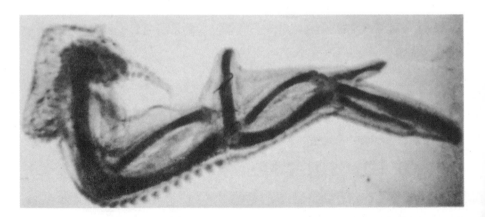

Figure 2. A limb in which the cartilaginous elements, humerus, radius and ulna, are repeated. This results from the grafting of a young progress zone of an older limb bud. The grafted zone behaves autonomously.

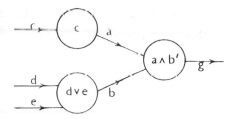

Figure 3. Circles stand for genes, and arrowed lines for control connections. Beside the circle for each gene we write its name, and inside the circle the logical formula for its state in terms of its control inputs. For example, gene b will be on if either d or e is on, or both are.

of combinations of our basic elements, and many ways of matching states of the network to the cell states perceived by the embryologist. An important and ingenious attempt on a particular problem of this type has, however, been made by Kauffman (20). He has shown in detail how to interpret transdetermination and homeotic mutation of the imaginal discs of *Drosophila* in terms of changes in the combination of genes active; and he has suggested how the pattern of determination may be related to position in the early embryo.

We too propose to treat cell behavior in terms of gene switching networks, genes being either on or off. The distinct states of the network correspond, in conventional embryological terms, to distinct states of determination. To describe our networks, we borrow a simple notation from formal logic (Table 1). We can combine the symbols $(\vee, \wedge, ', =)$ to describe any logical dependence; for instance, $g = a \wedge b'$ means that gene g is on if, and only if, gene a is on and gene b is off. We use this notation to mark logical dependences on our network diagrams (see Fig. 3), which will be used to illustrate some simple basic functions.

For cytodifferentiation, a cell must activate a particular battery of structural genes coding for enzymes or structural proteins. The members of the battery must somehow be co-ordinated, and Britten and Davidson (2) suggest that for each battery there is an 'integrator' gene, whose activity stimulates the activity of all the structural genes in the battery; the structural genes could be connected to their integrator in parallel (Fig. 4a), in series (Fig. 4b), or in some more elaborate hybrid fashion.

If a particular state is to be both stable and inherited, then a further feature is required: the control system must be capable of memory. If a switching network is to be capable of long-term memory, it must contain a closed feedback circuit. For proof of this elementary theorem, see (24). One sort of simple scheme is shown in Fig. 5a. The feedback loop need not be direct; Fig. 5b shows a slightly more complex scheme (18). One could perhaps do without such feedback loops by storing memories instead as heritable structural changes in the DNA (3).

We now consider how, in a many-celled organism, the genome can select for the cell a determined heritable state according to a cue. We suppose this cue to be simply the local value, c, of a graded chemical concentration. We demand that there

TABLE 1

Symbol	Read as	Meaning
g	g	g on
g'	not g	g off
$g \wedge h$	g and h	both g and h are on
$g \vee h$	g or h	either g or h is on, or both are on
$g = h$	g equals h	g is on if and only if h is on

should be a single threshold concentration c_o, such that the cells adopt one state in regions where $c < c_o$ and another where $c > c_o$. These could correspond to muscle and cartilage in the limb, or humerus cartilage as opposed to ulna cartilage. It is first necessary to have at least one gene directly controlled by the cue. But if we have only that, the cue will leave no permanent trace of its effect. A mechanism is required to record the effect of the cue, and this is simply done by triggering a feedback loop (Fig. 6). To register more detailed information about position using just one chemical gradient as the signal, we could have several homologous genes, each with its own feedback loop, triggered at different threshold concentrations c_o, c_1, c_2, . . .

It will, however, usually be necessary to restrict the sensitivity of the cell, so that it can respond to the signal only during some particular

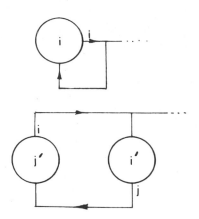

Figure 5. *a*, upper; *b*, lower. In each case, the gene *i* will stay off if it is off at first, and on if it is on at first.

time interval. For example, in the limb bud, only cells in the progress zone respond to the signal from the polarizing region (32). As the tradi-

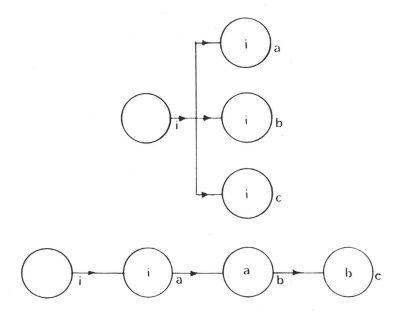

Figure 4. *a*, upper diagram; *b*, lower diagram. In each diagram, *i* is the integrator gene, and *a*, *b* and *c* are the structural genes that it controls.

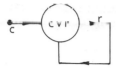

Figure 6. • denotes the source of the cue c, and r is the gene whose state records its effect.

tional embryologist would put it, the period of competence must be limited. Otherwise it will be possible to upset the cell's specification at any time by triggering a still untriggered feedback loop. Figure 7 shows how to impose the restriction: the feedback circuit is triggered only if the cue c is supplied at the same time as a competence marker m—most often generated internally as the product of another gene (6).

This brings us to the temporal aspect of the behavior of our gene network. If we let a finite switching network start from some given state, and follow its development in time, we must obtain one of two possible outcomes. The network may tend to a final equilibrium state, or it may enter a stable cyclic mode, i.e., its state may oscillate. We shall not try to give a general discussion of the very complicated temporal behavior of arbitrarily connected switching nets. (See Kauffman (19) for an illuminating analysis of the special case of the random net in which all elements have one and the same delay time.) But there are two aspects of temporal behavior that any model for the genetic control development must take account of. The first is memory, which, as we have already seen, depends on positive feedback loops. The second is oscillation, and, in particular, one supremely important oscillation the cell division cycle. In fact Holtzer and his co-workers (17) have very

strongly emphasized the possible importance of what they have termed 'quantal' mitosis. They suggest, in our terminology, that heritable changes in cell state can only occur in association with mitosis. A possible mechanism could be that large proteins only gain access to the genome when the nuclear membrane breaks down at mitosis (13). Thus mitosis could be a gate, which opens once in every cycle, exposing genes, during the cycle that follows, to control by the genes that were active in the cycle that came before. This would neatly link growth with the steps of developmental change. In our theory for the chick limb, cell divisions may be used to measure time in the progress zone, and hence to establish the positional value. Figure 8 shows how a chain of genes may serve to count cell divisions for this purpose. There is quite good evidence for a change in state associated with cell division in a variety of systems, such as insect epidermis (23), transdetermination (20), myogenesis, and chondrogenesis (17). On the other hand, there is no reason to believe that all transitions depend on cell division (4, 16, 25).

More generally, a chain of genes connected via delays can be used to define the developmental stage of the cell. Successive genes in the delay chain can operate as competence

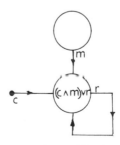

Figure 7. The gene m controls the competence of r to be triggered by c.

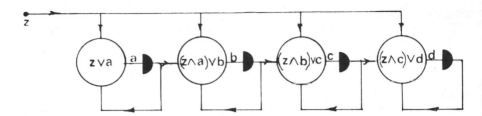

Figure 8. The control connections marked with a ⟩ in place of an arrow are those where transmission involves a delay (linked to cell division). The external signal Z may indicate, for example, whether the cell is in the progress zone, and so should continue counting division cycles. If Z acts for only one cycle, gene a will be left on, and genes b, c and d off; if Z acts for two cycles, gene b will also be left on, and so on.

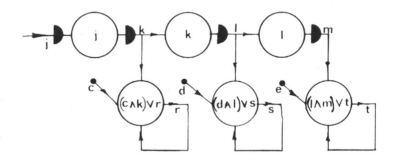

Figure 9. The delay chain consists of genes k, l and m: these in turn make genes r, s and t competent to respond to signals c, d and e respectively.

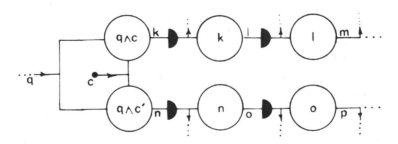

Figure 10. The external cue c directs which of the two delay chains shall be activated by the stimulus q.

markers for the triggering of a succession of different feedback loops by external cues (Fig. 9). The major branch-points in development, such as the determination of ectoderm versus mesoderm, may correspond to the activation of one or other of two alternative delay chains, and hence of

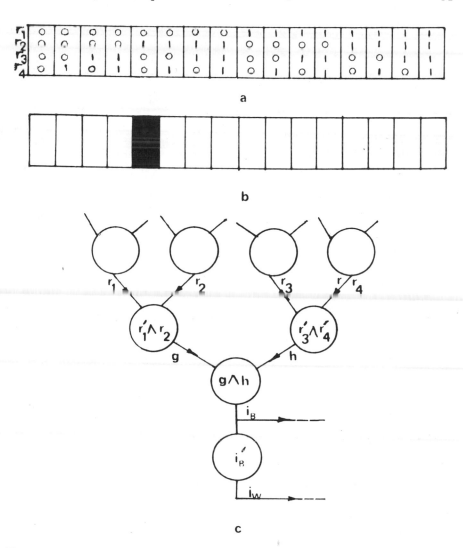

Figure 11. *a*: The boxes stand for cells. The figures in each box stand for the states of the record genes r_1 to r_4. Where a gene is on we write *1* and where it is off, *0*. *b*): The pattern given by the interpretation network shown in *c* acting on the pattern of record gene assignments.

one or other of two quite separate sequences of genes rendered competent to respond to external signals (Fig. 10).

We have finally to consider how the history of the gene switching network determines the part that

the cell plays in forming the final pattern of tissues. During development, a cell line will be exposed to several, probably less than 10, different signals at different times (38). Cells in different places will receive different signals. Thus the combined record of the signals and cues received and autonomously processed by the cell—that is, its state of determination—amounts to a specification of its position. The cell must use this specification to select from the repertoire one or other of the 200-odd modes of cytodifferentiation. There may be vastly more than 200 positional specifications, but different specifications can lead to the same mode of differentiation. As a simple illustration, suppose that we have a line of 16 cells, each containing 4 genes r_1, r_2, r_3 and r_4 that carry the record of the positional specification, and that the states of these record genes have been assigned as shown in Fig. 11a, perhaps by some sequence of signals associated with successive subdivision of the field. We might now, for example, want the 5th cell from the right hand end to differentiate by turning black, while the other 15 cells stay white (Fig. 11b). To achieve this, we link the integrator gene i_B for blackness to the record genes in such a way that it is governed by the condition $i_B = r_1' \wedge r_2 \wedge r_3' \wedge r_4'$. The integrator gene i_W for whiteness we govern by the condition $i_W = i_B'$. A small network of intermediate 'interpretation' genes may be used to implement the linking function, as shown in Fig. 11c. In this combinatorial fashion it can be shown that intricate spatial patterns can be generated by quite small networks as will be discussed in detail elsewhere (Lewis, ms in preparation).

CONCLUSION

We have stressed the idea that in development a cell receives simple signals, and makes complex responses. The system of genes controlling a cell provides it with a memory, and governs its behavior according to past as well as present circumstances.

We have set out to examine the logic of that control system, and have listed some basic features that it must incorporate. These are no more than first hesitant steps towards a theory of development. At the least they force one to formally define, for example, such concepts as competence and determination, and may thus give new insights into them. The global organization of the genetic control network has yet to be analyzed: that is the problem of how such simple circuits can be put together to provide an entire program for development. But we think that the task is feasible, and that a relatively simple network, involving perhaps less than a hundred control genes, may suffice to generate the whole complexity of, for example, the vertebrate limb, by suitable orchestration of the basic cellular activities of cell division, movement, and cytodifferentiation.

We believe, furthermore, with Kauffman (20) that we must understand the function of the genome at this level of abstraction, if we are to understand how a mutation like aristopedia can cause a fruitfly to grow legs where it should have antennae, or how evolution works its marvelous variations on the basic pattern of the vertebrate limb.

REFERENCES

1. APTER, M. J., AND L. WOLPERT. Cybernetics and development. *J. Theoret. Biol.* 8: 244–257, 1965.
2. BRITTEN, R. J., AND E. H. DAVIDSON. Gene regulation for higher cells: a theory. *Science* 165: 349–359, 1969.
3. COOK, P. R. Hypothesis on differentiation and the inheritance of gene superstructure. *Nature* 245: 23–25, 1973.
4. COOKE, J. Morphogenesis and regulation in spite of continued mitotic inhibition in *Xenopus* embryos. *Nature* 242: 55–57, 1973.
5. DAVIDSON, E. *Gene activity in early development.* New York: Academic, 1967.

6. DAVIDSON, E. H. Note on the control of gene expression during development. *J. Theoret. Biol.* 32: 123–130, 1971.

7. GARBER, B. B., AND A. A. MOSCONA. Reconstruction of brain tissue from cell suspensions. I. Aggregation patterns of cells dissociated from different regions of the developing brain. *Develop. Biol.* 27: 217–234, 1972.

8. GARCIA-BELLIDO, A., P. RIPOLL AND G. MORATA. Developmental compartmentalization of the wing disk of *Drosophila*. *Nature New Biol.* 245: 251–253, 1973.

9. GAZE, R. M., AND M. J. KEATING. The visual system and neuronal specificity. *Nature* 237: 375–378, 1972.

10. GOODWIN, B. C. *The Temporal Organization in Cells*. London: Academic, 1963.

11. GOULD, R. P., L. SELWOOD, A. DAY AND L. WOLPERT. The mechanism of cellular orientation during early cartilage formation in the chick limb and regenerating amphibian limb. *Exptl. Cell Res.* 83: 287–296, 1974.

12. GUERRIER, P. Les caractères de la segmentation et la détermination de la polarité dorsoventrale dans le développement de quelques Spiralia. I. Les formes à premier clivage égal. *J. Embryol. Exptl. Morphol.* 23: 611–637, 1970.

13. GURDON, J. B., AND H. R. WOODLAND. On the long term control of nuclear activity during cell differentiation. *Curr. Top. Develop. Biol.* 5: 39–70, 1970.

14. GUSTAFSON, T., AND L. WOLPERT. Cellular movement and contact in sea urchin morphogenesis. *Biol. Rev.* 42: 442–498, 1967.

15. HERTH, W., AND K. SANDER. Mode and timing of body pattern formation (regionalization) in the early embryonic development of cyclorrhaphic dipterans (*Protophormia, Drosophila*). *Wilhelm Roux' Arch. Entwicklungsmech. Organismen* 172: 1–27, 1973.

16. HICKLIN, J., AND L. WOLPERT. Positional information and pattern regulation in hydra: the effect of Y-irradiation. *J. Embryol. Exptl. Morphol.* 30: 741–752, 1973.

17. HOLTZER, H., H. WEINTRAUB, R. MAYNE AND B. MOCHAN. The cell cycle, cell lineages and cell differentiation. *Curr. Top. Develop. Biol.* 7: 229–256, 1972.

18. JACOB, F., AND J. MONOD. Genetic repression, allosteric inhibition, and cellular differentiation. In: *Cytodifferentiation and macromolecular synthesis*, edited by M. Locke. New York: Academic, 1963.

19. KAUFFMAN, S. Gene regulation networks: a theory for their global structures and behaviours. *Curr. Top. Develop. Biol.* 6: 145–182, 1971.

20. KAUFFMAN, S. Control circuits for determination and transdetermination. *Science* 181: 310–318, 1973.

21. LAWRENCE, P. A. The development of spatial patterns in the integument of insects. In: *Developmental Systems. Insects*, edited by S. J. Counce and C. H. Waddington. London: Academic, 1973, p. 157–211.

22. LAWRENCE, P. A. A clonal analysis of segment development in *Oncopeltus* (Hemiptera). *J. Embryol. Exptl. Morphol.* 30: 681–699, 1973.

23. LAWRENCE, P. A., F. H. C. CRICK AND M. MUNRO. A gradient of positional information in an insect, *Rhodnius*. *J. Cell Sci.* 11: 815–854, 1972.

24. MINSKY, M. *Computation: finite and infinite machines*. Englewood Cliffs, N. J.: Prentice-Hall, 1963.

25. RUTTER, W. J., R. L. PICTET AND P. W. MORRIS. Toward molecular mechanisms of developmental processes. *Ann. Rev. Biochem.* 42: 601–646, 1973.

26. SAUNDERS, J. W. Developmental control of three-dimensional polarity in the avian limb. *Ann. N.Y. Acad. Sci.* 29–41, 1971.

27. SAUNDERS, J. W., J. M. CAIRNS AND M. T. GASSELING. The role of the apical ridge of ectoderm in the differentiation of the morphological structure and inductive specificity of limb parts in the chick. *J. Morphol.* 101: 57–88, 1957.

28. SAXEN, L., AND S. TOIVONEN. Primary embryonic induction. London: Logos, 1962.

29. SPOONER, B. S. Microfilaments, cell shape changes, and morphogenesis of salivary epithelium. *Am. Zool.* 13: 1007–1022, 1973.

30. STEINBERG, M. S. Does differential adhesion govern self-assembly processes in histogenesis? Equilibrium configurations and the emergence of a hierarchy among populations of embryonic cells. *J. Exptl. Zool.* 173: 395–434, 1970.

31. STERN, C. *Genetic mosaics and other essays*. Cambridge, Mass.: Harvard Univ. Press, 1968.

32. SUMMERBELL, D. Interaction between the proximo-distal and antero-posterior coordinates of positional information in the early development of the

chick limb bud. *J. Embryol. Exptl. Morphol.* In press.

33 SUMMERBELL, D., J. H. LEWIS AND L. WOLPERT. Positional information in chick limb morphogenesis. *Nature* 244: 492–496, 1973.

34. SUMMERBELL, D., AND L. WOLPERT. Precision of development in chick limb morphogenesis. *Nature* 244: 228–230, 1973.

35. TILNEY, L. G., AND J. R. GIBBONS. Microtubules and filaments in the filopodia of the secondary mesenchyme cells of *Arbacia punctulata* and *Echinarochinus parma. J. Cell Sci.* 5: 195–210, 1969.

36. TURING, A. M. The chemical basis of morphogenesis. *Phil. Trans. Roy. Soc. London, Ser. B* 641: 37–72, 1952.

37. WADDINGTON, C. H. The morphogenesis of patterns in *Drosophila.* In: *Developmental Systems: Insects,* edited by S. J. Counce and C. H. Waddington. London: Academic, 1973, p. 499–535.

38. WOLPERT, L. Positional information and pattern formation. *Curr. Top. Develop. Biol.* 6: 183, 1971.

39. WOLPERT, L., A. HORNBRUCH AND M. R. B. CLARKE. Positional information and positional signalling along hydra. *Am. Zool.* 14: 647–663, 1974.

Gene regulation in differentiation and development

Introductory remarks

MICHAEL POTTER

Laboratory of Cell Biology, National Cancer Institute
National Institutes of Health, Bethesda, Maryland 20014

In multicellular systems the differentiation process has two interrelated but often separately studied components; the activation of special genes and the development of cellular specialization. The immune system, the model under consideration in this symposium, is no exception. Antibodies (or immunoglobulins) are controlled by a large number of structural genes that are expressed in perhaps the most highly specialized cellular system in the vertebrate organism. The elucidation of mechanisms whereby this differentiated function develops presents intriguing problems for both immunologist and developmental biologist. Many immunologists and, I am sure, biologists outside this field have been impressed with the seemingly new and exceptional mechanisms of cellular and gene differentiation in the immune system: e.g., clonal (V_L, V_H) specialization, the 2 gene:1 polypeptide chain relationship for immunoglobulin polypeptide chains, autosomal allelic exclusion, clonal selection, cell cooperation. These unusual mechanisms may have made the immune system at first an unattractive model for the developmental biologist; however as these processes become more familiar they can be appreciated for what they are: evolutionary exploitations of biological processes that have been modified to create a genetic and cellular system of defense for the vertebrate organism.

IMMUNOGLOBULIN GENE DIFFERENTIATION

The basic molecular unit of a functional immunoglobulin is a four chain structure with two identical light (L) chains and two identical heavy (H) chains. (For reviews, see ref 11, 20). Structural and genetic evidence has now amply confirmed the hypothesis of Dreyer and Bennett (7, 8) that two structural genes control a single immunoglobulin L or H chain. Each chain type has two continuous polypeptide segments—hereafter called regions—a C (constant) region and V (variable) region. These terms have grown out of the empirical serological and structural observations that within a species there are a relatively few varieties of species-specific C regions and a very much larger number of V regions. Functionally the V regions interact to form the part of the immunoglobulin molecule that contains the antigen-binding site while the C regions interact to form carrier parts of the molecule that interact physiologically with other components of the immune system, e.g., complement or cellular receptors.

The C regions contain amino acids that determine the polymerization of the 4-chain units, the interactions with J chains (IgA, IgM) and transport pieces (IgA secretory immunoglobulin). Thus, nature has designed a molecule that has maintained its physiological capacity to interact with other components in the organism but which also incorporates through its V regions a great diversity to interact with structures that are hostile to the organism, i.e., the antigens of microorganisms, viruses, and the like.

Immunoglobulin structural genes for C_L and V_L, C_H and V_H regions appear to be located in complex loci (see ref 15). Genetic analyses so far possible in only a few species suggest at least three complex loci per haploid set, one for heavy chains and two (kappa and lambda) for light chains (see R. Mage, p. 40, for ref). Each complex locus contains V and corresponding C genes (4, 14, 19). Structural evidence has indicated that characteristic sets of V genes associated with a given C locus do not participate with C genes of another complex locus (see 13, 20). There is no simple formula for the arrangement of genes in the complex locus. In some such as the mouse kappa there appears to be a single C gene and multiple V genes based on sequence findings (13). The mouse, rabbit and human heavy chain loci contain four or more C genes

(14) and a set of V genes each of which can interact with any one of the C_H genes.

In man, mouse and rabbit where genetic (allotypic) markers are available, immunoglobulin is produced in a single cell from only one of the two autosomal loci (12, 15, 21). This pertains to both L and H chain synthesis. In addition in the rabbit where markers for both C_H and V_H can be studied it has been found that the *cis* arranged genes cooperate in heavy chain production (see R. Mage, p. 40). The activation of C and V genes for immunoglobulin synthesis appears then to be monosomic. All of these characteristics suggest that the differentiation of an immunoglobulin chain requires the close linkage of C and V structural genes. V genes associated with a given C gene appear to be multiple as exemplified by the number of V_{kappa} regions that have been isolated from a single genome (i.e., the inbred BALB/c strain of mouse (13)) and from the RNA:DNA hybridization studies (21) utilizing H-chain mRNA that A. Williamson will discuss in this symposium. A critical step in immunoglobulin differentiation appears to be the bringing together of the two DNA elements controlling V and C regions that are linked but not apparently continuous on the chromosome. The mechanism whereby this event is achieved has not yet been elucidated.

The IgC_H class associated with immunoglobulin produced by the earliest cells in the B cell lineage is IgM. This immunoglobulin is associated with the cell membrane and is involved in the processes of "clonal selection" whereby specific immunoglobulin-producing cells are activated to proliferate and form clones of immunoglobulin-secreting cells. However, during the subsequent developmental steps, occurring probably during mitotic expansion of B cells,

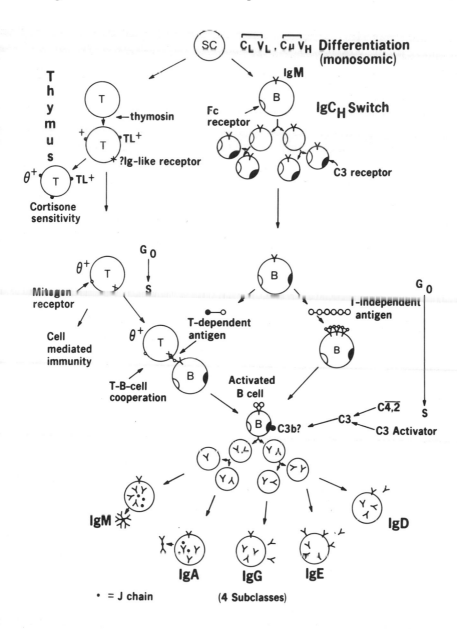

Figure 1. Hypothetical scheme, depicting the two main pathways of lymphocyte development: the thymus-derived lymphocytes (T lymphocytes) and the nonthymus-derived lymphocytes (B lymphocytes). The two cell lines are ultimately derived from the same precursor stem cell (SC). In the B-cell lineage two known pre- and postantigen clonal expansion points are depicted by divisions (small circles). The IgC_H switch appears to be related to mitosis and while it is shown with the preantigen divisions it may not be phenotypically manifest until the postantigen divisions. Abbreviations: θ = theta antigen, TL = thymus leukemia antigen; $G_0 \rightarrow S$ symbolizes activation from nondividing cell to mitotically active cell.

immunoglobulin-producing cells may switch the IgC$_H$ class from IgCμ to another class. (See discussions by A. Lawton, p. 33 and N. Klinman, p. 47). The IgC$_H$ switch could occur during the preantigen expansion phase or during the cell divisions stimulated by antigen. IgC$_H$-V$_H$ association in a mature immunoglobulin-secreting cell, e.g., plasmacytoma, appears to be a highly stable arrangement, persisting during innumerable cell divisions.

CELLULAR DIFFERENTIATION

During the cellular differentiation process immunoglobulin-producing cells develop: special cell surface receptors (Fc and C3), changes in mitotic potential, and finally the cytoplasmic elements for immunoglobulin secretion. Cells capable of interacting with antigens originate from undifferentiated cells (lymphocytes). They develop in two major pathways; one occurs in the thymus, and the other in extrathymic tissues—bursa of Fabricius in avians, bone marrow and fetal liver in mammals (see discussion by A. Lawton, p. 33) (Fig. 1).

The thymus-derived lymphocytes acquire several characteristic cell surface markers, θ, TL (see E. Boyse, p. 24). These cells (T cells) ultimately participate in various forms of cell-mediated immunity and cooperation with B lymphocytes (10, 16).

Thymocytes and their daughter cells released into the circulation as T lymphocytes apparently do not acquire subsequently the capacity to secrete immunoglobulin. The nature of the T-cell antigen binding component, including its genetic relationship to immunoglobulin, is not yet clear.

The lymphocytes originating in extrathymic tissues acquire special cell surface receptors; Fc receptor, C3 receptor and the specific antigen-binding immunoglobulin receptor (1, 3, 17). These cells are determined very early to produce only single V$_L$-V$_H$ regions, and hence are specialized so they can combine with only a very restricted number of antigens.

The immune potential depends on the differentiation of many specialized cell types. Quantitative expansion of the potential is brought about by several rounds of division of the differentiated lymphocytes. During these divisions the cells acquire new receptors, and probably undergo the IgC$_H$ switching process. The cells are apparently released in a G$_0$ state of mitosis, and do not undergo mitosis and further maturation until triggered by antigens, and other mitogenic signals. (5, 6, 9, 18). When B lymphocytes mature to Ig-secreting cell types they appear to lose their Fc and C3 receptors but may retain some immunoglobulin in the membrane (2, 17, 22).

REFERENCES

1. BASTEN, A., J. MILLER, J. SPRENT AND J. PYE. A receptor for antibody on B lymphocytes. I. Method of detection and functional significance. *J. Exptl. Med.* 135: 610–626, 1972.

2. BASTEN, A., N. L. WARNER AND T. MANDEL. A receptor for antibody on B lymphocytes. II. Immunochemical and electron microscopy characteristics. *J. Exptl. Med.* 135: 627–647, 1972.

3. BIANCO, C., R. PATRICK AND N. NUSSENZWEIG. A population of lymphocytes bearing a membrane receptor for antigen-antibody-complement complexes. I. Separation and characterization. *J. Exptl. Med.* 132: 702–720, 1970.

4. BLOMBERG, B., W. R. GECKLER AND M. WEIGERT. Genetics of the antibody response to dextran in mice. *Science* 177: 178–180, 1972.

5. COUTINHO, A., E. GRONOWICZ, W. W. BULLOCK AND G. MÖLLER. Mechanisms of thymus independent immunocyte triggering. Mitogenic activation of B cells in specific immune responses. *J. Exptl. Med.* 139: 74–92, 1973.

6. COUTINHO, A., AND G. MOLLER. B-cell mitogenic properties of thymus independent antigens. *Nature New Biol.* 245: 11–14, 1973.

7. DREYER, W. J., AND J. D. BENNETT. The molecular basis of antibody formation: a paradox. *Proc. Natl. Acad. Sci. U.S.* 54: 864–869, 1965.

8. DREYER, W. J., W. R. GRAY AND L. HOOD. The genetic, molecular and cellular basis of antibody formation: some facts and a unifying hypothesis. *Cold Spring Harbor Symp. Quant. Biol.* 32: 353–368, 1967.

9. DUKOR, P., AND K. U. HARTMANN. Hypothesis. Bound C3 as the second signal for B-cell activation. *Cell. Immunol.* 7: 349–356, 1973.

10. FELDMANN, M., AND G. J. V. NOSSAL. Tolerance enhancement and the regulation of interactions between T cells, B cells and macrophages. *Transplant. Rev.* 13: 3–34, 1972.

11. GALLY, J. A. Structure of immunoglobulins. In: *The Antigens*, edited by M. Sela. New York: Academic, 1973, p. 161–298.

12. HARBOE, M., C. K. OSTERLAND, M. MANNIK AND H. G. KUNKEL. Genetic characters of human γ-globulins in myeloma proteins. *J. Exptl. Med.* 116: 719–738, 1962.

13. HOOD, L., D. McKEAN, V. FARNSWORTH AND M. POTTER. Mouse immunoglobulin chains. A survey of the amino terminal sequences of κ chains. *Biochemistry* 12: 741, 1973.

14. LIEBERMAN, R., M. POTTER, E. B. MUSHINSKI, W. HUMPHREY, JR. AND S. RUDIKOFF. Genetics of a new IgV$_H$ (T15 idiotype) marker in the mouse regulating natural antibody to phosphorylcholine. *J. Exptl. Med.* 139: 983–1001, 1974.

15. MAGE, R., R. LIEBERMAN, M. POTTER AND W. D. TERRY. Immunoglobulin allotypes In: *The Antigens*, edited by

M. Sela. New York: Academic, 1973, p. 299–376.

16. MITCHISON, N. A., R. TAYLOR AND K. RAJEWSKY. Cooperation of antigenic determinants in the induction of antibodies. In: *Development aspects of antibody formation and structure*, edited by J. Sterzl. Prague: Czech. Acad. Sci. 1970, p. 547.

17. MÖLLER, G. Effect of B-cell mitogens on lymphocyte subpopulations possessing C3 and Fc receptors. *J. Exptl. Med.* 139: 969–982, 1974.

18. MÖLLER, G., O. SJÖBERG AND J. ANDERSSON. Immunogenicity, tolerogenicity and mitogenicity of lipopolysaccharides. *J. Infect. Diseases* 128: Suppl, S52–S56, 1973.

19. PAWLAK, L. L., E. B. MUSHINSKI, A. NISONOFF AND M. POTTER. Evidence for the linkage of the IgC$_H$ locus to a gene controlling the idiotypic specificity of anti-*p*-azophenylarsonate antibodies in strain A mice. *J. Exptl. Med.* 137: 22–31, 1973.

20. POTTER, M. Immunoglobulin-producing tumors and myeloma proteins of mice. *Physiol. Rev.* 52: 631–719, 1972.

21. PREMKUMAR, E., M. SHOYAB AND A. R. WILLIAMSON. Germline basis for antibody diversity IgV$_H$ and C$_H$ gene frequencies measured by DNA:RNA hybridization. *Proc. Natl. Acad. Sci. U.S.* 71: 99–103, 1974.

22. SHEVACH, E., R. HERBERMAN, R. LIEBERMAN, M. M. FRANK AND I. GREEN. Receptors for immunoglobulin and complement on mouse leukemias and lymphomas. *J. Immunol.* 108: 325–328, 1972.

23. WARNER, N. L., L. A. HERZENBERG AND G. GOLDSTEIN. Immunoglobulin isoantigens (allotypes) in the mouse. II. Allotype analysis of three γG2-myeloma proteins from (NZB × BALB/c) F$_1$ hybrids of normal γG2-globulins. *J. Exptl. Med.* 123: 707–721, 1966.

Surface reorganization as an initial inductive event in the differentiation of prothymocytes to thymocytes[1,2]

E. A. BOYSE AND J. ABBOTT

Memorial Sloan-Kettering Cancer Center

New York, New York 10021

For several years my colleagues and I have been studying the question of how the constitution of cell surfaces may be determined by selective gene action, according to the various pathways of cellular differentiation, in the same way that the specialized functions of differentiated cells are evidently governed by the selective expression of particular genes (4, 8). This has involved a great deal of work on membrane components that are expressed exclusively on the surface of mouse thymocytes, because these cells are especially favorable for immunogenetic studies. While elucidating the details of thymocyte differentiation, it has always been uppermost in our minds that similar principles of differentiation may be involved in developmental processes, and that valuable inferences regarding embryonic development may transpire from the study of cellular differentiation in adult systems.

Recently Komuro and I developed a simple assay whereby one of the steps in the differentiative history of the T lymphocyte can be induced and observed in vitro. This T-cell induction assay, as we shall call it, offers several possible applications, notably of course immunological ones. These will doubtless all be assessed in due course, but in this paper we shall offer some speculations of a more general kind concerning the possible value of the T-cell induction system as a model for studying the regulation of phenotype during certain types of differentiation.

Cellular differentiation clearly ranks among the foremost topics of

[1] From Session II, *Gene Regulation in Differentiation and Development*, of the FASEB Conference on *Biology of Development and Aging*, presented at the 58th Annual Meeting of the Federation of American Societies for Experimental Biology, Atlantic City, N. J., April 9, 1974.

[2] Supported by National Cancer Institute Grant CA 08748 and National Institutes of Health Grant RO-1-08415-01.

41

modern biology, for a better under-standing of its mechanisms would no doubt shed light on important ques-tions as diverse as the regulation of embryogenesis at one extreme and the nature of cancer at the other. The formation of the embryo pro-vides spectacular exhibitions of dif-ferentiation and diversification of cells. By a series of transitions that are little understood, the zygote gen-erates the complete range of organ-ized differentiated cell types that con-stitute the mature organism. It is believed to do so by unlocking cor-responding sets of genetic informa-tion according to a master plan. We have no notion of what informa-tion might be comprised by any one such set of genetic instructions, but it is in tune with contemporary thought that much of it should relate to cell surface structure. This is be-cause it is difficult to conceive of the orderly deployment of billions of diversified cells without invoking pre-cisely controlled systems of surface discrimination. Therefore we look to the plasma membrane especially for acquisition of unique or char-acteristic displays of surface mole-cules, regulated by the genome during specific stages of differentia-tion, whose function in the embryo would be to receive relevant environ-mental signals including those for inductive events as well as those to guide the processes of cellular migra-tion and tissue organization.

To approach such embryological questions directly is not quite so remote as it might seem, and current work we are doing on mutants af-fecting early developmental stages of the mouse (3) is already promising in that direction (5, 25); but even here the prospect of defining a set of genes whose products would become manifest on the cell surface in re-sponse to a particular inductive signal is not yet within sight. But this is what we seem to be seeing in the T-cell induction system, although the cells induced come from the adult mouse rather than the embryonic mouse.

I repeat that it is no more than a reasonable expectation that those processes of cellular differentiation that continue throughout life, whose purpose is to allow for the replace-ment of expendable cells such as those of the hemopoietic systems, are in fact similarly governed. But we hope this is justified, and that by studying the life history of such adult cells we may learn something about the conspicuous examples of differen-tiation that take place during develop-ment.

The T-cell induction assay is fo-cused on a single differentiative step in the intermediate development of the T lymphocyte, and concerns what we shall refer to as the conversion of a prothymocyte into a thymocyte, the latter being defined for this pur-pose as a cell whose surface exhibits numerous components that are rec-ognized and commonly referred to as the T-cell antigens or surface mark-ers. The phenotype of the mouse thymocyte, in respect exclusively of these surface components that are not apparent on the prothymocyte, is: TL^+ (IX), $Thy-1^+$ (II), $Ly-1^+$ (XII), $Ly-2/Ly-3^+$ (XI), $Ly-5^+$ (?), G_{IX} (I and IX), $MSLA^+$.

From the linkage groups, indicated (where known) in parentheses, it is clear that conversion of the pro-thymocyte to a thymocyte involves manifestation of the products of at least six gene loci, and taking into account other incompletely-analyzed systems the number is certainly greater.

The technical details of the induc-tion procedure in vitro involve density gradient centrifugation of spleen or bone marrow populations to enrich the proportion of prothymocytes (14).

Cells of the enriched layer are incubated with an inducing agent for 2 hours or more. In a strongly positive test, up to 30% of the appropriate fraction now express the markers named in sufficient quantity to render them susceptible to lysis by the respective antisera in the complement-dependent cytotoxicity assay. The induction assay has also been carried out with unfractionated cells by Basch and Goldstein (2) using antibody absorption as the positive criterion, in which case the relatively low proportion of induced cells is not a particular disadvantage.

The first point to note is that this conversion occurs before cell division. It may well be, judging from the high rate of mitosis in the thymic cortex where this event presumably takes place under physiological conditions, that conversion is automatically followed by proliferation of the induced thymocyte, which is not yet a functionally competent immunocyte, and hence by the evolution of fully functional lymphocytes, which have the phenotype: TL^-, $Thy\text{-}1\downarrow$, $Ly\text{-}1^+$, $Ly\text{-}2/Ly\text{-}3^+$, $Ly\text{-}5^+$, G_{IX}^-, $MSLA^+$ (7) and are found in peripheral lymphoid organs; but this is conjecture and is outside the scope of this present discussion.

Second, there is no reason to assume that this rapid induction of a new set of surface components is peculiar to the thymocyte. It is perhaps equally probable that the same would be found to be true for similar differentiative steps of other cell types, when acted on by their particular inducers, if the same wealth of data were available regarding the genes selectively involved in specifying their surfaces. There are numerous embryonic induction systems where cell division appears to be a required step before expression of specialized function (13) but nothing

is known about intervening molecular changes at the cell surface. The thymocyte induction assay may simply happen to be the first system for which we have enough information to reveal in the inductive process an essential early stage that involves surface reorganization prior to cell division and functional maturation. In embryonic systems so far studied, the interval between induction and expression of function may be several days, a period of which we have little knowledge with respect to regulatory steps. If more data were available regarding the genes selectively involved in specifying cell surfaces in these systems, we might expect to find early surface reorganization similar to that observed in the thymocyte induction system.

In summary therefore, a generalization worth considering for inductive steps of this kind, in the embryo as well as in adult life, is that cell division may be required for expression of the functional phenotype, but that the initial consequence of induction is reconstitution of the cell surface by an earlier-expressed set of genes.

However, whether this phenomenon of surface renovation is exceptional or commonplace we have the same provocative and potentially instructive problem of understanding the transition of the prothymocyte to a thymocyte. The first question is: Does induction itself involve establishment of the genetic program expressed by the thymocyte, or is the program already decided beforehand? In our early study with Allan Goldstein it was soon apparent that the latter is true, because several materials in addition to products of the thymus were seen to be capable of inducing prothymocyte conversion (18). These include extracts of tissues other than thymus, endotoxin and the synthetic polynucleotide poly

A:U which perhaps significantly are both known to act as immunoadjuvants in vivo, and also the "second messenger" cyclic AMP. It is therefore evident that the prothymocyte, before its migration to the thymus, already bears the instructions that will decide its phenotype, and which it will express in response to a signal from the thymus.

We see that prothymocyte induction can be initiated in vitro by a variety of agents, whereas plainly under physiological conditions only the thymic agent is active in vivo. In so-called 'nude' mice that have no thymus there is no lack of prothymocytes, as is indicated by the fact that their spleens and bone marrow are as rich a source of inducible cells as the spleen and bone marrow of normal mice (15, 18). Yet T lymphocytes are not normally found in these mice and in consequence they are immunologically crippled. Ostensibly therefore, under physiological conditions in vivo, it is the thymus and only the thymus that mediates prothymocyte conversion. The likelihood is that whatever fortuitous inductions of prothymocytes may take place in thymus-deprived mice, from chance circumstances such as exposure to endotoxin from intestinal flora, are not sufficient to yield a demonstrable population of thymocytes or mature T cells. It must be admitted that this conclusion is not entirely satisfactory, because the thymocyte phenotype is evidently transitional, and the ensuing stages of cell division and functional maturation that result in functional T cells are neither well understood nor yet readily amenable to study in vitro. Therefore to equate the lack of T lymphocytes in thymus-deprived mice with failure of prothymocyte induction is open to question. Until and unless agents capable of inducing prothymocytes are shown to restore the immune capacity of thymus-deprived mice, it seems unsafe to rule out that prothymocyte induction may occur fortuitously in thymus-deprived mice but is neither maintained nor progresses, and so escapes detection. Accepting this necessary reservation we can take the uncomplicated view that an essential differentiative step which in vivo displays a high degree of specificity (i.e., is dependent on a functional thymus) can be triggered in vitro by a variety of agents of no seeming relevance to thymic function.

It is in this respect that the circumstances of prothymocyte induction bear a possibly significant resemblance to some accounts of embryonic induction systems that have been studied in vitro. The essence of embryonic induction is that at given times, and in given locations in the developing embryo, sets of cells are differentiated, according to prescribed morphogenetic patterns, in a way that suggests they are responding to signals emitted by other tissues, supposedly the source of inducers. Test systems designed to provide models for the study of embryonic induction in vitro fit in a general way the description of the T-cell induction assay, in that they concern exposure of target cells to an inducer of some kind, or to a tissue that is the putative source of the inducer, in order to bring about under controlled conditions the expression of the new phenotype which the target cells were destined to exhibit in vivo.

As illustrated in Table 1, it has been a perplexing aspect of some such experimental systems that the differentiative step in question can apparently be triggered not only by the putatively relevant tissue or a product of it, but also by a variety of other agents (1, 10-12, 20, 21, 24). How might the T-cell induction system help in resolving the dilemma of precisely programmed morphogenetic processes that surely must in vivo be regulated by specific signals, yet which in vitro can sometimes be initiated by what seem to be physiologically irrelevant or inappropriate stimuli? Here of course it may be highly significant that most embryonic inductive systems are thought to involve preprogrammed target cells, as we have already inferred to be the case for the conversion of prothymocytes to thymocytes.

In the T-cell induction system we know that the inductive process, seemingly so indiscriminate in vitro, is mediated specifically in vivo. We can determine this because in vivo, in the absence of a thymus, the differentiative sequence of the T lineage of cells is blocked at a particular step. So we start with a clear picture that induction in vivo under physiological conditions is specific, regardless of what may be the case in vitro. Since the prothymocyte is a 'preprogrammed' or 'determined' cell, we can infer that the specificity of the thymus in this connection must lie in its capacity to induce the differentiation of prothymocytes exclusively, as distinct from other pre-

programmed cells such as B lymphocytes, which are not lacking from thymus-deprived mice. Undoubtedly there is much to be gained by drawing comparisons with peptide hormone systems, particularly in regard to two striking differences in the known consequences of the interaction of the hormone and inducer with their target cells. These refer in the case of thymopoietin, first to the initial prompt manifestation of a set of well-defined genes for surface composition and second, from what we can infer at the moment, to the presumed attainment of an irreversible differentiated state that will be maintained independently of the inducer. It is the latter that particularly invites the suggestion of general relevance of the T-cell induction system to differentiation-induction processes, including those in the embryo, which evoke the manifestation of a predetermined set of genes.

To substantiate that the function of the thymus in regard to prothymocyte induction is the provision of a specific signal for the prothymocyte, an additional parameter should be added to the T-cell induction procedure in vitro to distinguish specific from nonspecific induction.

TABLE 1. Some induction systems that respond to multiple inducing agents

Induction system	Natural inducer	Other inducing agents	Ref.
Gastrula ectoderm → neural tissue	Archenteron roof	Guinea pig liver or kidney tissue or extracts; yeast nucleoprotein; ionic changes	(1,11,20, 21,24)
Neurula ectoderm → lens	Optic vesicles head mesoderm	Liver and heart tissue, living or dead	(12,21)
Metanephrogenic mesenchyme → epithelial tubules	Ureteric bud	Dorsal spinal cord	(10)

TABLE 2. Specificity of thymopoietin for prothymocyte induction

	T-cell assay (acquisition of thymocyte antigens)	B-cell assay (acquisition of complement receptors)
Thymopoietin I and II	+	−
3rd polypeptide	+	+

Otherwise, although the assay would be useful in such practical applications as the enumeration of prothymocytes in clinical immune-deficiency states (22), it would be of only limited value in elucidating thymic function. The added parameter which my colleagues Scheid and Hammerling have decided to investigate is the induction of B-lymphocyte differentiation. Of several criteria that might be used to signify B-cell differentiation the one that they find most serviceable at the moment is the appearance of the complement receptor which causes B cells to form rosettes on exposure to red cells sensitized by antibody plus nonlytic complement (6). The precursor cells for this assay, representing committed members of the B-cell lineage, are also derived from spleen and bone marrow. With this dual assay we are in a better position to assess whether a given inducer prepared from thymus is physiologically relevant, for if so, it should be active in the T-cell but not the B-cell assay. On the other hand, the class of inducers that does not constitute primary physiological signals may not distinguish between the two types of precursor cells to which they are presented in the combined assay.

Results we are obtaining with polypeptides isolated from thymus by

Gideon Goldstein seem to vindicate this proposition and to illustrate the value of the dual assay (Table 2). The history of these polypeptides is an interesting story in itself: In the course of investigating the relation of the thymus to the human disease myasthenia gravis, Gideon Goldstein found that the thymus secretes substances which affect neuromuscular transmission (9). Using these neuromuscular effects in mice as an assay he isolated from thymus two closely related 7,000-molecular-weight polypeptides now termed thymopoietin I and II which have similar biological properties in the tests so far used (2, 9). Both are present only in thymus, according to the neuromuscular criterion. Both we now find to be highly active in T-cell induction but not in B-cell induction (Table 2). Thymopoietin therefore has a good claim to be the physiological inducer which causes prothymocytes to differentiate into thymocytes.

On the other hand a third polypeptide isolated from thymus had no neuromuscular effects. This polypeptide has a molecular weight of 8,500 and is active in both the T-cell and B-cell assays (Table 2). It comes as no great surprise therefore that this third polypeptide, which is a potent inducer of T- and B-cell differentiation in our assay systems, has since been identified by Gideon Goldstein in a wide variety of other tissues (personal communication).

Whatever the function of this very widely represented polypeptide may be, it certainly does not generally function as a prothymocyte inducer in vivo for it is found in the tissues of thymus-deprived as well as normal mice; it could well be the agent responsible for the inducing activity of tissue extracts other than those from thymus. So in regard to the theme of drawing inferences that may be generally useful in studying induction systems it can be pointed out that even a highly purified agent that can act as an inducer in high dilution in vitro may be physiologically irrelevant to the system under study. One way of distinguishing such an agent from the physiological inducer is to use more than one induction system, thereby establishing specificity. A second criterion, satisfied for thymopoietin, is that the physiological inducer is obtainable only from the tissue that is the natural source of the inductive signal.

A reasonable hypothesis for the T-cell induction system, which can serve as a basis for experimental verification, is that the specific thymic polypeptide engages a specific receptor on the prothymocyte and initiates expression of the thymocyte phenotype via adenylate cyclase and cyclic AMP, as some polypeptide hormones are known to act on their target organs. Preliminary results obtained in collaboration with colleagues at Sloan-Kettering support this hypothesis (17). Concerning the complexity of the phenotype expressed by prothymocytes in response to thymopoietin, it may be especially relevant that the interaction of polypeptide hormones with cell-surface receptors may engender pleiotypic responses involving activation of several different membrane enzymes (19).

Commitment or programming of the stem cell for the T-lymphocyte program must be an earlier step that takes place elsewhere. For cells of the erythroid, myeloid and megakaryocytic lines there is evidence that commitment occurs in discrete specific "hematopoietic-inductive microenvironments" in spleen and bone marrow, each of which will specifically commit the same previously indifferent stem cell to one or another program (See reviews by McCulloch (16) and Trentin (23)). Thus for example a stem cell committed to the erythroid pathway by the respective microenvironment will if subsequently acted on by erythropoietin, produce progeny expressing only the erythroid phenotype. For the prothymocyte we have no corresponding evidence of the site of commitment, except to say this is not in the thymus itself.

The nature of programming— the manner in which such sets of instructions are retained by committed cells and can even be stably transmitted to descendant cells without obvious expression—is a well-known and crucial puzzle in regard to cells of many different kinds. Whether manifestation of the programmed phenotype is controlled by transcription or translation, or in some other way, is not known, nor whether what we see in T-cell induction may be an amplification or revelation of components that were already subliminally or covertly expressed in the noninduced committed precursor cell.

But inasmuch as the T-cell induction process offers a special opportunity to study the institution of such a program in a simple system in vitro, without the intervention of cell division, it may provide an unusually favorable model for tackling precisely those questions.

Note added in proof: The "third inductive polypeptide" activates adenylases and has a wide species distribution; it has been named ubiquitous immunopoietic polypeptide (UBIP) (Goldstein, G., et al., *Proc. Natl. Acad. Sci. U.S.* In press).

REFERENCES

1. BARTH, I. G. *Biol. Bull.* 131; 415, 1966.
2. BASCH, R. S., AND G. GOLDSTEIN. *Proc. Natl. Acad. Sci. U.S.* 71: 1474, 1974.
3. BENNETT, D. *Science* 144: 263, 1964.
4. BENNETT, D., E. A. BOYSE AND L. J. OLD. In: *Cell Interactions,* edited by L. G. Silvestri. Amsterdam: North-Holland, 1972, p. 247.
5. BENNETT, D., E. GOLDBERG, L. C. DUNN

AND E. A. BOYSE. *Proc. Natl. Acad. Sci. U.S.* 69: 2076, 1972.

6. BIANCO, C., R. PATRICK AND V. NUSSEN-SWEIG. *J. Exptl. Med.* 132: 702, 1970.

7. BOYSE, E. A., AND D. BENNETT. In: *Cellular Selection and Regulation in the Immune Response*, edited by G. M. Edelman. New York: Raven, Vol. 29, 1974, p. 155.

8. BOYSE, E. A., AND L. J. OLD. *Ann. Rev. Genet.* 3: 269, 1969.

9. GOLDSTEIN, G. *Nature* 247: 11, 1974.

10. GROBSTEIN, C. *Exptl. Cell Res.* 13, 575, 1972.

11. HOLTFRETER, J. *Wilhelm Roux' Arch. Entwicklungsmech. Organismen* 127: 584, 1933.

12. HOLTFRETER, J. *Wilhelm Roux' Arch. Entwicklungsmech. Organismen* 133: 367, 1934.

13. HOLTZER, H. In: *Control Mechanisms in the Expression of Cellular Phenotypes*, edited by Padykula. New York: Academic, 1970, p. 69.

14. KOMURO, K., AND E. A. BOYSE. *Lancet* 1: 740, 1973.

15. KOMURO, K., AND E. A. BOYSE. *J. Exptl. Med.* 138: 479, 1973.

16. MCCULLOCH, E. A. In: *Regulation of Hematopoiesis*, edited by A. S. Gordon, New York: Appleton-Century-Crofts, 1970, p. 132.

17. SCHEID, M. P., G. GOLDSTEIN, U. HAMMERLING AND E. A. BOYSE. *Thymus Factors in Immunity*. New York: Ann. N.Y. Acad. Sci. In press.

18. SCHEID, M. P., M. K. HOFFMANN, K. KOMURO, U. HAMMERLING, J. ABBOTT, E. A. BOYSE, G. H. COHEN, J. A. HOOPER, R. S. SCHULOFF AND A. L. GOLDSTEIN. *J. Exptl. Med.* 138: 1027, 1973.

19. SONENBERG, M., N. I. SWISLOCKI, R. S. BOCKMAN, Y. AIZONO, M. C. POSTEL-VIMAY, M. RUBIN AND J. ROBERTS. *J. Supramolecular Structure* 1: 356, 1973.

20. SPEMANN, H., AND H. MANGOLD. *Arch. Mikrosk. Anat. Entwicklungsmech.* 100: 599, 1924.

21. TOIVONEN, S., AND T. KUUSI *Ann. Zool. Soc. Zool. Botan. Fennicae Vanamo* 13: 1, 1948.

22. TOURAINE, J. L., G. S. INCEFY, F. TOURAINE, Y. M. RHO AND R. A. GOOD. *Clin. Exptl. Immunol.* In press.

23. TRENTIN, J. J. In: *Regulation of Hematopoiesis*, edited by A. S. Gordon. New York. Appleton-Century-Crofts, 1970, p. 159.

24. YAMADA, T. *Embryologia* 3: 69, 1966.

25. YANAGISAWA, K., D. BENNETT, E. A. BOYSE, L. C. DUNN AND A. DIMEO. *Immunogenetics* 1: 57, 1974.

Germ line basis
for antibody diversity[1,2]

A. R. WILLIAMSON[3], E. PREMKUMAR[4] AND M. SHOYAB

Department of Microbiology and Immunology
University of California, Los Angeles School of Medicine
Los Angeles, California 90024

ABSTRACT

Each antibody polypeptide chain is the product of a gene pair comprising one constant (C) gene coding for that portion of the chain common to all chains of the same type and one variable (V) gene coding for the sequence unique to each chain. Previous evidence indicates that the haploid genome has a single copy of each distinct C gene and that for expression a gene pair is formed with any one of a family of V genes present in the same haploid genome. Hybridization of purified mRNA coding for immunoglobulin heavy chain (mRNA-H) with a vast excess of DNA confirms the existence of a single C gene of each type and multiple V genes. A large number (of the order of 10^4) of V genes would be consistent with the hybridization results. This suggests considerable V gene redundancy which is a predictable property of a multiple V gene family maintained by expansion and contraction mechanisms. The mRNA-H used in these hybridization studies was isolated by a specific interaction with immunoglobulin. The same method has also been used to isolate a nuclear precursor of mRNA-H. Identification of this precursor strengthens the evidence for the direct joining of the V and C gene pair at the DNA level prior to transcription.— WILLIAMSON, A. R., E. PREMKUMAR AND M. SHOYAB. Germ line basis for antibody diversity. *Federation Proc*. 34: 28–32, 1975.

All vertebrates possess the ability to make a set of protein molecules (antibodies) sufficiently similar to have once passed for a single protein, yet each subtly different such that there appears to be at least one molecule that will bind any chemical determinant.

Antibodies present a sufficient variety of combining sites such that for any antibody molecule there is another molecule (or more than one) which will specifically recognize the binding site of the first. This leads

[1] From Session II, *Gene Regulation in Differentiation and Development*, of the FASEB Conference on *Biology of Development and Aging*, presented at the 58th Annual Meeting of the Federation of American Societies for Experimental Biology, Atlantic City, N.J., April 9, 1974.

[2] Part of the work described in this article was supported by National Institutes of Health Grant CA12800 to Dr. John L. Fahey.

[3] Present address: Department of Biochemistry, University of Glasgow, Glasgow G12 8QQ, Scotland.

[4] Present address: Lab. of Cell Biology, National Cancer Institute, NIH, Bethesda, Md. 20014.

one to the position that the extent of antibody diversity must be governed by an 'uncertainty principle' such that we can never exactly define the extent of diversity.

Attempts to measure the number of antibody molecules experimentally support the uncertainty principle. The number of variable region sequences so far obtained for myeloma proteins points to a very large number of possible variable region sequences for mouse kappa chains (15). Even a minimal estimate of the number of V_{kappa} genes based on amino acid sequence differences outside of the hypervariable regions is about 240 (3). One experimental approach has been made to the question of the number of different antibodies binding a simple hapten. In inbred CBA/H mice the number of distinct $V_L V_H$ pairs binding 5-iodo-4-hydroxy-3-nitrophenylacetyl (NIP) was in the range of 5,000 (18).

Despite these daunting numbers several individual genetic loci coding for particular specificities have been defined in the mouse (4, 9, 16, 19, 28). These V-region loci behave as single Mendelian genes and it should soon be possible to draw a map of their relative positions.

The proposal of separate genes for V and C regions of L and H chains was made nine years ago by Dreyer and Bennett (8). Subsequently accumulated evidence has brought wide acceptance of the idea of two genes— one polypeptide chain. This remains a basic assumption for any hypothesis requiring multiple V genes, and any tenable hypothesis must now allow multiple V genes.

Faced with this fascinating novel genetic system we wish to know how it works. This article presents our recent approaches to the molecular genetics of antibody diversity. A range of techniques, developed mainly in studies of prokaryotic systems, is available. Here we present the use of one such technique, that of RNA hybridization to a vast excess of DNA. These experiments are made easier and more amenable to interpretation by the isolation of purified mRNA coding for immunoglobulin heavy chain (mRNA-H) using a specific method (31). One of the immediate questions concerns the mode of integration of V- and C-gene information. The available evidence points to the DNA or RNA level with a weighting towards interaction of DNA molecules. The specific isolation (32) of a nuclear precursor to mRNA-H is, as discussed below, a further strong piece of evidence for direct joining of V and C genes. The questions as to when, during development, joining occurs and whether joining leads to a stable V-C gene or whether there is reversibility, remain open.

The question most frequently posed is "how many V genes constitute the multiple V gene family?" If the family is small then one needs to search for mechanisms for generating diversity in each genome at the level of the somatic cell. If the family is large, which is the conclusion drawn from our present data, then in defining the size we may be answering the question of the extent of antibody diversity. However here again a veil of uncertainty is present in the form of gene redundancy which, as discussed below, is most probably a feature of the V gene family.

ISOLATION OF mRNA-H AND ITS NUCLEAR PRECURSOR

The interaction between mRNA-H and immunoglobulin was initially

---

Abbreviations: NIP = 5-iodo-4-hydroxy-3-nitrophenylacetyl.

postulated from the finding of a translational control in mouse myeloma 5563 cells (33, 34). It was then shown that 5563 myeloma protein (IgG₂ₐ) binds to mRNA-H from 5563 cells and that precipitation of the complex with rabbit anti-5563 IgG₂ₐ provides a

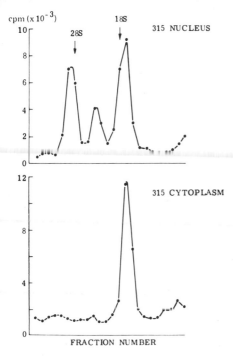

Figure 1. Electrophoretic patterns of mRNA-α isolated from the cytoplasm and nucleus of MOPC315 myeloma cells. Cultured 315 cells were incubated with [³H]-uridine for 3 hours at 37 C. Total polyA containing RNA was prepared separately from nuclei and cytoplasm as described previously (26). mRNA-α was isolated by precipitation with 315 myeloma protein and rabbit anti-315 myeloma protein as described for mRNA-γ₂ₐ (31) with the exception that the reaction was carried out in 150 mM NaCl-1.0 mM MgCl₂-20 mM phosphate buffer (pH 7.6). Analysis by polyacrylamide gel electrophoresis was performed as previously described (31). The positions of 28S and 18S ribosomal RNA markers are indicated.

specific route for the purification of mRNA-H (31). Further studies (Premkumar, Stevens and Williamson, ms in preparation) have shown interclass and interspecies binding of immunoglobulin to mRNA-H. This led to the proposal that there are conserved complementary binding sites on all immunoglobulin molecules and on all mRNA H molecules (35). Proof of this proposal would imply an important role for this binding. One interesting possibility would be a function for these binding sites in the induction of antibody synthesis.

Stevens (ms submitted for publication) has quantitated the interaction and finds it to be very tight. For rabbit IgG and 5563 mRNA-H he found an equilibrium constant K, $2-3 \times 10^{-13}$M at 24 C and 150 mM Na⁺. This value is within the range of the binding constants found for *lac* and λ-phage repressor-DNA interactions. The strength of the binding is another factor which suggests that it plays some important role. In addition knowing the strength of binding explains the high selectivity of the interaction and the fact of the isolation of highly purified mRNA-H by precipitation of the complex.

The purity of the mRNA-α isolated from MOPC315 cells by the immunoglobulin precipitation method (31) is illustrated in Fig. 1. The lower panel shows the monodisperse RNA molecule isolated from the cytoplasm. A closely similar component is present in the nucleus of MOPC315 cells and in addition two other RNA molecules are isolated from the nucleus. The RNA molecule with the highest molecular weight (>28S) is almost certainly equivalent to the large precursor to mRNA-γ₂ₐ isolated from the nucleus of 5563 cells (32). The intermediate-size RNA molecule probably represents a stage in the processing of the pre-mRNA-α to the 17S cyto-

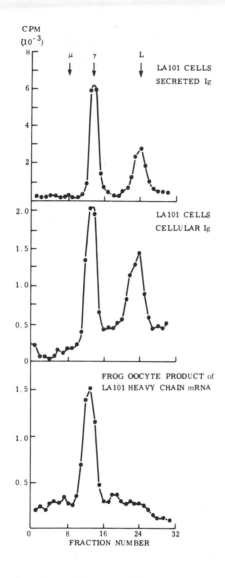

Figure 2. Comparison between the heavy and light chains synthesized and secreted by LA101 cells and the translation product of LA101 mRNA-H in *Xenopus laevis* oocytes. Top and middle panels: Cultured LA101 human lymphoid cells were incubated at 10^6 cells/ml in leucine-free medium with [^{3}H]-leucine for 6 hours. The cells and medium were separated by centrifugation. The cells were lysed with 1% NP-40, the nuclei removed at 2,000 *g* × 5 min and a clear supernatant prepared at 20,000 *g* × 30 min. Immunoglobulins were precipitated from both intracellular supernatant (cellular Ig) and from the growth medium (secreted Ig) with rabbit antihuman immunoglobulin. The precipitates were washed, dissolved in 2% SDS, reduced, alkylated and analyzed on polyacrylamide gels (36). Bottom panel: LA101 mRNA-H, isolated as described under Fig. 1, was injected, together with [^{35}S]-methionine, into oocytes from *Xenopus laevis* as previously described (36). Incubation was overnight at room temperature. The oocytes were disrupted, and radioactively labeled immunoglobulin was precipitated and analyzed as described above. The positions of marker μ and γ heavy chains and light chain (L) are indicated.

plasmic mRNA-α. The finding that the whole H chain is encoded in a single nuclear pre-mRNA-H greatly strengthens the previous evidence supporting the proposal that the joining of V gene and C gene information occurs at the level of DNA.

Human mRNA-γ has been isolated from a lymphoid cell line LA101, using the IgG-anti-IgG precipitation method. Cell line LA101, one of a series established in culture by M. Jobin, in the laboratory of Dr. J. L. Fahey, produces and secretes an IgG (Fig. 2, top and middle panels). The RNA extracted from the IgG-anti-IgG precipitate of the cytoplasm of ^{3}H-uridine labeled LA101 cells is a single component (Fig. 3). Translation of this RNA in *Xenopus laevis* oocytes yields γ chain with no detectable L-chain synthesis (Fig. 2, bottom panel).

FREQUENCY OF GENES CODING FOR mRNA-H

The frequency of genes coding for a given RNA molecule can be estimated by hybridization of that RNA (radioactively labeled) with a vast excess of DNA (2, 20). To achieve the required vast excess of DNA the concentra-

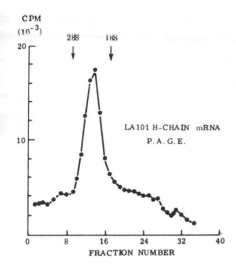

Figure 0. Radioactively labeled mRNA-γ isolated from the cytoplasm of LA101 cells by precipitation with human immunoglobulin and rabbit anti-human immunoglobulin. Exponentially growing LA101 cells were incubated with [³H]-uridine (1 mCi/ml) for 14 hours at 37 C. Isolation and analysis of mRNA-γ was similar to that described for mRNA-α (Fig. 1). The specific activity of mRNA-γ was 2 × 10⁶ cpm/μg.

reiteration frequency is estimated by comparison of the midpoint of the C_ot curve with that of a standard C_ot curve (20); in these experiments *Escherichia coli* cRNA, made by copying *E. coli* DNA with DNA-dependent RNA polymerase, was hybridized to homologous DNA giving a standard for unique sequence hybridization (26).

Meaningful interpretation of the experimental C_ot curve requires that the purity of the labeled mRNA be high. This condition is met by the mRNA-H used in these experiments. The required high specific of the mRNA was achieved by labeling cell cultures with ³H nucleosides (uridine alone or together with cytidine) at 1 mCi/ml culture. The mRNA-α from MOPC315 cells was labeled to a specific activity of 1.2×10^6 cpm/μg (26).

The C_ot curve for hybridization of murine mRNA-α to whole mouse embryo DNA is shown in Fig. 4. This curve is most simply interpreted as a biphasic curve, though it may be more complex. A multiphase curve

tion of radioactive RNA must be low and so for detection purposes the specific activity of the RNA must be high. It is usual to fragment the DNA to be used in the reaction and in our experiment the radioactive mRNA-H was also sheared by sonication. After this treatment the DNA and mRNA-H were mixed, denatured together at 100 C and allowed to hybridize at 65 C. At intervals samples were removed and treated with ribonuclease to determine the proportion of labeled RNA in nuclease-resistant RNA–DNA hybrids. This value is plotted as a function of the logarithm of C_ot (concentration of DNA as nucleotides in mole/liter multiplied by the time of reaction in seconds) (5). The gene

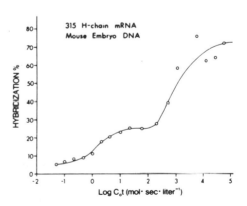

Figure 4. Kinetics of hybridization of 315 mRNA-α with DNA from whole mouse embryos. Details have been described elsewhere (26). (From Premkumar et al. (26) with permission).

can be analyzed in terms of the proportion of the RNA hybridizing to complementary DNA sequences of different reiteration frequency. The major portion of the C_0t curve (Fig. 4) accounts for 65% of the total hybridization achieved up to C_0t 50,000. The $C_0t_{\frac{1}{2}}$ value for this major transition is 10^3 which gives a calculated reiteration frequency of 8 genes. The accuracy in this region of high C_0t values is such that this major transition, i.e., 65% of mRNA-α, should be regarded as being encoded by 'unique' genes. The remaining 35% of the mRNA-α molecule is complementary to highly reiterated DNA sequences. Approximately 6% of mRNA-α hybridizes by C_0t 0.1 and a further 29% hybridizes by C_0t 100. The midpoint of this transition $C_0t_{\frac{1}{2}}$ = 1.5 corresponds to a reiteration frequency of 5,300 genes.

An interpretation of these data in terms of the coding regions of mRNA-α is shown in Fig. 5. The cytoplasmic mRNA-α_{315} contains about 1,800 nucleotides of the original transcript from the V_{315}-C_α gene. The number of nucleotides needed to code for the V and C regions is shown as 350 and 1,000

respectively. This leaves 450 nucleotides apparently untranslated, though an indeterminate portion of this sequence (indicated by the dashed line at the 5'-end of the V region) probably codes for a precursor peptide with which translation is initiated but which is subsequently cleaved. The ribosome binding site for initiation of translation is shown schematically as is the binding site for immunoglobulin which is assumed on the basis of present evidence (30) to be at or near the ribosome binding site. The assignment of untranslated sequences to the 5'- and 3'-ends of the mRNA is on the basis of the C_0t curve. The C region (55% of mRNA) is expected, from the extensive genetic data, to be encoded by a unique gene so this accounts for 85% of the unique C_0t transition. The remainder of the unique C_0t transition, 10% of total hybridization, appears to be insufficient to account for the V region (19.5% of mRNA) and so is assigned to untranslated sequence between the C region and the poly A. The V region and the remainder of the untranslated sequence, including the two binding sites, are assigned to the low C_0t transition.

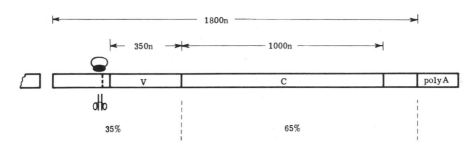

Figure 5. Schematic representation of 315 mRNA-α showing the putative positions of the coding regions for V and C sequences relative to the untranslated regions based on the data shown in Fig. 4. The binding sites for the ribosome initiating translation and for the immunoglobulin molecule controlling that initiation step are indicated appropriately. Both sites are assumed to lie to the 5'-end of the codon for the N-terminal amino acid of the isolated α-chain to allow for the probable existence of a precursor α-chain with an additional N-terminal sequence.

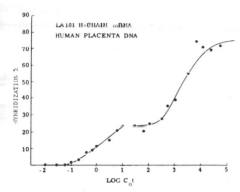

Figure 6. Kinetics of hybridization of LA101 mRNA-γ with DNA from human placenta. The mRNA-γ described under Fig. 3 was hybridized with excess DNA under similar conditions to those used for Fig. 4.

An alternative model to that shown in Fig. 5 would be to assign both V and C regions (74.5% of mRNA) to the unique transition and to account for the low $C_o t$ transition entirely in terms of untranslated sequence. This does not fit the experimental curve (Fig. 4) as well as the model shown in Fig. 5.

The hybridization results using human mRNA-γ should be considered together with the above results before discussing them further. The mRNA-γ was labeled with ^{3}H-uridine to a specific activity 2×10^6 cpm/μg. The $C_o t$ curve obtained by hybridizing this mRNA-γ with human placental DNA is shown in Fig. 6. The curve, like that shown in Fig. 4, is essentially biphasic. The unique transition (calculated reiteration frequency = 4) accounts for 68% of the total hybridization achieved. The low $C_o t$ transition with a midpoint at 1.4 is broader than expected for the hybridization of a single sequence to identical reiterated genes. The reiteration frequency for this transition is 7,800.

Both sets of data, and indeed either of the two types of interpretation

offered above, fit a scheme with multiple V_H genes and a set of C_H genes comprising one copy for each class and subclass of H chain. Most variations on these interpretations point to a large pool of V_H genes. Models which consider that only untranslated nucleotide sequences are involved in the low $C_o t$ transition are plausible. The simplest explanation of such highly reiterated sequences coding for the untranslated part of mRNA-H would be that they represent a sequence common to all V_H genes. The reiteration frequency determined from the low $C_o t$ transition would thus be a maximum size for the V_H-gene pool.

Taking the more attractive interpretation of the data in which V_H-region sequence of the mRNA-H is included in the low $C_o t$ transition (e.g., model shown in Fig. 5) it is harder to estimate the size of the V_H gene pool. The most extreme, and unlikely, form of this model is one which says that mouse and human DNA have 5,300 and 7,800 copies of genes V_{H-315} and V_{H-101} respectively.

Another interpretation is that these reiteration frequencies represent cross-hybridizing V_H genes similar in basic sequence, but not identical to the probe sequences V_{H-315} and V_{H-101}. The constancy of amino acid sequences for human V_H regions of the same subgroup (1, 7) could be consistent with extensive cross-hybridization of one mRNA with genes of the same V_H subgroup. However, the possibility of base changes in the third position of each codon without alteration of the encoded amino acid sequence makes such predictions hazardous (10). The amino acid sequence of the V region of MOPC315 α chain is known (12). It does not show extensive homology with other known mouse V_H regions but the available data are limited. Consistent with the idea of cross-homology between the probe mRNA and a diverse set of V_H genes is the breadth of the low $C_o t$ transition, especially noticeable in Fig. 6. This transition may be a complex curve made up of various fractions of the V_H region and untranslated nucleotide sequences, some of which are common to many or all V_H genes, while others are shared by a smaller number of V_H genes. In this interpretation the sequence specifying the binding site for immunoglobulin would be an example of a region shared between all V_H genes. The number of V_H genes represented by such a complex curve could be in excess of 20,000. This interpretation does not comment on how many different V_H are carried in the germ-line pool. The number of different V_H genes might be considerably less than the total number of V_H genes since gene redundancy, i.e., multiple copies of each gene, is a predictable property of such a multigene system (see below).

EVOLUTION AND MAINTENANCE OF MULTIPLE V-GENE SYSTEM

The assumption will now be made, on the basis of the arguments cited above, that a large number of V_H genes are present in the germ-line DNA. It is then pertinent to ask how this set of genes has been acquired and how and to what degree it is stabilized. These questions are discussed briefly in this section with the conclusion that, for a multiple V gene system to supply a sufficiently large set of V regions to account for antibody diversity, there would inevitably be extensive V-gene redundancy.

Any model for the evolution of the immune response is required to introduce the capacity for extensive antibody diversity as an early property

of the system. If antibody diversity has always depended mainly on a sufficient set of germ-line V genes this implies a rapid initial expansion of the number of V genes with subsequent introduction of diversity among the genes. For sufficient diversity to be generated without the need for special mutation rates a very large number of V genes must be generated in the initial expansion. The processes whereby rapid amplification of V genes can occur were not operative only at one time during evolution but rather they are continually functional. The existence of V_H-region allotypes, characteristic of most but not all V_H sequences of a given rabbit haplotype (39), of V-region subgroups (23, 25) and of phylogenetically associated amino acids (7, 11) all testify to recent V gene amplification.

Rapid gene amplification occurs in other multiple gene systems (27, 37). The need for such amplification can be seen in terms of the need to offset the tendency to eliminate genes from multigene systems (21, 22, 27). Expansion and contraction of the ribosomal RNA genes can occur by unequal crossing-over between homologous chromosomes or between sister chromosomes. Regulation of the number of V genes by unequal crossing-over would have to be restricted to exchanges between sister chromatids in order to account for the low recombination frequency observed with V_H allotypes in the rabbit. Tartof (38) has shown that unequal mitotic sister chromosome exchange is the method by which ribosomal gene amplification proceeds in *Drosophila melanogaster*. Unequal recombination would tend to transmit mutations 'horizontally' (6) and would naturally lead to the known patterns of amino acid sequence conservation in V regions (allotypes, subgroups and phylogenetically associated residues). The entire multigene family can remain essentially homogeneous depending on the frequency of recombination relative to the rate of mutation and the number of genes in the family (38). For the multiple V genes it would be necessary to have mutations accumulating at a rate exceeding the tendency towards a homogeneous set of genes: here of course selection may be the crucial event.

Unequal recombinational events would result in a certain level of V gene redundancy being maintained. Gene redundancy would also result from alternative amplification mechanisms in which multiple tandem copies of any V gene can be generated, by, for example, a "rolling circle" mode of DNA replication (13). In this saltatory replication model the steady-state level of redundancy might be higher than in the recombinational model.

The idea that expansion and contraction might apply to the V gene family (14, 24, 29) seems to have been introduced to explain the patterns of V-region amino acid sequence. It can be seen that fluctuation of the composition of the V-gene family by concurrent amplification of some genes and elimination of others would probably be an inherent feature of the maintenance of a multiple V-gene family. As a consequence of this fluctuation redundant copies of many V genes will probably exist at any one time. The large number of V_H genes estimated from our RNA-DNA hybridization data is consistent with the maintenance of a sufficient population of different V_H genes to account for reasonable estimates (17, 40) of the antibody repertoire.

REFERENCES

1. BIRSHTEIN, B. K., AND J. J. CEBRA. *Biochemistry* 10: 4930, 1971.
2. BISHOP, J. O. Gene transcription in reproductive tissue. *Karolinska Symposia on Research Methods in Reproductive Endocrinology*, 5th Symposium, p 247.
3. BLOMBERG, B., M. COHN, W. GECKELER, W. RASCHKE, R. RIBLET AND M. WEIGERT. In: *The Immune System: Genes, Receptors, Signals*, edited by C. F. Fox, E. E. Sercarz and A. R. Williamson. New York: Academic, 1974.
4. BLOMBERG, B., W. R. GECKELER AND M. WEIGERT. *Science* 177: 178, 1972.
5. BRITTEN, R. J., AND D. E. KOHNE. *Science* 161: 529, 1968.
6. BROWN, D. D., P. C. WENSINK AND E. JORDAN. *J. Mol. Biol.* 63: 57, 1972.
7. CAPRA, J. D., R. L. WASSERMAN AND J. M. KEHOE. *J. Exptl. Med.* 138: 410, 1973.
8. DREYER, W. J., AND J. C. BENNETT. *Proc. Natl. Acad. Sci. U.S.* 54: 864, 1965.
9. EICHMANN, K., AND C. BEREK. *European J. Immunol.* 3: 599, 1973.
10. FARQUHAR, M. N., AND B. J. McCARTHY. *Biochemistry* 12: 4113, 1973.
11. FRANEK, F. *FEBS Letters* 8: 269, 1970.
12. FRANCIS, S. H., R. G. Q. LESLIE, L. HOOD AND H N EISEN. *Proc. Natl. Acad. Sci. U.S.* 71: 1123, 1974.
13. GILBERT, W., AND D. DRESSLER. *Cold Spring Harbor Symp. Quant. Biol.* 33: 473, 1968.
14. HOOD, L., K. EICHMANN, H. LACKLAND, R. M. KRAUSE AND J. J. OHMS. *Nature* 228: 1040, 1970.
15. HOOD, L., D. McKEAN, V. FARNSWORTH AND M. POTTER. *Biochemistry* 12: 741, 1973.
16. IMANISHI, T., AND O. MÄKELÄ. *European J. Immunol* 3: 323, 1973.
17. INMAN, J. K. In: *The Immune System: Genes, Receptors, Signals*, edited by C. F. Fox, E. E. Sercarz and A. R. Williamson. New York: Academic, 1974.
18. KRETH, H. W., AND A. R. WILLIAMSON. *European J. Immunol.* 3: 141, 1973.
19. KUETTNER, M. G., A. L. WANG AND A. NISONOFF. *J. Exptl. Med.* 135: 579, 1972.
20. MELLI, M., C. WHITFIELD, K. V. RAO, M. RICHARDSON AND J. O. BISHOP. *Nature New Biol.* 231: 8, 1971.
21. MILLER, L., AND J. B. GURDON. *Nature* 227: 1108, 1970.
22. MILLER, L., AND J. KNOWLAND. *J. Mol. Biol.* 53: 329, 1970.
23. MILSTEIN, C. *Nature* 216: 330, 1967.
24. MILSTEIN, C., AND J. R. L. PINK. *Progr. Biophys. Mol. Biol.* 21: 211, 1970.
25. NIALL, H. D., AND P. EDMAN. *Nature* 216: 262, 1967.
26. PREMKUMAR, E., M. SHOYAB AND A. R. WILLIAMSON. *Proc. Natl Acad. Sci. U.S.* 71: 99, 1974.

27. RITOSSA, F. M. *Proc. Natl. Acad. Sci. U.S.* 60: 509, 1968.

28. SHER, A., AND M. COHN. *European J. Immunol.* 2: 319, 1972.

29. SMITH, G. P., L. HOOD AND W. M. FITCH. *Ann. Rev. Biochem.* 40: 969, 1971.

30. STEVENS, R. H. *European J. Biochem.* 42: 553, 1974.

31. STEVENS, R. H., AND A. R. WILLIAMSON. *Proc. Natl. Acad. Sci. U.S.* 70: 1127, 1973.

32. STEVENS, R. H., AND A. R. WILLIAMSON. *Nature New Biol.* 245: 101, 1973.

33. STEVENS, R. H., AND A. R. WILLIAMSON. *J. Mol. Biol.* 78: 505, 1973.

34. STEVENS, R. H., AND A. R. WILLIAMSON. *J. Mol. Biol.* 78: 517, 1973.

35. STEVENS, R. H., AND A. R. WILLIAMSON. *Contemporary Topics in Molecular Immunology* In press.

36. STEVENS, R. H., AND A. R. WILLIAMSON. *Nature* 239: 143, 1972.

37. TARTOF, K. D. *Science* 171: 294, 1971.

38. TARTOF, K. D. *Proc. Natl. Acad. Sci. U.S.* 71: 1272, 1974.

39. TODD, C. W., AND F. R. INMAN. *Immunochemistry* 4: 407, 1967.

40. WILLIAMSON, A. R. *Biochem. J.* 130: 325, 1972.

Sequential expression of germ line genes in development of immunoglobulin class diversity[1,2]

A. R. LAWTON, P. W. KINCADE AND M. D. COOPER

Spain Immunology Laboratories
Departments of Pediatrics and Microbiology
University of Alabama in Birmingham
Birmingham, Alabama 35294

ABSTRACT

Differentiation of B cells occurs in two discontinuous stages. Primary differentiation of stem cells to B lymphocytes in birds occurs exclusively in the lymphoepithelial bursa of Fabricius; the fetal liver may serve this function in mammals. In chickens both the size of the B-lymphocyte pool and the generation of precursors for cells secreting different immunoglobulin classes is controlled by the bursa. The latter process involves the sequential expression of genes coding for heavy chain constant regions in the order μ, γ, α. The second stage of B-cell differentiation is antigen-driven, and involves proliferation and maturation of B lymphocytes to plasma cells. Ontogenetic development of different classes of B lymphocytes in mammals is orderly, independent of exogenous antigens, and occurs in the sequence μ, γ, α. A developmental switch in expression of C_H genes, beginning with μ, has been experimentally verified. We favor the hypothesis that generation of class diversity of B lymphocytes occurs during the antigen-independent first stage of differentiation, and that the genetic switch in C_H gene expression follows the sequence $\mu \rightarrow \gamma \rightarrow \alpha$, but evidence of these points remains inconclusive.—LAWTON, A. R., P. W. KINCADE AND M. D. COOPER. Sequential expression of germ line genes in development of immunoglobulin class diversity. *Federation Proc.* 34: 33–39, 1975.

[1] From Session II, *Gene Regulation in Differentiation and Development,* of the FASEB Conference on *Biology of Development and Aging*, presented at the 58th Annual Meeting of the Federation of American Societies for Experimental Biology, Atlantic City, N. J., April 9, 1974.

[2] Original work from the authors' laboratory has been supported in part by Public Health Service grants CA-13148 and AI 11502, and by the American Cancer Society. Dr. Lawton is recipient of a Public Health Service Research Career Development Award, AI 70780.

The following abbreviations are used in reference to the structural genes coding for immunoglobulins. Variable (V) genes specify the amino-terminal portion of the light (V_L) and heavy (V_H) polypeptide chains which determine antibody specificity. Constant (C) genes code for the carboxy-terminal portions of the chains which determine light chain type (C_k or C_λ) and heavy chain class (C_μ, C_γ, C_α, C_δ, C_ϵ).

Some of the content of this symposium will be devoted to the evidence that has established the conceptual validity of the clonal selection hypothesis (4) at the level of individual lymphocytes. Included in the theory was the idea that the specificity of antibodies was encoded in the genome rather than determined by antigens, and that the mechanism by which antigen stimulated an immune response was to select and cause to proliferate the appropriate preexisting clones of immunocompetent cells. From the standpoint of cell differentiation, this hypothesis had two very important implications. First, it meant that at some point in differentiation prior to contact with a particular environmental antigen, individual lymphocytes must become restricted with respect to the specificity of antibody they are destined to secrete. Second, the process of differentiation was divided into two discontinuous stages. In order to be selected on by antigens, clones of lymphocytes expressing the proper receptors must be generated; this could be considered the first stage of lymphoid differentiation. The second stage would then comprise all of the differentiative events that follow the selection of a particular clone, or clones, by a specific antigen. In other words, the second stage is synonymous with the immune response. We know that the immune system is divided into two developmentally independent pathways of lymphoid differentiation (7). T lymphocytes, derived from the thymus, are responsible for functions called cell-mediated immunity, while B lymphocytes are the precursors of antibody-secreting cells.

In this paper we will review a series of studies dealing with the primary events of B-lymphocyte differentiation[3]. As a marker for differentiation we have used the expression of genes coding for the constant regions of heavy chains of the major immunoglobulin classes, IgM, IgG, and IgA. The picture emerging from these studies suggests that the primary generation of B lymphocytes is an orderly, genetically programmed process depending on influences provided by a specific inductive microenvironment rather than random contact with environmental antigens. We will present evidence suggesting that during this stage of differentiation there is a sequential switch in expression of C_H genes in the order $\mu \rightarrow \gamma \rightarrow \alpha$ without any necessary change in expression of genes for light chains or for the variable regions of the heavy chains. Finally, we will suggest that, at least in the chicken, restriction with regard to the class of antibody to be secreted by individual B cells and their progeny is accomplished during this stage of differentiation.

PRIMARY B-CELL DIFFERENTIATION IN CHICKENS

The inductive microenvironment for B-cell differentiation in birds is a lymphoepithelial diverticulum of the cloaca called the bursa of Fabricius. Hemopoietic stem cells, originating in the yolk sac, first enter the epithelial bursa via the circulation on about the 13th day of embryonation (27, 28). By the 14th day, lymphoid cells can be identified within epithelial buds projecting from the luminal surface.

Bursal lymphopoiesis occurs at a very rapid rate during this period of development. The mean generation time for bursal lymphocytes in 15-day embryos was estimated to be be-

---

[3] A more comprehensive review of the early events in lymphoid differentiation is contained in ref 17.

tween 7 and 9 hours (36). These rapidly dividing cells assume a distinct follicular organization bounded by a basement membrane. Subsequent to hatching at 20–21 days, a cuff of lymphocytes develops on the mesenchymal side of the basement membrane, forming the cortex of the bursal follicle.

The first recognizable event of functional differentiation in this site is the synthesis of IgM by small clusters of cells within developing follicles. This was detected in cytoplasm and on the surface of bursal lymphocytes as early as the 14th day using direct immunofluorescence (15, and Kincade and Cooper, unpublished observations); in vitro biosynthesis of IgM was found in 18-day bursal lymphocyte cultures by Thorbecke et al (40). Immunoglobulin synthesis was not detected in other tissues of these early embryos (13, 40).

The first cells containing IgG were found in bursal follicles 7 days later, at about the time of hatching but not necessarily associated with this event. These cells were found in the larger follicles which already contained many IgM producers; they tended to occur individually rather than in clusters. During the first week following hatching there was a further increase in the size and number of follicles accompanied by development of a distinct follicular cortex. At this stage the medullary areas of most follicles were stained for both IgM and IgG in a reticular pattern, although a few follicles contained only IgM producers. The cortical areas of follicles had only rare immunoglobulin-containing cells; these were generally more intensely stained than the medullary cells and most had plasma cell morphology (13). The distribution of IgA in the bursa was quite similar to that of IgG; medullary areas of some but not all follicles exhibited a reticular staining pattern (14).

The ontogeny of immunoglobulin synthesis in peripheral lymphoid tissues closely paralleled that in the bursa, but was delayed for several days. IgM-containing cells were detected in spleen and cecal tonsils as early as 17–19 days gestation but were not found in all chicks until 3–4 days after hatching. IgG-containing cells were not seen in extrabursal sites until after hatching (13). Functional studies indicated that IgA producers were seeded even later (14).

Immunoglobulin synthesis by bursal lymphocytes does not appear to be influenced to any degree by external antigens. Thorbecke et al. found no difference in IgM synthesis by bursal cultures from 8-day old gnotobiotic and normal chicks (40). Kincade and Cooper observed (13) that intentional antigenic stimulation of embryos did not alter the development of IgM- or IgG-containing cells in the bursa. In contrast, antigens stimulated, while maintenance in germfree conditions retarded, the development of peripheral immunoglobulin-containing cells in young chickens.

EVIDENCE FOR A SWITCH FROM IgM TO IgG

When serial sections of bursa from young chickens were treated alternately with fluorescein-tagged antibodies to IgM or to IgG, the distribution of staining for the two classes appeared identical in most follicles. A minority stained only for IgM, but none stained exclusively for IgG. Examination of bursal cell suspensions indicated that more than half of the cells containing γ determinants also were stained by anti-μ, while "double producers" were rare in control suspensions of spleen cells (13). These observations suggested that the temporal development of IgM- and

IgG-synthesizing cells in the bursa might reflect an intraclonal switch in expression of heavy chain constant region genes. The alternative possibilities seemed to be: *1*) that stem cells precommitted to μ or γ synthesis arrive in the bursa in successive waves, or *2*) that the bursal environment alters with time, so that stem cells arriving early are induced to synthesize IgM and later arrivals begin to synthesize IgG. If either of the latter possibilities were correct, interference with IgM synthesis should not impair development of cells synthesizing IgG.

Thirteen-day embryos were given a single intravenous injection of purified goat antibodies specific for μ chains, while control embryos received a similar quantity of normal goat IgG. On the day of hatching, both experimental and control birds were surgically bursectomized to remove the source of further B-cell differentiation. In a series of experiments, it was found that this treatment results in permanent elimination of all morphological elements and functional capacities of the B-cell line, while cell-mediated immune functions remain intact (14–16). Most importantly for this discussion, these birds fail to synthesize IgG and IgA (14, 15, 23). An important control was provided by chickens that were bursectomized at hatching and then treated with anti-μ antibodies during the first week of life. IgM levels in serum of these birds was significantly depressed, but IgG concentrations were, if anything, higher than those in bursectomized birds given normal goat globulin (15). This experiment demonstrated that the suppression of IgG synthesis by anti-μ antibodies was primarily dependent on the bursa, since the IgG precursors that had already escaped from the bursa were not suppressed by subsequent anti-μ injections. Another indication of the

importance of the bursa in suppression was provided by a group of birds given anti-μ as embryos but not bursectomized. These animals showed only transient suppression of serum levels of IgM and IgG. Using a prolonged anti-μ treatment schedule it is possible in both chickens (23) and mice (20, 25, 29) to produce in vivo suppression of IgG and IgA synthesis while the bursa (or its mammalian equivalent) remains intact. The experiments in mice will be discussed in a subsequent section.

BURSAL CONTROL OF IMMUNOGLOBULIN SYNTHESIS

The capacity of chickens to synthesize different classes of immunoglobulins is regulated by the bursa. This conclusion arises from observations on the effects of early bursectomy. Removal of the bursa at the time of hatching does not produce agammaglobulinemia. Birds so treated show a delay in the buildup of IgM and IgG concentrations in serum for the first few weeks of life, but eventually most develop significantly higher levels than controls (18). Many of these birds will, however, lack detectable IgA (14). Bursectomy at an earlier stage, 16–17 days of embryonation, may result in complete agammaglobulinemia (5). Birds that have been bursectomized at some time between 17 days and hatching may develop a dysgammaglobulinemia, characterized by very high levels of serum IgM, low or absent IgG, and absent IgA (5, 18). These birds provide a valuable source for chicken IgM, and so several have been followed up to 1 yr. During this time, despite intentional hyperimmunization, the pattern of elevated IgM and very low IgG has persisted (18). In other words, birds capable of making large amounts of IgM antibodies could not be induced to switch to

IgG production. It would appear that the bursa is the exclusive site for generation of class heterogeneity, and that the cells which have left the bursa are committed with respect to the class of antibody that they and their progeny can produce.

In addition to regulating the production of different classes of immunoglobulins, the bursa apparently controls the size of the B-lymphocyte pool. Removal of the bursa at the time of hatching or before results in a greatly reduced proportion of lymphocytes bearing surface IgM or IgG in the circulation and spleen. This effect persists at least 8 mo, in spite of the fact that the same birds develop supernormal concentrations of circulating IgM and IgG (18). This observation clearly indicates that generation of B lymphocytes and subsequent terminal differentiation to antibody-producing cells are subject to different control mechanisms, and emphasizes the discontinuity of B-cell development. A

possible explanation is that early bursectomy limits the number of clones, and this is reflected in the absolute number of B lymphocytes. The clones that have seeded peripheral lymphoid tissue prior to bursectomy may not expand to fill the gap since their proliferation is controlled by feedback from the antibodies their progeny produce. Preliminary evidence supporting this view has come from a study of the immune response to phosphorylcholine, an antigen which induces an antibody response of limited heterogeneity in mice (8). It has been found that early bursectomy causes a permanent loss of response to this antigen in some birds (Cozenza and Cooper, unpublished observations).

Figure 1 presents a schematic outline of the ontogeny of B lymphocytes in chickens. The sequential development of precursors for IgM, IgG, and IgA during embryonation, and their subsequent emigration from the bursa to peripheral lym-

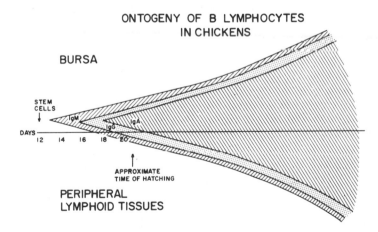

Figure 1. The horizontal scale indicates the approximate time at which development of B lymphocytes expressing different classes of immunoglobulin occurs in the bursa. The intercepts with the time scale indicate roughly when cells committed to synthesis of different classes emigrate to peripheral lymphoid tissues. The time of origin of IgA precursors has not been carefully studied. Surgical bursectomy at a given point may result in normal or increased synthesis of immunoglobulin classes with intercepts to the left, and low or absent synthesis of those to the right, of that time.

phoid tissues are indicated on a rough time scale. We have attempted to show how bursectomy at a particular time can result in deficiency of IgA, or of IgG and IgA, or of all three major classes.

A MODEL FOR B-LYMPHOCYTE DIFFERENTIATION

These observations on the ontogeny of B lymphocytes in chickens led to proposal of a general model for B-lymphocyte differentiation (6). The diagram shown in Fig. 2 outlines the development of a clone of B lymphocytes. The differentiation process is divided into two discontinuous stages. The first stage, which is designated "clonal development," begins with the migration of stem cells to a specific microenvironment, the bursa or

bursa equivalent. Differentiation begins with the synthesis of IgM antibodies, most of which become incorporated into the cell membrane. Under the influence of the microenvironment, the original lymphocyte undergoes a series of divisions giving rise to identical daughter cells, most of which migrate to peripheral lymphoid tissues. At some point a few of the daughter cells undergo a second differentiation step: they switch from expression of the gene specifying IgM, C_μ, to expression of C_γ.

The switch in expression of C_H genes does not necessarily involve alteration of the three other genes involved in immunoglobulin synthesis, so that the specificity of the clone, and its light chain type, remain unaltered. The model further pro-

STAGES OF B CELL DIFFERENTIATION

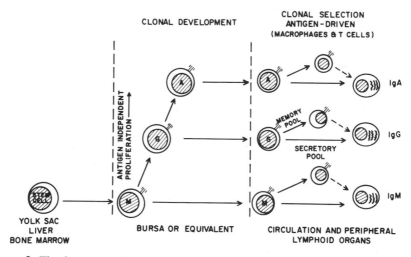

Figure 2. The first stage of differentiation is antigen-independent and occurs in a specific microenvironment. Diversity of both class and specificity of immunoglobulins is believed to be generated during this stage. The second stage occurs in peripheral lymphoid tissues and comprises all of the events that follow introduction of a specific antigen. (Reproduced from Cooper, M. D., R. Keightley, L. Y. F. Wu, and A. R. Lawton, *Transplant. Revs.* 16: 51, 1973, with permission of Munksgaard, Copenhagen.)

poses that precursor cells committed to IgA synthesis arise by a switch from expression of C_γ to C_α. Presumably, precursors for IgE and IgD arise in a similar manner, but we have no information as regards their place in the sequence.

It should be emphasized that there is no requirement that each B lymphocyte committed to IgA synthesis, for example, has undergone a switch in its life history. The switch is rather a characteristic of the life history of a clone, and may occur in only a few of its members. The end result of this process is the migration to peripheral lymphoid tissues of a clone of B lymphocytes having members committed to synthesis of IgM, others destined to make IgG, and still others, IgA.

To this point differentiation has been genetically programmed and driven through inductive influences of the bursa or its equivalent. Subsequent steps are dependent on contact of members of the clone with the antigenic determinants that its immunoglobulin receptors recognize. This second stage of differentiation, called clonal selection in the diagram, comprises all of the differentiation events of the immune response. With appropriate cooperation of macrophages and T lymphocytes, the B lymphocytes are stimulated to proliferate to form memory cells and to undergo terminal differentiation to antibody-secreting plasma cells.

There is now precise immunochemical evidence supporting involvement of a C_H gene switch in the generation of antibodies of the same specificity and light-chain type, but of different classes (37, 41). The model presented here differs from most others with respect to the stage of differentiation during which the switch occurs and the nature of the signals that drive it. Based primarily on the evidence for the bursa-de-pendence of the switch in chickens, we have proposed that it is independent of contact with exogenous antigens[4]. Having left the bursa, B lymphocytes are committed to synthesis of a single species of antibody.

B-LYMPHOCYTE DIFFERENTIATION IN MAMMALS

Studies of primary development of B cells in mammals have been hampered by lack of knowledge about where these events take place. The leading candidates for the bursa equivalent have been the bone marrow and the gut-associated lymphoid tissues. Recent experiments suggest that neither of these sites are the exclusive bursa equivalent, and point instead towards the fetal liver. Removal of the gut from fetal lambs prior to the appearance of B lymphocytes in the circulation did not effect the subsequent development of B lymphocytes (Dawes, G., R. Patrick, K. Ritchie, W. Gathings, and M. Cooper, unpublished observations). These results confirm earlier observations by Silverstein and Pendergast (38), and indicate that the gut-associated lymphoid tissue cannot be the exclusive site of B-lymphocyte development. Similar evidence is forthcoming with respect to the bone marrow. Destruction of bone marrow of adult mice with ^{89}Sr is followed by a shift in myelopoiesis and hematopoiesis to spleen. When such animals are lethally irradiated and treated with fetal liver cells, B-cell development occurs despite failure of bone marrow recovery. Also, B-lympho-

---

[4] The involvement of endogenous histocompatibility antigens in the primary differentiation of either B or T lymphocytes, as proposed in Jerne's negative selection hypothesis (12), is compatible with this model.

cyte development is not impaired in neonatal mice treated in utero with [89]Sr (Kincade and Moore, unpublished observations). Recent experimental results have implicated the fetal liver as a bursa equivalent in mammals. Owen, Cooper, and Raff have shown (32) that lymphocytes bearing surface immunoglobulin are generated in organ cultures of 14-day mouse embryo liver. IgM-positive cells and rare IgG$_2$-bearing cells were found by the 4th day of culture. Their numbers increased rapidly over the next few days, and IgA-bearing cells were found by the 7th day. Future experiments using this in vitro model should help to resolve some of the controversies to be mentioned later.

Since mammals lack a bursa which can be easily manipulated, it is necessary to identify other characteristics of B-cell differentiation that may be used in making comparisons. Incorporated into our model are two predictions that can be studied. First, the primary development of B lymphocytes should be genetically programmed and not dependent on random contact with external antigens. In other words, this process should be analogous to differentiation of erythrocytes, myeloid cells, or any other organ system. A related prediction is that the differentiation of different classes of B lymphocytes, as regards their genetic commitment to synthesize different immunoglobulin classes, should occur in the sequence $\mu \rightarrow \gamma \rightarrow \alpha$ at a particular time in embryogenesis.

The ontogeny of B lymphocytes, identified by the expression of membrane-bound immunoglobulin, has been studied in several mammalian species. In man, B-lymphocyte development begins at about the 9th week of gestation, when a few lymphocytes bearing membrane-bound IgM can be found in fetal liver. Cells bearing IgG are present at very

close to the same time, while IgA cells appear by about the 11th week. By 15 weeks gestation, the proportion of lymphocytes in fetal spleen or blood which stain for each of these classes is similar to that found in normal adults (22). These observations provided a particularly striking example of the discontinuous nature of B-cell differentiation. Although adult proportions of the three major classes of B lymphocytes were present early in the second trimester, there were very few mature antibody-secreting plasma cells. The long delay between the development of adult concentrations of B lymphocytes and of circulating immunoglobulins suggests that the two steps of differentiation are under separate control.

Similar examples of the dissociation between primary B-lymphocyte development and terminal differentiation to antibody secreting cells are found in mice. Spleen cells from germfree mice, examined by direct immunofluorescence, have similar proportions of B lymphocytes bearing μ, γ_2, and α determinants as conventionally raised animals of the same strain, although serum IgG$_2$ and IgA levels may be very low or undetectable[5] (1, and Lawton and Asofsky, unpublished observations). A second example occurs in athymic nude mice. These animals have a defect in synthesis of IgG$_2$ and IgA immunoglobulins (9), yet they have very high proportions of lymphocytes bearing μ, γ, and α determinants (2). Thus neither T cells nor exogenous antigens appear to be required for

---

[5] E. S. Vitetta and J. W. Uhr could not detect synthesis of IgG by splenocytes from axenic mice using in vitro incorporation of ^{3}H tyrosine or cell surface iodination (personal communication). We believe that this discrepancy is quantitative, but further studies are required for its resolution.

primary development of different classes of B lymphocytes.

Early and regular development of different classes of B lymphocytes prior to birth has been observed in mice (32), guinea pigs (10), and pigs (3, 39). In fetal guinea pigs μ-bearing B lymphocytes are the first class to appear, but by the time of birth the majority of B lymphocytes, and of antigen-binding cells, bear γ_2 determinants (10). The pig is a particularly important model, since fetuses are shielded from external antigens, and most maternal serum proteins, by an impermeable six-layered placenta. Despite the fact that piglets are virtually agammaglobulinemic at birth, lymphocytes bearing μ or γ determinants are present more than a month prior to this time (3, 39).

Evidence for a sequential expression of C_H genes in mammalian B-cell differentiation has come from a series of experiments in which newborn mice were treated with heterologous heavy-chain specific antibodies. These experiments were based on our previous observations in chickens that an embryonic injection of a single dose of anti-μ antibody, followed by bursectomy at hatching, resulted in permanent agammaglobulinemia (15). Since removal of the source of

newly differentiated B lymphocytes in the mouse is not feasible, the experimental design was altered to include repeated injections of antibody from the day of birth to approximately 3 months of age. We have employed goat antibodies to myeloma proteins of the IgM, IgG$_1$, IgG$_2$, and IgA classes which were purified and rendered specific on solid immunoadsorbent columns. Details of several experiments have been published and most of the series has been recently reviewed (1, 20, 21).

Approximately 60 germfree BALB/c mice have been treated from birth with purified antibodies to μ chain. Similar experiments have been done in other laboratories using conventionally raised mice and different antibody preparations, with generally concordant results (25, 29). With a single exception (1), the result of this treatment has been a nearly complete elimination of B-cell development, as summarized in Table 1. Morphologically, lymphoid tissues from these mice contain few or no germinal centers. Fewer than 2% of their spleen cells bear the surface immunoglobulin marker for B lymphocytes as compared to about 45% in controls. Serum concentrations of all classes of immunoglobulin are significantly

TABLE 1. Effects of in vivo treatment with heterologous anti-μ chain antibodies on lymphoid development of germfree mice

Groups	B-cell development						T-cell development		
	Germinal centers	Spleen weight	Ig-bearing lymphocytes	Serum Ig	IgA cells in gut	Antibody response	T-dependent areas	GvH activity	Helper activity
Anti-μ, full[a]	↓↓	↓	↓↓	↓[e]	↓↓	↓↓	N	↑	N
Anti-μ, lag[b]	↑	↑	↑[d]	↑	N	↑	N		
Anti-μ, short[c]	N	N	N	N	N	N	N		
Goat IgG control	↑	↑	N	↑	N	N	N		

Data on which this summary is based are presented in refs 1, 21 and 22. N is normal with respect to untreated germ-free mice, ↑ indicates an increase, and ↓ is a decrease.   [a] Treated from birth to maturity.   [b] Treated from 1 week to maturity.   [c] Treated from birth to 1 week.   [d] IgG$_1$-bearing B lymphocytes increased in frequency.   [e] IgG$_1$ levels higher than normal controls, but lower than goat IgG controls.

depressed with respect to controls treated with similar amounts of normal goat IgG. One of the most striking observations has been the nearly complete absence of IgA-secreting plasma cells in the guts of these animals (20, 29). As in chickens treated with anti-μ but not bursectomized (15, 23), complete agammaglobulinemia has been exceptional. It has occurred, however, in one mouse.

These mice have been incapable of producing humoral antibodies following immunization with ferritin or ovalbumin, with or without Freund's adjuvant, and to sheep erythrocytes (20, 21, 25, 29). Their spleens lacked cells capable of binding ^{125}I ferritin or of adoptively transferring a secondary response to irradiated recipients (1). Consistent with the incomplete suppression of IgG synthesis, we have detected low titers of antibodies to goat serum proteins in approximately half of the anti-μ treated mice (20, 21). These antibodies presumably are the products of a few cells that have escaped anti-μ suppression and have been stimulated by the constant presence of goat antigens in the anti-μ preparation.

T-cell function does not seem to be significantly affected by anti-μ treatment. Manning and Jutila showed that these animals rejected allogeneic skin grafts as well as controls (26). Spleen cells from anti-μ treated mice were approximately twice as effective, in terms of cell numbers, as control cells in inducing graft-versus-host reactions. This increase in activity probably reflects the absence of a diluting population of B lymphocytes (1). More recently we have found that spleen cells from anti-μ treated mice primed with ovalbumin are capable of T-lymphocyte "helper" function. These cells were mixed with spleen cells from normal animals primed to dinitrophenyl-keyhole limpet hemo-

cyanin and transferred to irradiated recipients which were then challenged with DNP-ovalbumin. The anti-μ treated cells were somewhat less effective than primed cells from normals in promoting an anti-DNP response at a dose of 100×10^6 cells, but were equally effective at a dose of 20×10^6 cells (Lawton, A. R., C. A. Janeway, and R. M. Asofsky, unpublished observations).

The mechanism of anti-μ suppression is unknown. There is some evidence to suggest that its effect occurs at a very early stage of B-cell differentiation. If the first anti-μ injection is delayed until 1 wk of age, suppression of immunoglobulin synthesis does not occur. In fact, mice treated late with anti-μ have higher immunoglobulin levels and somewhat better antibody responses than normal goat IgG-treated controls (21).

If the proposed sequence of C_H gene expression during primary B-cell development were correct, then elimination of IgG precursors as they first appear should block IgA synthesis as well. This experiment is complicated by the transfer of maternal IgG from mother to infant. This screen of maternal IgG makes it difficult for injected antibodies to reach the appropriate target cells at the critical early stage of differentiation.

A total of six attempts to suppress IgG synthesis has been made, and only one has been successful. In the successful experiment we attempted to circumvent transplacental transfer of IgG in the following way: During the first week of life the mice were treated with 2.5 mg anti-μ in order to delay the development of B lymphocytes. Beginning on *day 5*, injections of antibody recognizing shared determinants of γ_1 and γ_2 heavy chains were begun and continued each week. Anti-μ was not given after *day 7*. In previous experiments we had shown that this brief treatment with anti-μ had no discernible effects on B-cell development studied at 8–10 wk of age.

Each of these 12 mice had high levels of IgM in their serum. In 6, neither IgG_1, IgG_2, or IgA could be detected. Two others had low levels of IgG_1, but lacked IgG_2 and IgA. The remaining mice that had detectable IgA also had substantial levels of IgG_1. Our confidence in this result was greatly increased by the observation that the intestinal lamina propria of 8 of the 12 mice showed strikingly diminished numbers of IgA-containing plasma cells. Although normal germfree mice, or mice treated for the first week of life with anti-μ, have a fairly high frequency of undetectable serum IgA, their guts invariably contain large numbers of IgA-positive plasma cells (19, 21).

Attempts to repeat this experiment, using the same protocol of early treatment with anti-μ, have been unsuccessful. However, a significant correlation still holds. Failure to suppress synthesis of IgA with injections of antibodies to IgG_1 and IgG_2, either together or independently, has invariably been associated with failure to suppress IgG synthesis. In five other experiments in which either anti-γ_1, anti-γ_2, or antibodies cross-reactive to both classes have been given, synthesis of IgG has not been blocked. A partial exception occurred in one study involving IgG_1 suppression, in which serum IgG_1 was undetectable in 16/17 mice (1). However, tissues from these mice synthesized substantial amounts of IgG_1, indicating that the antibody had simply removed IgG_1 from the circulation. Other workers have had similar difficulty in suppressing IgG synthesis using antibodies to γ chains, and have not observed suppression of IgA synthesis (25, 29).

Suppression of IgA synthesis with antibodies to IgA has been achieved (19, 24, 29). As with IgG suppression, the results have been somewhat variable, and recovery of IgA synthesis during the course of treatment has occurred. However, in some experiments it has been possible to eliminate both circulating IgA and the population of IgA-producing cells in the lamina propria. Most importantly as regards the proposed switch mechanism, IgA suppression does not affect synthesis of IgM or IgG.

CONCLUSION

The model for B-lymphocyte differentiation presented here is controversial in two major respects. First, we have proposed that class heterogeneity of B-lymphocyte clones, involving a switch in expression of C_H genes, develops independently of exogenous antigens. Second, we have suggested that the switch occurs in a specific sequence, $\mu \rightarrow \gamma \rightarrow \alpha$.

The concept that the switch from expression of IgM to expression of IgG occurs prior to antigen contact has been challenged by a number of studies in mice indicating that such a switch may occur during antigen-driven differentiation, either in vitro or in adoptive transfer experiments (11, 30, 31, 33–35). At the very least, these observations demonstrate that the B-lymphocyte precursors of IgG-producing cells may have IgM receptors. At most, they suggest that the process of B-lymphocyte differentiation in mice is distinctly different from that in chickens. This controversy will not be resolved until we have more information on the relationship of class of receptor immunoglobulin to the genetic potential of the cell. It is conceivable, for example, that a cell could synthesize IgM by way of a long-lived ribosomal message while committed at the DNA level to translation of IgG. Such a postulate could reconcile the apparent differences between chickens and mice. A more detailed analysis of this problem has been attempted in a recent review (21).

The question of the sequence of the switch also has not been resolved. Its potential importance may rest with the genetic mechanisms involved in switching. If, for example, it were determined that the genes for heavy chain constant regions were linked in the sequence μ, γ, α, a mechanism would be immediately suggested. Such a sequential readout of linked genes could also be involved in expression of V_H and V_L genes and could contribute to generation of diversity.

There is little doubt that the view of B-lymphocyte differentiation presented here is oversimplified and contains many gaps. Whatever its defects, we believe that this model illustrates the potential of using the lymphoid system as an experimental tool in studying the relationship between gene expression and specific events of differentiation.

We are particularly indebted to our collaborators, Drs. R. M. Asofsky, J. M. Davie, R. Tigelaar, C. A. Janeway, Jr., and Ms. Martha Hylton for permitting us latitude in interpretation of shared experiments.

REFERENCES

1. ASOFSKY, R. M., M. D. COOPER, J. M. DAVIE, M. B. HYLTON, A. R. LAWTON AND R. TIGELAAR. *Cell. Immunol.* In press.
2. BANKHURST, A. D., AND N. L. WARNER. *Australian J. Exptl. Biol. Med. Sci.* 50: 661, 1972.
3. BINNS, R. M., A. FEINSTEIN, B. W. GURNER AND R. R. A. COOMBS. *Nature New Biol.* 239: 114, 1972.
4. BURNET, F. M. In: *The Clonal Selection Theory of Acquired Immunity.* Nashville: Vanderbilt Univ. Press, 1959.
5. COOPER, M. D., W. A. CAIN, P. J. VAN ALTEN AND R. A. GOOD. *Intern. Arch. Allergy Appl. Immunol.* 35: 242, 1969.
6. COOPER, M. D., A. R. LAWTON AND P. W. KINCADE. *Clin. Exptl. Immunol.* 11: 143, 1972.
7. COOPER, M. D., R. D. A. PETERSON, M. A. SOUTH AND R. A. GOOD. *J. Exptl. Med.* 123: 75, 1966.
8. COSENZA, H., AND H. KÖHLER. *Proc. Natl. Acad. Sci. U.S.* 69: 2701, 1972.
9. CREWTHER, P., AND N. L. WARNER. *Australian J. Exptl. Biol. Med. Sci.* 50: 625, 1972.
10. DAVIE, J. M. AND W. E. PAUL. In: *Contemporary Topics in Immunobiology,* vol. 3, edited by M. D. Cooper and N. L. Warner. New York: Plenum. 1974, p. 171.
11. HERROD, H. G., AND N. L. WARNER. *J. Immunol.* 108: 1712, 1972.
12. JERNE, N. K. *European J. Immunol.* 1: 1, 1971.
13. KINCADE, P. W., AND M. D. COOPER. *J. Immunol.* 106: 371, 1971.
14. KINCADE, P. W., AND M. D. COOPER. *Science* 179: 398, 1973.
15. KINCADE, P. W., A. R. LAWTON, D. E. BOCKMAN AND M. D. COOPER. *Proc. Natl. Acad. Sci. U.S.* 67: 1918, 1970.
16. KINCADE, P. W., A. R. LAWTON AND M. D. COOPER. *J. Immunol.* 106: 1421, 1971.
17. KINCADE, P. W., AND M. A. S. MOORE. In: *The Lymphocyte: Structure and Function,* edited by J. J. Marchalonis. New York: Marcel Dekker. In press.
18. KINCADE, P. W., K. S. SELF AND M. D. COOPER. *Cell. Immunology* 8: 93, 1973.
19. LAWTON, A. R., R. M. ASOFSKY, J. M. DAVIE AND M. B. HYLTON. *Federation Proc.* 32: 1012, 1973.
20. LAWTON, A. R., R. ASOFSKY, M. B. HYLTON AND M. D. COOPER. *J. Exptl. Med.* 135: 277, 1972.
21. LAWTON, A. R. AND M. D. COOPER. In: *Contemporary Topics in Immunobiology,* vol. 3, edited by M. D. Cooper and N. L. Warner. New York: Plenum. 1974, p. 193.
22. LAWTON, A. R., K. S. SELF, S. A ROYAL AND M. D. COOPER. *Clin. Immunol. Immunopathol.* 1: 104, 1972.
23. LESLIE, G. A., AND L. N. MARTIN. *J. Immunol.* 110: 959, 1973.
24. MANNING, D. D. *J. Immunol.* 109: 1152, 1972.
25. MANNING, D. D., AND J. W. JUTILA. *J. Exptl. Med.* 135: 1316, 1972.
26. MANNING, D. D., AND J. W. JUTILA. *Nature* 237: 58, 1972.
27. MOORE, M. A. S., AND J. J. T. OWEN. *Nature* 208: 956, 1965.

28. MOORE, M. A. S., AND J. J. T. OWEN.
    Develop. Biol. 14: 40, 1966.
29. MURGITA, R. A., C. A. MATTIOLI AND
    T. B. TOMASI, JR. J. Exptl. Med. 138:
    209, 1973.
30. NOSSAL, G. J. V., A. SZENBERG, G. L.
    ADA AND G. M. AUSTIN. J. Exptl. Med.
    119: 485, 1964.
31. NOSSAL, G. J. V., N. L. WARNER AND
    H. LEWIS. Cell. Immunol. 2: 41, 1971.
32. OWEN, J. J. T., M. D. COOPER AND M. C.
    RAFF. Nature. 249: 361, 1974.
33. PIERCE, C. W., R. ASOFSKY AND S. M.
    SOLLIDAY. Federation Proc. 32: 41, 1973.
34. PIERCE, C. W., S. M. SOLLIDAY AND R.
    ASOFSKY. J. Exptl. Med. 135: 675, 1972.
35. PRESS, J. L., AND N. R. KLINMAN. J.
    Exptl. Med. 138: 300, 1973.
36. RUBIN, E., M. D. COOPER AND F. W.

KRAUS. Bacteriol. Proc. 71: 67, 1971.
37. SCORNIK, J., L. KLUSKENS AND H.
    KOHLER. Federation Proc. 32: 989a, 1973.
38. SILVERSTEIN, A. M., AND R. A. PENDER-
    GAST. In: Advances in Experimental Medi-
    cine and Biology, Vol. 12: Morphological
    and Functional Aspects of Immunity, edited
    by K. Lindahl-Kiessling, G. Alm and
    M. G. Hanna. New York: Plenum,
    1971, p. 37.
39. SYMONS, D. B. A., AND R. M. BINNS.
    Intern. Res. Commun. System (73-9)
    17-1-31, 1973.
40. THORBECKE, G. J., N. L. WARNER, G. M.
    HOCHWALD AND Ş. H. OHANIAN. Im-
    munology 15: 123, 1968.
41. WANG, A. C., S. K. WILSON, J. E. HOPPER,
    H. H. FUDENBERG AND A. NISONOFF.
    Proc. Natl. Acad. Sci. U.S. 66: 337, 1970.

Normal and altered phenotypic expression of immunoglobulin genes[1]

ROSE G. MAGE

Laboratory of Immunology

National Institute of Allergy and Infectious Diseases

National Institutes of Health, Bethesda, Maryland 20014

ABSTRACT

Genetically controlled intraspecific differences between immunoglobulins (allotypes) provide valuable markers for the study of the quantitative expression of allelic and nonallelic alternative forms of immunoglobulins (Igs) during the normal development of rabbits. Heterozygous rabbits are mosaics of cells expressing different Ig-genes since fully differentiated productive cells generally secrete only one of alternative forms of Ig. The proportions of cells that differentiate to produce allelic forms of immunoglobulins during normal development depend on the particular heterozygous genotype. The normal proportions of some markers can be drastically altered if the differentiation of lymphoid cells in the young rabbit occurs in a milieu of antibody specific for one form (allotype suppression). An initiating step in the establishment of persistent allotype suppression is probably the interaction of antiallotype antibody with allotype-bearing receptors on lymphoid cell surfaces, but the mechanism for the maintenance of a state of chronic suppression may well be more complex. Allotype suppression can be viewed as one example of numerous immunological phenomena that reflect specific and finely tuned regulatory mechanisms governing the differentiation and clonal expansion of lymphoid cells destined to secrete immunoglobulins.—MAGE, R. G. Normal and altered phenotypic expression of immunoglobulin genes. *Federation Proc.* 34: 40–46, 1975.

Genetically controlled structural differences between the immunoglobulins (Igs)[2] produced by different rabbits (allotypes) can be detected by serological techniques (34). Antiallotype antisera and the genetic

[1] From Session II, *Gene Regulation in Differentiation and Development*, of the FASEB Conference on *Biology of Development and Aging*, presented at the 58th Annual Meeting of the Federation of American Societies for Experimental Biology, Atlantic City, N.J., April 9, 1974.

markers which they detect, constitute a powerful tool for the study of the phenotypic expression of immunoglobulin genes, and the factors that regulate this expression.

GENETICS AND STRUCTURE

A summary of some allotypes whose quantitative expression we will be examining is given in Table 1. The a1, a2 and a3 allotypes, assigned to the *a* locus, behave in breeding studies as if controlled by simple Mendelian alleles, yet chemical studies support the localization of *a* locus antigenic determinants in the variable regions of rabbit heavy chains (17, 25, 37, 49). The *a*-locus allotypes, as well as other

TABLE 1. Some rabbit allotypes, their structural correlates, and localization

Heavy chains	Localization and chemical information
V_H a1, a2, a3	Associated with multiple amino acid interchanges within the variable region. Found in association with different constant regions ($C\gamma$, $C\alpha$, $C\mu$, $C\epsilon$).
x32 y33	Found in association with different constant regions
C_γ d11 d12	Methionine (position 225)[a] Threonine (position 225)[a]
e14 e15	Threonine (position 309)[a] Alanine (position 309)[a]
Light chains	
kappa-type b4, b5, b6, b9	Multiple amino acid interchanges, probably within the constant region.
lambda-type c7, c21	No chemical information available

[a] Eu numbering (10).

antigenically distinct markers on *a*-negative molecules, such as x32 and y33 (20), are found on IgG, IgA and IgM (21). Different classes of heavy chains share the same set of variable regions and this is one of the reasons why we consider these markers to be associated with genes controlling structures on the variable portion of the heavy chains (V_H). The kappa chain allotypes b4, b5, b6, and b9 also appear to be controlled by simple Mendelian alleles at a locus designated *b* which is not closely linked to the *a* locus. The constant regions of these kappa chains differ in sequence at a number of residue positions. There may also be some qualitative or quantitative differences between the variable regions associated with the different *b*-locus allotypes (2). There is little doubt that some of the antigenic determinants recognized by anti-*b*-locus allotype antisera are due to amino acid differences in the constant regions, but it is not ruled out that other determinants could be localized or at least influenced by sequence differences in the variable portions of kappa chains.

An unlinked locus designated *c* controls antigenically distinct forms of rabbit lambda-type light chains such as c7 and c21 (11). The chemical

[2] Abbreviations: Designations of rabbit allotypes and the genes controlling them have sometimes omitted the capital "A" for brevity (34). The variable and constant regions of immunoglobulins are termed V regions and C regions, respectively. V_H and C_H are generic terms for the corresponding regions of heavy chains: V_L and C_L for light chains. The symbol H is replaced by the symbol of the chain when specifying a particular heavy chain class or light chain type. Ig(s), Immunoglobulin(s); B cell, lymphocyte derived from the "mammalian bursal equivalent"; T cell, thymus-derived lymphocyte; PBL, peripheral blood lymphocyte; BL, blood; SPL, spleen; APP, appendix; and BM, bone marrow.

basis for the antigenic differences between c7 and c21 types is not known; they may be pseudoallelic rather than allelic forms, and the determinants have not been localized to the variable or constant regions of the chains. There are multiple amino acid differences between the alternative forms of a, b, and probably c allotypes. Therefore, it is clearly possible that the structural genes for the polypeptide chains characteristic of each allotype are not simple alleles. The apparent allelism could reflect, for example, allelic regulatory genes that determine which of a linked set of genes at a complex locus can be expressed.

There are also allotypes localized on the constant portions of rabbit heavy chains. The chemical basis for several serologically distinguishable forms of gamma chains has been investigated. Interchange of methionine and threonine at the position immediately N-terminal to the heavy chain interchain disulfide bridge correlates with the A11 and A12 allotypes (43). The A14 and A15 allotypes correlate with alternative residues threonine and alanine at position 309 on the same γ chain (1). These sets have been referred to as the group d and group e allotypes. It is likely that the d and e antigenic determinants are coded for by a single cistron: the structural gene for the constant portion of the γ heavy chain. Thus I shall represent them as products of a de locus with known alleles $de^{11,15}$, $de^{12,15}$, and $de^{12,14}$. Specificities inherited together may be on products of either single or closely linked cistrons. The genes controlling specificities on the constant regions of γ, α and μ heavy chains are closely linked to each other, and to the variable region genes of the a, x and y groups (34).

Figure 1 is a hypothetical representation of the three complex genetic regions or linkage groups that control the structure of kappa, lambda and heavy polypeptide chains of rabbits. We do not know the actual order of genes within each region, and can only hypothesize that they are clustered as shown. Dots have been placed between cistrons to represent our lack of knowledge of the total sizes of these regions and of what else might be included in the linkage group as regulatory information or untranslated spacer. Some examples of serologically distinguishable forms of the polypeptide chains are listed below them. Specificities listed along one line beneath the heavy chain linkage group are examples of some of the groups of markers that have been found inherited together in families (allo groups or haplotypes) (8, 26, 34). Although the entire allogroup is generally inherited together, inspection of the assortment of markers found on one chromosome in different populations suggests that recombinations may have occurred between cistrons within the heavy chain linkage group. In fact, apparent recombinations between V_H and C_γ markers have been observed in two different laboratories during experimental breeding (22, 35). Breeding studies utilizing markers such as those listed in Fig. 1 have also demonstrated that there is not close linkage between the kappa, lambda and heavy chain linkage groups (34). These linkage relationships are consonant with structural data which show that the sets of variable regions found associated with kappa chains, lambda chains and heavy chains are different (34).

LYMPHOID DIFFERENTIATION AND Ig GENE EXPRESSION

Cells which differentiate to secrete antibodies are highly specialized. A fully differentiated antibody-secreting cell appears to express only one V_H and one C_H gene from the array of genes in the heavy chain linkage group; and one V_L and one C_L gene from either the kappa or lambda light chain linkage groups. In addition, the product of only one homologous chromosome is expressed in any given cell although both allelic forms are expressed by different cells of heterozygotes at Ig loci. This high degree of specialization presumably provides the means by which the cell can produce an antibody with a unique combining site. Clonal selection theories speculate that the particular V_L-V_H pair expressed generates an antibody-combining site which is present in the form of membrane-bound Ig receptor on precursors of the productive cell. The site is capable of binding a variety of potential antigenic determinants with varying affinities. Differentiation of the precursor to an actively synthesizing cell probably requires several signals, one of which may be interaction with an antigenic determinant with a sufficiently high association constant.

In heterozygotes, two alternative allelic forms are often expressed in different proportions; that is, sera generally contain more of one allelic form than the other (33). The proportions in serum are a reflection of the proportions of cells secreting the alternative forms. Close correspondence is found between relative numbers of antibody-producing cells which stain with fluorescent antiallotype reagents, and relative numbers of molecules with two allelic allotypes in individual heterozygous rabbits (4, 41). The experimental facts have raised many questions which await answers. Why are alternative forms

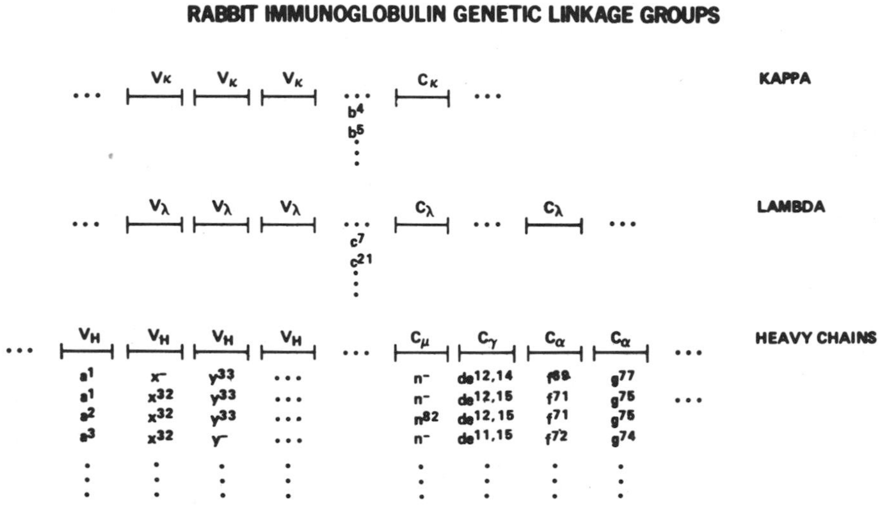

RABBIT IMMUNOGLOBULIN GENETIC LINKAGE GROUPS

Figure 1. Representation of a possible arrangement of the genes in the three complex regions controlling the structure of kappa, lambda and heavy polypeptide chains of rabbits. Neither the total number nor the order of genes is known. Additional examples of heavy chain allogroups (haplotypes) can be found in refs (8) and (34).

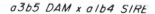

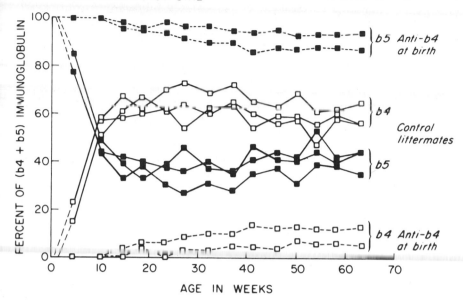

Figure 2. Proportions of kappa-positive Ig in developing b^4b^5 offspring of b^5b^5 nonimmunized dams and b^4b^4 sires. The treated animals received 2.5 ml of anti-b4 antiserum containing 2.2 mg anti-b4 on the day of birth. (From Mage (32), where additional information can be found).

expressed in unequal proportions? Is it possible that the earliest precursors of B cells of different types are not generated with equal frequency? If an early event in the differentiation of a B cell is the translocation of V-region information and its fusion with a constant-region gene, could the probability of such an event occurring on one chromosome compared to the other be a general reflection either of the total number of functional germline V genes, or the relative efficiency of the translocation event? Alternatively, could differentiation for the expression of alternative alleles occur with equal frequency, but factors affecting further clonal expansion such as suppressing or augmenting thymus-derived cells,

antigens, macrophages and soluble factors have differential effects on precursor cells with receptors of different allotypes?

Allotype suppression

Shortly after he discovered the rabbit allotypes (38, 39), Oudin showed that newborn rabbits have circulating immunoglobulins derived from their dams but secrete little or none of their own (40). During the first 8–10 weeks of life, the young rabbits catabolize the maternal Ig and begin to synthesize and secrete their own. In heterozygotes whose dam and sire differ in allotype, newly synthesized Ig can be identified by its content of paternal allotype (7). If newborn heterozygotes are offspring of mothers immunized against the father's allotype (7), or are injected with antiserum of the same specificity, an abnormally low expression of the type results, often lasting for the entire life of the animal (32, 33). For a period of time, allotype-suppressed rabbits produce no detectable Ig with paternal allotype whereas normal littermate controls can develop proportions of the same type that are higher than those inherited from the mother. In the example shown in Fig. 2, the father's b4 allotype typically constitutes 60% of the total kappa-positive Ig by 10–15 weeks of age whereas in suppressed animals, less than 10% of the total kappa-positive Ig is of paternal type at more than 1 year of age. Total immuno-

globulin levels are normal in these suppressed animals due to compensatory increased amounts of Ig with kappa-type light chains inherited from the mother.

We have found that although newborns do not secrete detectable amounts of Ig with paternal allotype, it is already present on the surface of lymphocytes as membrane-associated Ig (14). Figure 3 shows percentages of cells in various lymphoid organs of developing rabbits which had membrane Ig of maternal and paternal kappa chain allotype detectable by fluorescent staining. As shown in the previous figure, (Fig. 2), normal adult rabbits generally produce 1.5 times more b4 than b5 Ig. In neonatal offspring, whether of b4 or b5 sires,

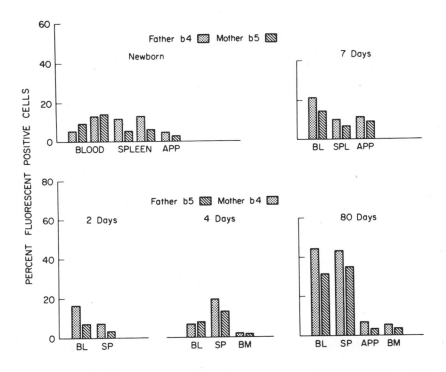

Figure 3. Percentages of cells in lymphoid organs of developing rabbits that had membrane-associated Ig of maternal and paternal kappa chain allotype detectable by fluorescent staining. The original data and details of methods used can be found in Harrison and Mage (14).

TABLE 2. Disappearance of lymphocyte membrane Ig of paternal b5 allotype after treatment of neonatal b^4b^5 rabbits with b9 anti-b5 antisera

				Percent fluorescent-positive cells[b]			
Treatment of neonatal b^4b^5 rabbits[a]			Organs examined	b4 cells (F_1 b5 anti-b4)	b5 cells (F_1 b4 anti-b5)	Cells coated with b9 (F_1 b4b5 anti-b9)
Newborn b^4b^5 rabbits	b9 anti-b5 5 ml i.p. at birth	24 hours later (age <2 days)	Blood	10.6	<0.2	<0.2
			Spleen	7.0	<0.2	<0.2
			Bone marrow	2.5	<0.2	<0.2
	No treatment	Same	Blood	16.4	6.7	<0.2
			Spleen	7.1	3.4	<0.2
			Bone marrow	2.0	1.4	<0.2

[a] Each group consisted of three to five neonatal rabbits. Cells from each organ were pooled to provide enough cells for examination.   [b] At least 500 cells were counted in each preparation. In animals treated with anti-b5 no b5-bearing cells were detected. b9 anti-b5 antibodies were not detectable on the surface of these cells by sensitive fluorescent staining with b4b5 and b9 antisera

cells with detectable membrane Ig of the b4 type were more numerous than those with b5 (with the exception of peripheral blood lymphocytes (PBL) of two litters of newborn offspring of b5 dams). In these probable precursors of primary antibody-producing cells, the b4 type was more prevalent than b5, either because differentiation to b4 actually occurred more frequently, or because even at this early stage, clones of b4 precursors had already developed which were of larger size (see Klinman, this symposium (24)). Cells with membrane-bound Ig of paternal type are potential targets for injected anti-allotype antiserum in newborns. Table 2 shows the results of an experiment in which lymphoid cells from newborn offspring of b5 sires and b4 dams were examined 24 hours after injection of anti-b5 allotype antiserum (14). The antiserum was made in a rabbit of b9 allotype to provide a specific means of identifying the injected antibody. Whereas the or-

gans of untreated control animals had cells with membrane Ig of both b4 and b5 allotypes, the treated animals had no cells with membrane Ig of the father's b5 type. The injected antibody was also not detectable on the surface of cells from the treated group using a sensitive fluorescent anti-b9 reagent. Thus in these animals, the injected antibody did not remain complexed to the Ig receptors on cells which could be examined in the organs by this time. We cannot be sure that the target cells were still present in the organs, but it is quite likely, based on in vitro studies, that the injection of anti-immunoglobulin antibody led to aggregation or patching of the immunoglobulin receptors on the cell. In vitro, this is followed by endocytosis, pinocytosis, or sloughing of complexes and clearing of membrane Ig from the cell surface in less than 1 hour (29, 30, 45). Regeneration of surface immunoglobulin can occur in such cells, but in the presence of excess antibody in vitro, the regeneration is not observed (30). The cells of rabbits exposed to anti-immunoglobulin in vivo may be affected in a manner similar to the in vitro events but their subsequent fate is not known. If sufficient amounts of antiallotype antiserum are administered to neonates to maintain an excess of antibody for several weeks, cells with membrane Ig of paternal allotype remain absent for weeks to months thereafter (Fig. 4) (3, 14). Recovery of some capability to produce Ig of paternal type is heralded by appearance of a few cells (0.5–1%) with membrane Ig of paternal type in bone marrow and peripheral blood. Soon after, small amounts (1–2 μg/ml) are found in the serum, but the proportion of suppressed type generally remains abnormally low for the rest of the animal's life (14). The suppressing effect of maternal or injected antiallotype antibody can be reversed even after rabbits have developed in a milieu of antiallotype for 1–2 weeks (31, 50). Neutralization of suppression can be obtained by injection of paternal type or by foster-nursing babies on mothers of the father's allotype (31, 50).

The phenomenon of suppression of expression of one allelic allotype can readily be obtained with all the various combinations of heterozygotes at the a and b loci. Total suppression of all a allotype or all b allotypes can also be achieved in homozygotes. Zygotes are transferred to immunized or normal mothers of a different genotype so that the serum allotype of the mother will not neutralize injected antibodies. The neonates can then develop in a milieu of antiallotype antibodies. When total suppression of a-locus allotype is achieved, compensatory production of the closely linked a-negative (x and y group) V_H regions is observed. When total suppression of kappa chains is achieved, there is compensatory production of Ig with lambda type light chains which as noted above are not closely linked to the kappa or heavy chain linkage groups (34). A group of rabbits totally suppressed for expression of b5 had no PBL with membrane-associated Ig of b5 type until they were 7 months

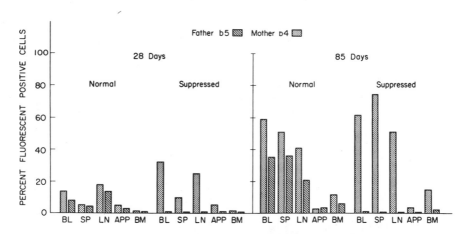

Figure 4. Percentages of b4- and b5-bearing cells in lymphoid organs of control and b5- suppressed littermates detectable by fluorescent staining. The original data and details of methods used can be found in Harrison and Mage (14).

of age (15). The PBL were detected shortly before circulating Ig with the b5 type was present. Animals with 4–7% b5-bearing PBL had less than 1 μg/ml of b5 Ig. The proportions of b5-bearing lymphocytes in peripheral blood developed toward normal but proportions of circulating Ig of the b5 type remained disproportionately depressed. It appears that a population of precursors reappeared but were not undergoing further differentiation to productive cells in proportion to their numbers. There are a number of possible explanations for this observation, but in some manner, extrinsic or intrinsic regulatory factors are interfering with the further normal differentiation of these probable precursors of the productive cells.

Expression of V_H and $C\gamma$ markers

The proportions of markers for the variable and constant portions of the heavy chains of IgG from rabbits of known genotype have been studied utilizing purified iodine-labeled IgG and cross-linked antiallotype antisera (27). From these and other similar studies (23) it became apparent that the great majority of differentiated cells that produce IgG are utilizing genetic information for variable and constant regions which are genetically linked on one parental chromosome. A small percentage (generally less than 2%) of "recombinant-type" cells and molecules, that is, ones that express the variable markers from one parent and constant region markers from the other parent, also appear to be present (28, 42). The quantitative data therefore suggest that the selection of the allele to be expressed at the a locus precedes or coincides with cellular differentiation for γ chain production. It can be seen in Table 3 that the proportion of a-locus allotype expressed

dictates the proportion of $C\gamma$ marker in doubly heterozygous rabbits. If the expression of an a-locus allotype is suppressed by exposing developing heterozygotes to antibody to the father's allotype (a1, in an a^1a^2 heterozygote, in Table 3), the genetically linked $C\gamma$ allotype (A14) inherited from the father is also suppressed. The proportions of V_H and $C\gamma$ markers in the IgG of an a1-suppressed rabbit at 11 months of age were the reverse of those in comparable normal IgG from a rabbit of the same genotype (top line, Table 3). We were interested in knowing whether exposure to antibody to a constant region marker would lead to its suppressed expression, and if so, would the linked variable region marker also be affected. So far, we have not obtained chronic suppressed expression of a $C\gamma$ marker. Since the concentrations of antibody in anti-A14 and anti-A15 antisera are generally lower than in anti-a or anti-b allotype antisera, we cannot rule out the possibility that an effect could be obtained by administration of more antibody. However, Lowe and co-workers (31) note similar negative results using a strongly precipitating anti-A11 antiserum with a titer comparable to effective anti-b allotype antisera. Maternal anti-A14 did not cause chronic suppressed expression of paternal A14 in two litters of an a1, A15/a2, A15 dam making anti-A11. By 14 weeks of age the doubly heterozygous offspring had ~80% paternal a1 and A14 and 20% maternal a2 and A15; the typical proportions found in normal sera. The a1 homozygous rabbits had proportions of A14 and A15 that were also indistinguishable from those in sera of normal adults of the same genotype. In view of these negative results, we next considered the possibility that the differentiation of cells destined to produce IgG might occur relatively late during lymphoid development and thus require prolonged administration of antibody. We therefore gave 4 of 6 offspring of a dam making anti-A15 additional injections of their mother's antibody (and antibody of identical specificity) until 8 or 9 weeks of age. The two rabbits that received only maternal anti-A15 had adult proportions of A15 by 8 weeks of age. A slight delay in reaching this level was seen in the sera of the four animals that were repeatedly injected with anti-A15. Elevation of the proportion of A14 caused by injection of A14 anti-A15 antiserum plus a simple removal of some synthesized A15 by the antibody probably accounts for the apparent delay. Clearly, no chronic suppression was established. The adult levels of V_H and $C\gamma$ allotypes in these animals are also summarized in Table 3. We are continuing with more experiments of this sort, but can tentatively state that total suppression of expression of $C\gamma$ markers is not readily attained, possibly because

TABLE 3. Proportions of V_H and $C\gamma$ allotypes in sera[a] of adult rabbits

Genotype	Description	Allotype; %				Description	Allotype, %			
		a1	A14	a2	A15		a1	A14	a2	A15
a1, A14 / a2, A15	Normal IgG[b]	80	81	20	20	IgG of a1[c] Suppressed	27	24	73	69
	Maternal[d] Anti-A14 I	83	84	17	16	Maternal[e] Anti-A14 II	79	78	21	22
	Maternal[f] Anti-A15 III-A	84	75	16	25	Maternal[g] Anti-A15 III-B	81	78	19	22
a1, A15 / a2, A14	Normal IgG[b]	75	18	19	68					
a1, A14 / a1, A15	Normal IgG[b]		52		46	Sera of[h] Normal Adults		62		38
						Maternal[i] Anti-A14 I + II		61		39

[a] Percentages of allotypes in purified IgG samples were determined by measuring the amount of binding of ^{125}I-labeled IgG to insolubilized antiallotype antisera (27). Percentages of allotypes in sera were measured by radial immunodiffusion and are expressed as follows: $\%a1 \text{ or } a2 = \dfrac{a1 \text{ or } a2 \text{ concentration}}{a1 + a2 \text{ concentration}} \times 100; \%A14 \text{ or } A15 = \dfrac{A14 \text{ or } A15 \text{ concentration}}{A14 + A15 \text{ concentration}} \times 100.$ [b] Purified IgG from a single rabbit of known genotype.   [c] Purified IgG from serum collected at 11 months of age from a single rabbit suppressed via maternal anti-a1.   [d] Mean proportions in sera of four a^1a^2 littermates collected at 14, 19, 23, 27, and 32 weeks of age.   [e] Mean proportions in sera of six a^1a^2 littermates collected at 17, 21 and 26 weeks of age.   [f] Mean proportions in the sera of two littermates that received maternal anti-A15 only. Sera were collected at 13, 19, 23, and 27 weeks of age.   [g] Mean proportions in the sera of four littermates that received additional anti-A15 until 8 or 9 weeks of age. Sera were collected at 13, 19, 23, and 27 weeks of age.   [h] Mean proportions in the sera of 11 normal adults.   [i] Mean proportions in sera of four a^1a^1 offspring in litters I and II collected after 12 weeks of age.

receptors with these determinants may be absent or inaccessible to antibody on the surface of cells that differentiate to produce these IgG molecules.

It is likely that an initiating step in the establishment of chronic allotype suppression is the interaction of antiallotype antibody with surface receptors carrying the antigenic determinants on differentiating lymphocytes. The long-term effect however, cannot be explained on the basis of simple interaction of injected antibody with precursors of Ig-producing cells. We know that chronic depressed expression of the affected type occurs long after circulating Ig has been catabolized and during a period when cells with membrane-associated Ig of the suppressed type and traces of circulating Ig are present. As we noted earlier, in animals totally suppressed for production of kappa-b5-type light chains, the proportion of PBL with membrane b5 approaches toward normal while circulating b5 Ig levels remain disproportionately depressed (15). We have also demonstrated that these b5-bearing lymphocytes synthesize the b5 Ig which appears on their membranes, since it reappears during in vitro culture after pronase stripping of the surface Ig (13). It is conceivable that such cells have an intrinsic functional defect which prevents their further differentiation after appropriate stimulation. We have indeed found that the capacity of PBL from these animals to transform into blast cells and synthesize DNA in response to anti-b5 antisera is markedly subnormal (12). Sell had similar observations on suppressed heterozygotes a number of years ago (44). Such experiments do not rule out the possibilities that cellular interactions are necessary to activate these putative precursors. T cells, for example, may be required to help trigger further

differentiation, or alternatively a suppressive action of T cells could be actively preventing their activation. Such suppressor T cells have been implicated as mediators of a long-term allotype suppression phenomenon which occurs in the F_1 offspring of BALB/c female mice mated to SJL sires (16). Recent experiments of Jacobson (18) suggest that the suppressive effect in this system is due to the production of a diffusible factor, rather than a direct cell–cell interaction. Introduction of allogeneic (parental strain) thymus cells into such suppressed F_1 animals has been found to abrogate the suppression (5). It seems quite likely to me that in both the murine and rabbit allotype suppression models, a complex regulatory network is present (19), and the final level of expression of a suppressed allotype represents the net result of antagonistic suppressive and stimulatory cells and mediators which normally govern the differentiation and clonal expansion of the lymphoid cells destined to secrete immunoglobulins.

REFERENCES

1. APPELLA, E., A. CHERSI, R. G. MAGE AND S. DUBISKI. Structural basis of the A14 and A15 allotypic specificities in rabbit immunoglobulin G. *Proc. Natl. Acad. Sci. U.S.* 68: 1341, 1971.
2. APPELLA, E., AND J. K. INMAN. The primary structure of rabbit and mouse immunoglobulin light chains: structural correlates of allotypy. In: *Topics in Molecular Immunology*, edited by R. A. Reisfeld and W. J. Mandy. New York: Plenum, 1973.
3. CATTY, D., L. CHAMBERS AND J. A. LOWE. Humoral aspects of immunoglobulin allotype suppression in the rabbit. II. Effect of *b* locus suppression on immunoglobulin receptor-bearing lymphocytes. *Immunology* 26: 331, 1974.
4. CEBRA, J. J., J. E. COLBERG AND S. DRAY. Rabbit lymphoid cells differentiated with respect to α-, γ- and μ-heavy polypeptide chains and to allotypic markers Aa1 and Aa2. *J. Exptl. Med.* 123: 547, 1966.

5. CINADER, B., S. W. KOH AND P. KUKSIN. Allotype levels in normal and allotype suppressed mice after allogeneic stimulation. *Cell. Immunol.* 11: 170, 1974.

6. DAVID, G. S., AND C. W. TODD. Suppression of heavy and light chain allotypic expression in homozygous rabbits through embryo transfer. *Proc. Natl. Acad. Sci. U.S.* 62: 860, 1969.

7. DRAY, S. Effect of maternal isoantibodies on the quantitative expression of two allelic genes controlling γ-globulin allotypic specificities. *Nature* 195: 677, 1962.

8. DRAY, S., B. S. KIM AND A. GILMAN-SACHS. Allogroups of rabbit Ig heavy chains. *Ann. Immunol. Paris* 125c: 41, 1974.

9. DUBISKI, S. Suppression of the synthesis of allotypically defined immunoglobulins and compensation by another subclass of immunoglobulin. *Nature* 214: 1365, 1967.

10. GALLY, J. A., AND G. M. EDELMAN. The genetic control of immunoglobulin synthesis. *Ann. Rev. Genetics* 6: 1, 1972.

11. GILMAN-SACHS, A., R. G. MAGE, G. O. YOUNG, C. ALEXANDER AND S. DRAY. Identification and genetic control of two rabbit immunoglobulin allotypes at a second light chain locus, the *c* locus. *J. Immunol.* 103: 1159, 1969.

12. HARRISON, M. R., G. J. ELFENBEIN AND R. G. MAGE. Defective activation of b5 bearing lymphocytes in rabbits recovering from b5 allotype suppression. *Cell. Immunology* 11: 231, 1974.

13. HARRISON, M. R., P. P. JONES AND R. G. MAGE. Endogenous synthesis of membrane b5 by lymphocytes from rabbits recovering from b5 allotype suppression. *J. Immunol.* 111: 1595, 1973.

14. HARRISON, M. R., AND R. G. MAGE. Allotype suppression in the rabbit. I. The ontogeny of cells bearing immunoglobulin of paternal allotype and the fate of these cells after treatment with antiallotype antisera. *J. Exptl. Med.* 138: 764, 1973.

15. HARRISON, M. R., R. G. MAGE AND J. M. DAVIE. Deletion of b5 immunoglobulin-bearing lymphocytes in allotype-suppressed rabbits. *J. Exptl. Med.* 137: 254, 1973.

16. HERZENBERG, L. A., E. L. CHAN, M. M. RAVITCH, R. J. RIBLET AND L. A. HERZENBERG. Active suppression of immunoglobulin allotype synthesis. III. Identification of T cells as responsible for suppression by cells from spleen, thymus, lymph node, and bone marrow. *J. Exptl. Med.* 137: 1311, 1973.

17. INMAN, J. K., AND R. A. REISFELD. Differences in amino acid composition of papain Fd fragments from rabbit γG-immunoglobulins carrying different H chain allotypic specificities. *Immunochemistry* 5: 415, 1968.

18. JACOBSON, E. B. In vitro studies of allotype suppression in mice. *European J. Immunol.* 3: 619, 1973.

19. JERNE, N. K. Towards a network theory of the immune system. *Ann. Immunol. Paris* 125c: 373, 1974.

20. KIM, B. S., AND S. DRAY. Identification and genetic control of allotypic specificities on two variable region subgroups of rabbit immunoglobulin heavy chains. *European J. Immunol.* 2: 509, 1972.

21. KIM, B. S., AND S. DRAY. Expression of the *a*, *x*, and *y* variable region genes of heavy chains among IgG, IgM, and IgA molecules of normal and *a* locus allotype-suppressed rabbits. *J. Immunol.* 111: 750, 1973.

22. KINDT, T. J., AND W. J. MANDY. Recombination of genes coding for constant and variable regions of immunoglobulin heavy chains. *J. Immunol.* 108: 1110, 1972.

23. KINDT, T. J., W. J. MANDY AND C. W. TODD. Association of group a with allotypic specificities A11 and A12 in rabbit immunoglobulin. *Biochemistry* 9: 2028, 1970.

24. KLINMAN, N. R., AND J. L. PRESS. Expression of specific clones during B-cell development. *Federation Proc.* 34: 47, 1975.

25. KOSHLAND, M. E. Location of specificity and allotypic amino acid residues in antibody Fd fragments. *Cold Spring Harbor Symp. Quant. Biol.* 32: 119, 1967.

26. LAMMERT, J. M., W. C. HANLEY, K. L. KNIGHT, E. A. LICHTER AND S. DRAY. Identification and characterization of additional rabbit IgA allotypes. *Federation Proc.* 33: 737, 1974.

27. LANDUCCI TOSI, S., R. G. MAGE AND S. DUBISKI. Distribution of allotypic specificities A1, A2, A14 and A15 among immunoglobulin G molecules. *J. Immunol.* 104: 641, 1970.

28. LANDUCCI TOSI, S., AND R. M. TOSI. Recombinant IgG molecules in rabbits doubly heterozygous for group *a* and group *e* allotypic specificities. *Immunochemistry* 10: 65, 1973.

29. LINTHICUM, D. S., W. MAYR, K. MIYAI AND S. SELL. Endocytosis of lymphocyte surface immunoglobulin in the absence of cap formation demonstrated by ultrastructural labelling. *Federation Proc.* 32: 983, 1973.

30. LOOR, F., L. FORNI AND B. PERNIS. The dynamic state of the lymphocyte membrane. Factors affecting the distribution and turnover of surface immunoglobulins. *European J. Immunol.* 2: 203, 1972.

31. LOWE, J. A., L. M. CROSS AND D. CATTY. Humoral and cellular aspects of immunoglobulin allotype suppression in the rabbit. I. Kinetics of neutralization of suppression.*Immunology* 25: 367, 1973.

32. MAGE, R. G. Quantitative studies on the regulation of expression of genes for immunoglobulin allotypes in heterozygous rabbits. *Cold Spring Harbor Symp. Quant. Biol.* 32: 203, 1967.

33. MAGE, R. G. Altered quantitative expression of immunoglobulin allotypes in rabbits. In: *Current Topics in Microbiology and Immunology,* vol. 63, edited by N. Jerne. Heidelberg: Springer-Verlag, 1974, p. 131.

34. MAGE, R., R. LIEBERMAN, M. POTTER AND W. D. TERRY. Immunoglobulin allotypes. In: *The Antigens,* vol. 1, edited by M. Seal. New York: Academic, 1973, p. 229.

35. MAGE, R. G., G. O. YOUNG-COOPER AND C. ALEXANDER. Genetic control of variable and constant regions of immunoglobulin heavy chains. *Nature New Biol.* 230: 63, 1971.

36. MAGE, R. G., G. O. YOUNG AND R. A. REISFELD. The association of the c7 allotype of rabbits with some light polypeptide chains which lack *b* locus allotype. *J. Immunol.* 101: 617, 1968.

37. MOLE, L. E., S. S. JACKSON, R. R. PORTER AND J. M. WILKINSON. Allotypically related sequences in the Fd fragment of rabbit immunoglobulin heavy chains. *Biochem. J.* 124: 301, 1971.

38. OUDIN, J. Reaction de precipitation specifique entre des serums d'animaux de meme espece. *Compt. Rend. Acad. Sci.* 242: 2489, 1956.

39. OUDIN, J. L'Allotypie de certains antigens proteidiques du serum. *Compt. Rend. Acad. Sci.* 242: 2606, 1956.

40. OUDIN, J. Allotypy of rabbit serum proteins II. Relationships between various allotypes: their common antigenic specificity, their distribution in a sample population; genetic implications. *J. Exptl. Med.* 112: 125, 1960.

41. PERNIS, B., G. CHIAPPINO, A. KELUS AND P. GELL. Cellular localization of immunoglobulins with different allotypic specificities in rabbit lymphoid tissues. *J. Exptl. Med.* 122: 853, 1965.

42. PERNIS, B., L. FORNI, S. DUBSKI, A. S. KELUS, W. J. MANDY AND C. W. TODD. Heavy chain variable and constant region allotypes in single rabbit plasma cells. *Immunochemistry* 10: 281, 1973.

43. PRAHL, J. W., W. J. MANDY AND C. W. TODD. The molecular determinants of the A11 and A12 allotypic specificities in rabbit immunoglobulin. *Biochemistry* 8: 4935, 1969.

44. SELL, S. Studies on rabbit lymphocytes in vitro. IX. The suppression of anti-allotype-induced blast transformation in lymphocyte cultures from allotypically suppressed donors. *J. Exptl. Med.* 128: 341, 1968.

45. TAYLOR, R. B., P. H. DUFFUS, M. C. RAFF AND S. DE PETRIS. Redistribution and pinocytosis of lymphocyte surface immunoglobulin molecules induced by antiimmunoglobulin antibody. *Nature New Biol.* 233: 225, 1971.

46. VICE, J. L., A. GILMAN-SACHS, W. L. HUNT AND S. DRAY. Allotype suppression in a^2a^2 homozygous rabbits fostered in uteri of a2-immunized a^1a^1 homozygous mothers and injected at birth with anti-a2 antiserum. *J. Immunol.* 104: 550, 1970.

47. VICE, J. L., W. L. HUNT AND S. DRAY. Zygote transfer to facilitate altered expression of immunoglobulin light chain phenotypes in homozygous rabbits.*Proc. Soc. Exptl. Biol. Med.* 130: 730, 1969.

48. VICE, J. L., W. L. HUNT AND S. DRAY. Allotype suppression with anti-b5 antiserum in b^5b^5 homozygous rabbits fostered in uteri of b^4b^4 homozygous mothers: compensation by allotypes at other loci. *J. Immunol.* 103: 629, 1969.

49. WILKINSON, J. M. Variation in the N-terminal sequence of heavy chains of immunoglobulin G from rabbits of different allotype.*Biochem. J.* 112: 173, 1969.

50. YOUNG-COOPER, G. O., AND R. G. MAGE. Neutralization of allotype suppression in rabbits. *Immunology* 26: 809, 1974.

Expression of specific clones during B cell development[1,2]

NORMAN R. KLINMAN[3] AND JOAN L. PRESS[4]

Department of Pathology

University of Pennsylvania Medical School

Philadelphia, Pennsylvania 19174

ABSTRACT

The expression of DNP- and TNP-specific B cells in spleens of neonatal BALB/c mice was analyzed by the in vitro splenic focus technique. B cells of these specificities were found to be present in slightly higher frequency in neonatal than in adult spleens. The parameters of stimulation of neonatal B cells were similar to those of adult B cells but the antibody-forming cell progeny of neonatal B cells produce predominantly γM rather than γG antibody and produce less antibody than the progeny of adult B cells. Isoelectric focusing analyses of monoclonal antibodies derived from neonatal B cells stimulated in vitro with DNP or TNP revealed that over 90% of the antibodies could be identified as belonging to one of six predominant clonotypes, three specific for DNP and three for TNP. While individual neonates rarely expressed all of the predominant clonotypes, B cells of each of the six clonotypes were found in several donors. When B cells of a given predominant clonotype were present in an individual many such B cells could be found and in many cases the entire DNP- or TNP-specific B cell population of an individual could be accounted for by B cells of a single clonotype. These findings are discussed in terms of the diversity of clonotype specificities available in neonates, the kinetics of development of cells within a clonotype, and factors that may play a role in controlling the expression of B cell clones.—KLINMAN, N. R. AND J. L. PRESS. Expression of specific clones during B cell development. *Federation Proc.* 34: 47–50, 1975.

---

[1] From Session II, *Gene Regulation in Differentiation and Development*, of the FASEB Conference on *Biology of Development and Aging*, presented at the 58th Annual Meeting of the Federation of American Societies for Experimental Biology, Atlantic City, N.J., April 9, 1974.

[2] Supported by Research Grant A1-08778 from the Public Health Service.

[3] Recipient of a Public Health Service Career Development Award (1-KO4-A1-33983) from the National Institute of Allergy and Infectious Diseases.

[4] Present address: Department of Medicine, Division of Immunology, Stanford University School of Medicine, Stanford, California 94305.

Abbreviations: B cell:antibody forming cell precursor; DNP:2, 4-dinitrophenyl; Fl:fluorescein; Hy:*Limulus polyphemus* hemocyanin; TNP:2, 4, 6-trinitrophenyl.

The immune mechanism represents a biological system whose components are extensively diverse yet exquisitely specific. An adult mouse, for example, contains 2×10^8 B cells (antibody-forming cell precursors) each of which, upon antigenic stimulation, may give rise to a clone of 10^3 progeny (15, 28). The clonal progeny of each such stimulated B cell synthesize a homogeneous population of antibody molecules that is both highly specific for the stimulating antigen and unique to that clone (2, 3, 11–17). Thus, while the mature immune system may have the capacity to express antibodies with as many as 10^7 distinct amino acid sequences (clonotypes), at any point in time, each B cell is apparently restricted or unipotential with regard to its specificity and cell receptors. As a biological system, the immune response must be characterized and

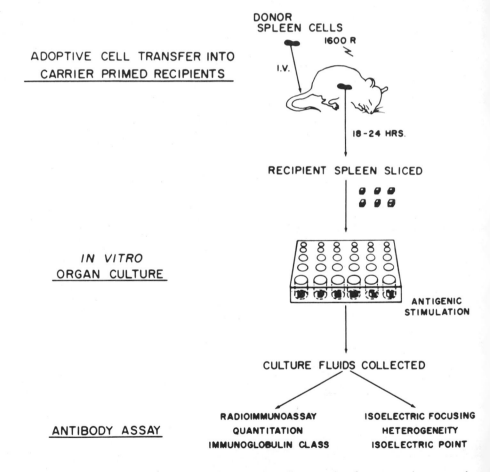

Figure 1. The fragment culture method for obtaining and analyzing antibody-forming cell clones. For analysis of neonatal B cells, the cell suspension from an entire neonatal spleen is injected intravenously into one or two recipients.

understood in terms of this unique specificity and diversity. It presents, therefore, an intriguing developmental system to study. For example, it is unlikely that all of the genetic information required to code for the vast array of specific antibodies found in the adult is present at any one time in a single cell, yet a great deal of biologically functional antibody specificity is present at a time in development when the total lymphoid cell content is considerably less than the number of potential antibody specificities (21, 26, 27). Alan Williamson has suggested earlier in this symposium that sufficient information indeed exists in the DNA of all cells, assuming that heavy and light polypeptide chains can be systematically shuffled (9, 20). Alternatively, the appearance of unique sequences may require the generation of new genetic information during embryonic or postnatal development (5, 7).

It is clear that a variety of pertinent questions may be asked of the developing animal to delineate mechanisms for antibody diversification, as well as elucidate those biological processes which eventually give rise to the mature immune system. These questions include: a) When do competent B cells first appear in development and what are the biological properties of neonatal B cells? b) Is the expression of individual clonotypes a systematic or a random process? c) What are the kinetics of the development of B cells within an individual clonotype? and d) What is the role of environmental factors, such as antigen, in the development process? Several laboratories have already approached some of these questions preliminarily in a variety of ways. To summarize: their findings indicate that B cells can be stimulated to produce antibody relatively early in development, i.e., by the second intrauterine trimester in the sheep

and days 17 to 19 of gestation in the mouse (1, 4, 8, 21, 25, 27). However, the expression of specific antibody appears restricted and reactivity to antigens may appear sequentially (18, 24, 27). In addition, in the mouse, cells bearing immunoglobulins on their surface (B cells) can be detected by day 16 of gestation (19, 26).

The approach of this laboratory to the questions posed above is based on the supposition that B cells from spleens of neonatal mice, if transferred to an adult environment in which all ancillary stimulatory mechanisms have been maximized, should be able to be stimulated to yield clones of antibody secreting cells. Figure 1 diagrams the general procedure used in these analyses. It should be noted that a great body of literature now exists for similar transfers of cells obtained from spleens of immune and nonimmune adult mice, where the clonal nature of the responses obtained has been verified (2, 3, 11–16). In addition the efficiency of clonal expression in the cell transfer and in vitro cloning procedures used in this laboratory has been determined to be 3–4%, which allows an absolute measure of the frequency of B cells of a given specificity in the donor cell suspension (15).

FREQUENCY AND BIOLOGICAL PROPERTIES OF PRECURSOR CELLS IN SPLEENS OF NEONATAL MICE

Preliminary experiments demonstrated that cell populations derived from the liver or spleen of fetuses in the 17th to 19th day of gestation contained cells that could respond in in vitro fragment cultures to 2, 4-dinitrophenylated hemocyanin (DNP-Hy) (21). Extensive analyses have now been carried out on cells obtained from spleens of neonates from the first to the fifth day after birth (23). Table 1 summarizes the data on the frequency of splenic B cells specific for the haptenic determinants DNP; 2, 4, 6-trinitrophenyl (TNP); and fluorescein (Fl) during this time of development as well as comparative data for B cells of these specificities in spleens of adult BALB/c mice. It can be seen that the frequency of B cells specific for DNP and TNP are at least as high in the neonate as in the adult while those specific for Fl are relatively quite low during the first several days after birth, as compared to the adult frequency for this specificity.

Table 2 summarizes the properties of clones derived from neonatal spleens and compares them to those derived from adult spleen cells. Monoclonal antibodies derived from adult spleen cells have been shown to be homogeneous by equilibrium dialysis, polypeptide chain recombination, and isoelectric focusing (11–14). Monoclonal antibodies derived from neonatal B cells appear equally homogeneous in isoelectric focusing (22). The population of clones derived from neonatal B cells differs, however, from those derived from adult B cells in several prop-

TABLE 2. Properties of neonatal and adult splenic DNP-specific B cells

	Adult	Neonatal
Range of haptenic determinant concentration giving stimulation	10^{-5} to 10^{-13} M	10^{-5} to 10^{-13} M
Requirement for carrier recognition, %	>99	>98
Overlap stimulation of DNP-specific B cells by TNP, %	<5	<10
Inhibition of stimulation by 10-fold excess of free DNP-lysine, %	60–80	60–80
Maximum average amount of antibody produced, ng/day	3	1.5
In vitro half-life of clone, days	12–14	7–9
Clones producing antibody of only μ heavy chain class, %	16	50–70

erties. Neonatal B cells give a greater preponderance of clones producing antibody with heavy chains only of the μ class (15). Clones derived from neonatal precursor cells generally make less antibody than adult clones and have a shorter duration of antibody production (15, 21). However, most of the parameters of stimulation of neonatal B cells are quite similar to those of adult B cells, including antigen dose response characteristics and ease of inhibition of stimulation with free hapten (13, 15, 21). In addition, the stimulation of neonatal B cells seems as specific as that of adult B cells since for both neonatal and adult B cells, stimulation with a mixture of DNP-Hy and TNP-Hy yields as many clones as the sum of clones stimulated by these determinants separately (15, 16). The additivity of primary stimulation indicates that these determinants stimulate separate sets of precursor cells even though the anti-DNP and anti-TNP antibodies produced are highly cross-reactive (16). Thus, early in

TABLE 1. Frequency of specific B cells in spleens of neonatal and adult BALB/c mice

Donor	Haptenic determinant used for stimulation		
	DNP,[a] clones per 10^4 B cells[b]	TNP, clones per 10^4 B cells	FL, clones per 10^4 B cells
8- to 12-week-old adult	2.0[c]	1.8	1.2
0- to 5-day-old neonate	2.5	2.5	0.4

[a] All stimulation at 10^{-6} M hapten on hemocyanin.
[b] B cells enumerated as immunoglobulin-bearing cells.
[c] Clonal frequency calculated using an in vitro cloning efficiency determined as 3.4%.

development, the neonatal spleen contains a population of TNP-precursor cells and a population of DNP-precursor cells which can be differentially and specifically stimulated.

EXPRESSION OF SPECIFIC CLONES DURING NEONATAL DEVELOPMENT

Several laboratories have demonstrated that mice of an inbred strain may express antibodies of identical idiotype or isoelectric focusing patterns (6, 10). Thus it may be anticipated that the B cell populations of syngeneic mice are, at least in part, identical. While the frequency of B cells specific for DNP and TNP in spleens of neonatal mice is at least as high as the frequency in adult spleens, the total number of B cells in neonatal spleens is considerably smaller. This has permitted a detailed analysis and comparison of the DNP- and TNP-specific B cells expressed in the

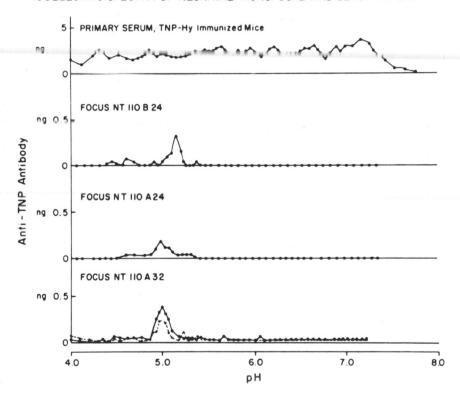

ISOELECTRIC SPECTRA OF NEONATAL "MONOFOCAL" AND SERUM ANTIBODY

Figure 2. Isoelectric focusing patterns of anti-TNP antibody from the serum of an adult BALB/c mouse primarily immunized with 0.1 mg of TNP-Hy in complete Freund's adjuvant 2 weeks previously (top panel), and three monoclonal antibodies derived from the stimulation of neonatal B cells. Analyses were carried out in 1 ml sucrose density gradients. Points represent quantitation by radioimmunoassay of collected drops plotted against the measured pH of the drop on the abscissa. The bottom panel represents duplicate runs of the same monofocal antibody.

spleens of neonatal BALB/c mice. Although the method of isoelectric focusing utilized to compare neonatal clones cannot fully delineate antibodies of closely similar net charge, it can nevertheless give minimum estimates of diversity (22). Figure 2 shows the isoelectric spectra of primary serum anti-TNP antibody obtained in an adult BALB/c mouse (top panel) and three monoclonal antibodies obtained from neonatal B cells stimulated in fragment cultures. Antibodies were suspended in ampholines on a 1 ml sucrose density gradient and antibody peaks were detected in collected fractions by a radioimmunoassay (12, 13, 22). The patterns in the bottom panel represent duplicate runs of the same monoclonal antibody. The pattern above this is of a monoclonal antibody derived from a B cell of the same neonatal donor. Both of these monoclonal antibodies focus at an isoelectric point (*pI*) of 5.00. The third monoclonal antibody was derived from a different donor and has a *pI* of 5.15. Table 3 presents a summary of isoelectric focusing analyses of monoclonal antibodies obtained from B cells of neonates during the first 3 days of life and stimulated in fragment culture with TNP-Hy. It can be seen that neonatal monoclonal antibodies specific for TNP display at least five distinctly different isoelec-

TABLE 4. Isoelectric focusing patterns of monoclonal anti-DNP antibody derived from 0- to 3-day-old neonatal BALB/c mice

Isoelectric point	No. of monofocal antibodies of each *pI*	No. of donor mice expressing each clonotype
5.05	16	8
5.25	7	5
5.55	13	9
5.35	1	1
5.95	1	1

tric points. It should be noted, however, that more than 90% of the neonatal B cells in BALB/c mice that are specific for TNP give rise to three predominant clonotypes, that is, monoclonal antibodies that are identifiable by isoelectric points of 5.00, 5.15 or 5.40. Table 3 also presents data indicating the number of donor mice in which each of the clonotypes was found. While each of the predominant clonotypes was found in several donors, a donor that expressed a given predominant clonotype usually exhibited two or more such clonotype precursors and only rarely expressed a precursor of a different clonotype. Thus, while on the average neonatal mice have a frequency of 2.5 TNP-specific precursors per 10^4 splenic B cells, in any given neonate, this number can usually be accounted for by B cells of only one of the predominant clonotypes. Individual neonates, therefore, expressed different predominant clonotypes at differing frequencies. Table 4 presents data from a similar analysis of monofocal antibodies produced by B cells stimulated with DNP-Hy. Again three predominant clonotypes are noted. The three predominant DNP clonotypes occur with frequencies and donor distributions similar to those observed for predominant TNP clonotypes. Careful

TABLE 3. Isoelectric focusing patterns of monoclonal anti-TNP antibody derived from 0- to 3-day-old neonatal BALB/c mice

Isoelectric point	No. of monofocal antibodies of each *pI*	No. of donor mice expressing each clonotype
5.00	10	6
5.15	14	7
5.40	8	5
5.70	1	1
5.90	1	1

analysis indicated that the predominant clonotypes produced in response to TNP and DNP are different, corroborating the finding that there is little or no overlap stimulation of neonatal B cells by these two determinants. Thus, it would appear that BALB/c neonates have available relatively limited sets of precursors specific for DNP or TNP. However, any two neonates may express different elements of these sets at different times. Thus, the expression of specific clones during neonatal development has a significantly random element.

KINETICS OF CLONAL DEVELOPMENT

If it is assumed that monoclonal antibodies of the same pI are indeed identical, then the data presented in Tables 3 and 4 on the occurrence of predominant clonotypes can be utilized to delineate the cell repertoire available in neonatal spleens and the kinetics of expansion of any given clone. Given the fact that 3–4% of specific B cells in a transferred cell population can be detectably stimulated in splenic fragment cultures, the frequency of occurrence of any given precursor can be calculated. Results from such calculations indicate that precursors of each of the six predominant DNP- or TNP-specific clonotypes represent on the average 1/12,000 of the total B-cell pool in spleens of 1- to 3-day-old BALB/c neonates. In any given individual neonate, however, some of these clones will not be expressed or will be minimally expressed, while others may be represented by as much as 1/3,000 of that neonate splenic B-cell population. Furthermore, by the second or third day of neonatal life, as many as 100–200 B cells of a single clonotype may be present. If clonal precursors are first present at days 16–17 of gestation, then a doubling time of approximately 24 hours could account for the kinetics of appearance of such precursor cell clones. This doubling time is similar to that of the B cell population as a whole in neonates (19, 26). Thus, in the first days of neonatal life, individual mice appear to express perhaps 3–5,000 different clonotypes, each represented by clones of as many as 50–200 B cells. The neonatal mouse population as a whole, however, may express more than 12,000 distinct specificities and those which are expressed in any individual may be determined by random processes.

Similar analyses have been carried out with 4- to 6-day-old neonatal donors whose spleens have as many as 10^7 B cells. While the frequencies of DNP- and TNP-specific B cells are somewhat lower in these mice, the same predominant clonotypes can be detected. In this case, however, the frequency of these clonotype precursors is diminished and they are often found in the presence of precursors of clones producing antibodies with a different pI. Thus it would seem that the clones that predominate early do not expand much beyond the third day and other clones may begin to be expressed with greater frequency. By day 9 the predominant clonotypes represent a small minority of the DNP- or TNP-specific B cells. The presence of DNP- and TNP-specific B cells that are not of the predominant clonotypes even in the first 3 days of life may be of great importance since these clones may be products of events that occur at relatively low frequencies.

ROLE OF EXTRINSIC FACTORS ON B CELL DEVELOPMENT

It is unlikely that antigen plays a significant role in the generation of the precursor cells present in nonimmune mice. This has been concluded from the observation that precursor cells generated as the result of antigenic contact are qualitatively different from those present before antigen contact and the observation that germfree mice have specific B-cell frequencies similar to conventionally reared mice (13–16, 23). In addition, Sterzl and Silverstein (27) and recently Sherwin and Rowlands (25) have demonstrated that the presence of antigen during development does not affect the time at which an animal is capable of responding to that antigen. However, other factors in the intrauterine environment may play a role. In the studies presented here it was noted that while different individual neonates expressed one or another of the predominant DNP or TNP clonotypes in a relatively random fashion, littermates had a tendency to express the same clonotype. This finding may indicate a maternal or intrauterine influence on the selection of the antibody clones that are expressed.

CONCLUDING REMARKS

These studies indicate that the B cells of neonatal mice, if placed in a proper environment, are capable of responding to antigenic stimulation by giving rise to a clone of antibody-forming cells. A detailed analysis of the antibody produced by such clones should eventually allow a greater understanding of the mechanisms responsible for immunological diversity. While, to date, this analysis has been carried out only by isoelectric focusing, it has been possible to generate minimal estimates of the diversity present at different stages of development. Even these minimal estimates permit a preliminary definition of the early events that give rise to an immunocompetent cell population. Figure 3 presents a schematic diagram of several stages of develop-

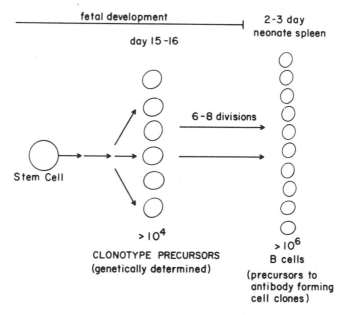

Figure 3. Schematic representation of the early stages of murine B cell development.

ment of fetal and neonatal B-cell populations. By day 15–16 of gestation it would appear that BALB/c neonates have the capacity to exhibit more than 10^4 clonotypes. This is ascertained by the finding that in the population of neonates six clonotypes have been identified that display similar rates of occurrence averaging 1/12,000 B cells. In any individual approximately one-third of these clonotypes is expressed by a burst of 6–8 divisions characterized by a doubling time of 1 day and yielding perhaps 200 daughter B cells by the 2nd or 3rd day of neonatal life. Subsequently, other clonotypes are expressed and eventually predominate. It is difficult as yet to ascertain whether these events reflect basically random or systematically regulated processes. While the presence of sporadically occurring clonotypes early in development and the inconsistent expression of predominant clonotypes appear to support random mechanisms, the repeated recurrence of the same predominant clonotypes clearly indicates that these specificities are genetically determined. Equally intriguing is the evidence of regulation of specificities within littermates which may indicate that many of the observed phenomena are the result of regulatory events affecting clonotype precursors and thus the ultimate expression of B-cell clones.

REFERENCES

1. ARRENBRECHT, S. European J. Immunol. 3: 506, 1973.
2. ASKONAS, B. A., A. R. WILLIAMSON AND B. E. G. WRIGHT. Proc. Natl. Acad. Sci. U.S. 67: 1398, 1970.
3. BOSMA, M., AND E. WEILER. J. Immunol. 104: 203, 1970.
4. CHISCON, M. O., AND E. S. GOLUB. J. Immunol. 108: 1379, 1972.
5. COHN, M. In: The Biochemistry of Gene Expression in Higher Organisms, edited by S. K. Pollack and J. W. Lee. Dordrecht, Holland: D. Reidel Publishing Co., 1973, p. 574.
6. CRAMER, M., AND D. G. BRAUN. J. Exptl. Med. 138: 1533, 1973.
7. GALLY, J. A., AND G. M. EDELMAN. Nature 227: 341, 1970.
8. GOIDL, E. A., AND G. W. SISKIND. Federation Proc. 33: 735, 1974.
9. HOOD, L., AND D. W. TALMAGE. Science 168: 325, 1970.
10. HOPPER, J. E., AND A. NISONOFF. Advan. Immunol. 13: 58, 1971.
11. KLINMAN, N. R. Immunochemistry 6: 757, 1969.
12. KLINMAN, N. R. J. Immunol. 106: 1345, 1971.
13. KLINMAN, N. R. J. Exptl. Med. 136: 241, 1972.
14. KLINMAN, N. R., AND G. ASCHINAZI. J. Immunol. 106: 1338, 1971.
15. KLINMAN, N. R., J. L. PRESS, A. R. PICKARD, R. T. WOODLAND AND A. F. DEWEY. In: The Immune System: Genes, Receptors, Signals, edited by E. Sercarz, A. Williamson and C. F. Fox. New York: Academic. 1974, p. 357.
16. KLINMAN, N. R., J. L. PRESS AND G. P. SEGAL. J. Exptl. Med. 138: 1276, 1973.
17. LUZZATI, A. L., I. LEFKOVITS AND B. PERNIS. European J. Immunol. 3: 636, 1973.
18. MONTGOMERY, P. C., AND A. R. WILLIAMSON. J. Immunol. 109: 1036, 1972.
19. NOSSAL, G. S. V., AND B. L. PIKE. Advan. Exptl. Med. Biol. 29: 11, 1972.
20. PREMKUMAR, E., M. SHUYAB AND A. R. WILLIAMSON. Proc. Natl. Acad. Sci. U.S. 71: 99, 1974.
21. PRESS, J. L., AND N. R. KLINMAN. J. Immunol. 111: 829, 1973.
22. PRESS, J. L., AND N. R. KLINMAN, Immunochemistry. 10: 621, 1973.
23. PRESS, J. L., AND N. R. KLINMAN. European J. Immunol. 4: 155, 1974.
24. ROWLANDS, D. T., D. BLAKESLEE AND E. ANGALA, J. Immunol. 112: 2148, 1974.
25. SHERWIN, W. K., AND D. T. ROWLANDS. Federation Proc. 33: 735, 1974.
26. SPEAR, P. G., A. WANG, U. RUTISHAUER AND G. M. EDELMAN. J. Exptl. Med. 138: 557, 1973.
27. STERZL, J., AND A. M. SILVERSTEIN. Advan. Immunol. 6: 337, 1967.
28. WOODLAND, R. T. Federation Proc. 33: 807, 1974.

Growth and death of diploid and transformed human fibroblasts

ROBIN HOLLIDAY

Division of Genetics
National Institute for Medical Research
Mill Hill, London NW7 1AA, England

ABSTRACT

Three possible explanations are presented for the differences in growth potential between human diploid fibroblasts of finite life-span and permanent transformed lines: *1)* Only diploid cells have a molecular clock mechanism which counts cell divisions prior to senescence. Two hypothetical examples of such mechanisms are described; however, the available evidence argues against a clock mechanism for aging in fibroblasts. *2)* Cells become committed with a given probability to a slow buildup in protein errors, which leads after many divisions to a lethal error catastrophe. It can be shown that speeding up the rate at which the error catastrophe develops, as may occur in transformed cells, can convert a population of finite life-span to one with infinite growth. *3)* The growth rate of diploid cells may not depend on the limiting concentration of any one protein. If so, cells with a low level of errors will not have a reduced generation time, and there will be no selection against them. On the other hand the uncontrolled growth of transformed cells may be reduced in rate by the presence of faulty proteins, so that there is continuous selection for those with the fewest errors. Finally, the analogous problem of the mortality of somatic cells and the immortality of the germ line is also briefly discussed.— HOLLIDAY, R. Growth and death of diploid and transformed human fibroblasts. *Federation Proc.* 34: 51–55, 1975.

I t is now well established that diploid human fibroblasts have a defined life-span in culture. Starting with a primary culture of cells from a sample of tissue (phase I), the cells multiply at a constant rate for many cell generations (phase II), but finally enter a senescent condition (phase III) which culminates in death of the culture (3, 4). On the other hand, heteroploid cultures that have arisen from diploid cells treated with a virus, such as SV 40, or from tumor tissue, can be grown indefinitely in culture (3).

However, it is not established that all heteroploid strains with the morphological characteristics of transformed cells can be grown indefinitely. There are reports that some cells of this type, or variants from them, die out in the same way as diploid ones (18, 26).

In this paper I will discuss some possible reasons for the difference in growth potential between diploid cells and permanent heteroploid lines, and comment briefly on the analogous problem of the mortality of somatic cells and the immortality of the germ line in higher organisms. Two general theories of aging will be considered: either that it is determined by a defined genetic program, or that it is the result of accumulated errors or damage in macromolecules. At the outset it must be made clear that although aging must be under genetic control, this does not by itself imply that a program is involved, since the frequency of mutation or the fidelity of protein synthesis is also strongly influenced or determined by the genotype. A program for aging is assumed to be some kind of clock mechanism that either counts cell divisions or measures some other recurrent or sequential cellular process.

PROGRAMMED AGING

It is not only whole organisms or populations of cells in culture that age, as, in addition, groups of cells or whole tissues degenerate and die during normal development (2, 19). The example often quoted is that of the tadpole's tail, but more subtle and less obvious changes also occur. For instance, in the growth of the chick limb bud, a group of cells known as the posterior necrotic zone undergoes autolysis at a very precise time during the development of the bud. One possibility is that these cells have an organizing or regulatory role at an early developmental stage, but must be eliminated before a subsequent stage can be initiated. The mechanism of this cell death is unknown, but there is little doubt that it is in some way genetically programmed. A less well-defined, but probably equally valid example of a program can be seen in the clonal growth of protozoa such as *Paramecium* (21). After conjugation, during which meiosis and fertilization occur, the separated cells initiate a defined sequence of changes that is related to the number of asexual binary fissions. During the early growth of the clone the cells are not sexually mature, but after a given number of divisions they become fertile and can conjugate with cells of opposite mating type. Subsequently their fertility declines, although they may still be capable of the self-fertilization process known as autogamy. At this stage their rate of division is still normal, but later on growth rate declines, senescence sets in, and the cells eventually die. These observations strongly suggest that the whole cycle of changes in *Paramecium* and other ciliate protozoa depends on a program or clock based on the number of cell divisions, although this does not imply that the final senescent phase is not due to the accumulation of genetic or cytoplasmic damage.

Two molecular mechanisms for counting cell divisions have been proposed. One depends on the failure to complete the replication of DNA at the very end of chromosome arms, and leads to progressive terminal deletion of genetic material with continued cell division (13). It is illustrated in Fig. 1. The other depends on the sequential modification of bases in repeated sequences of DNA by specific enzymes. The number of divisions counted is directly related to the number of repeats in the sequence (5a). The mechanism is shown in Fig. 2. The running out of either of these clocks could trigger one of several possible lethal events. The activity of a single indispensable gene may be turned off, leading to the dilution out of its product; DNA replication might be blocked; or lysosomal enzymes may be released. Alternatively, there might simply be a loss of cellular control or homeostasis, which is followed by the accumulation of defects in various macromolecules (16).

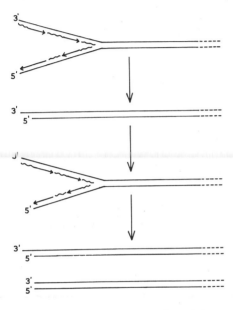

Figure 1. The progressive loss of DNA from the ends of chromosomes, based on the scheme of Olovnikov (13). According to current evidence, DNA polymerase acts on a short RNA primer adding deoxyribonucleotides from the 3' end. The RNA, indicated by wavy lines in the figure, is removed by an endoribonuclease specific for RNA/DNA hybrids, and the gap is filled by DNA synthesis from the adjacent Okazaki DNA fragment. This cannot happen at the very end of one arm of the replication fork, therefore during successive divisions pieces are progressively removed from the 5' terminus (for a full discussion of this problem see Watson (25)). The clock mechanism depends on the quantity of redundant or nonessential DNA at the end of the chromosome arm; as soon as indispensable genetic information is deleted, the cell loses viability. A special additional mechanism must, of course, maintain the integrity of chromosomes in the germ line.

The hypothesis that aging is based on a clock mechanism has appeal because it suggests a basis for the difference between cultured diploid fibroblasts and heteroploid lines. We simply say that the integrated cellular functions and normal genotype of the differentiated fibroblasts allows a clock that has been started in vivo to run its course in vitro, whereas the abnormal transformed cells have lost essential controlling mechanisms and/or genetic material and the clock mechanism is inactivated or bypassed.

Several observations suggest that the life-span of diploid cells is more closely related to the number of cell or population doublings than to chronological time. By studying individual colonies of human glial cells, Ponten (17) was able to show that cells at the quiescent center of old colonies retain capacity for further divisions, whereas those at the edge had become senescent. This difference bears no relationship to the cells' chronological age. In addition, a population of fibroblasts which is subcultured with a 1:2 split ratio spends relatively more time in lag or stationary phase and less in logarithmic phase than one which is subcultured with a 1:10 split ratio. Yet in terms of population doublings their longevities are the same (3). Parallel cultures of cells grown under identical conditions often do vary in their longevity. Nevertheless, in some cases such populations do show a striking synchrony in their aging. For instance, 10 populations of MRC-5 fibroblasts grown at 34 C all died out between passages 56 and 61 (24).

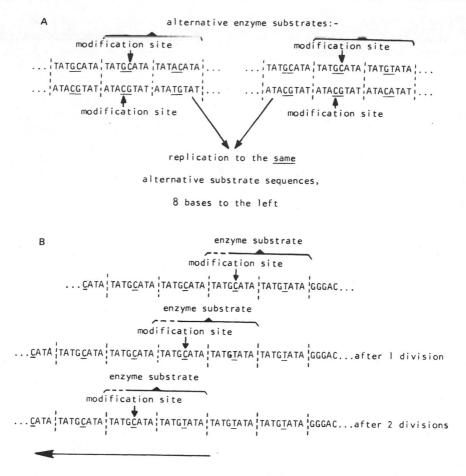

Figure 2. *A*) (top) A clock mechanism for aging based on the sequential modification of repeated sequences of DNA. Scarano (20) has suggested that a CG base pair can be changed to TA by the methylation of cytosine at the 5 position, followed by deamination at the 6 position; replication then establishes a new TA base pair. The modification enzyme(s) that do this may be highly specific for base sequences, as are modification enzymes in bacteria (5a). The modification enzyme recognizes the first sequence of 8 bases, because it contains T at the 4th position, together with the whole or some part of the sequence to its left. The C at the 4th position of this second sequence is changed to T. On replication the new TA base pair produces a new recognition sequence 8 bases to the left. When all the sequences have been suc-

cessfully modified, an essential structural gene at the extreme left of the repeated sequences (not shown here) is inactivated, or its transcription is blocked by the modification of an operator or promoter region adjacent to it. *B*) (bottom) If the aging is to be synchronized, modification of both strands of DNA must occur. The enzyme recognizes a sequence that has a CG pair at either the 4th *or* 5th position (note that if each sequence forms a short palindrome, the recognition sequences can be structurally identical, as shown here). In both cases it modifies C at the 4th *and* 5th position of the sequence to the left. Both these modified sequences then become recognition sequences after replication. Modifications therefore move progressively from right to left and count cell divisions as in Fig. 2*A*.

TABLE 1. Life-span of fetal lung fibroblasts, strain MRC-5, cultured in medium containing concentrations of 5-fluorouracil that do not reduce growth rate

	From passage 24		From passage 21	
	Control	FU (0.125 μg/ml)	FU (0.25 μg/ml)	Control
	60	50	51	61
	66	50	53	61
	68	60	53	61
	68	60	55	63
	70	64	55	63
Mean ± SD	66.4 ± 3.85	56.8 ± 6.42	53.4 ± 1.67	62.2 ± 1.79
		0.01 < 0.05		<0.001
P (t test)			>0.05	

The cells were grown under the conditions described by Holliday and Tarrant (6) and split 1:4 when they became confluent. FU = 5-fluorouracil.

However, results of this type are deceptive; they must be interpreted with caution, owing to what has been termed the "concertina effect." The death of cells during phase III means that the remaining viable cells have to divide many times in order to achieve confluency. Therefore the growth during the last few passages is probably based on many small subpopulations of cells undergoing very different numbers of cell divisions.

There are, in fact, several compelling reasons for believing that the life-span of diploid fibroblasts is not related to a clock based on cell divisions:

1) MRC-5 fibroblasts grow quite vigorously at 40 C, and can be routinely subcultured at the normal rate. Nevertheless, their life-span in comparison to parallel cultures at 37 C is reduced by about half (24). The premature slowing down and cessation of growth at 40 C is due to an irreversible process like phase III, as switching cultures to 37 C a few passages before death does not lead to their recovery. If a simple environmental treatment can severely shorten life-span, then a rigid clock mechanism based on cell divisions is unlikely to be operating.

2) The same argument applies to other environmental treatments that reduce life-span. For instance, growth of MRC-5 in low concentrations of 5-fluorouracil (5-FU), which do not reduce growth rate, significantly shortens their life-span, as is shown in Table 1. 5-FU is incorporated into RNA and is known in other systems to reduce the fidelity of transcription and/or translation (10).

3) Cristofalo and Sharf (1) have shown that the number of cells entering S phase declines fairly gradually during phase II and more rapidly in phase III. This observation is not what one would expect for a synchronous or programmed aging process.

4) Finally, Smith and Hayflick (22) isolated individual cells from an early passage WI-38 culture and recorded the number of generations that elapsed before the individual clones died out. Their results show that there is considerable heterogeneity in

growth potential even in "healthy" populations. Thirty to forty percent of the cells divided no more than eight times before the clones died. This result is much more compatible with error theories than with a programmed theory of aging.

I conclude that it is unlikely that the aging of fibroblasts is based on a clock mechanism, although such mechanisms may well operate in other aging systems, and in particular in the programmed death of cells during the development of an organism.

ERROR THEORIES OF AGING

Two types of error theory have been proposed to explain fibroblast aging, although it is now realized that the distinction between them is not as clear as was previously thought (6, 16). The somatic mutation theory suggests that during growth genetic damage accumulates and that after a given number of defects have occurred the cells enter phase III (3). This theory can only account for the limited lifespan if two conditions are met. First, there must on average be at least one defect per division, i.e., not less than half the daughter cells must carry a new mutation, otherwise the mutations will be diluted out by growth. Second, the mutations that initially accumulate must have no effect on growth rate, otherwise those cells with the fewest mutations would be continually selected. To explain the difference between diploid and transformed cells one either has to suppose that there is a lower mutation rate in the latter, which seems unlikely, or a difference in cellular selection. This will be discussed in a later section. On the whole the somatic mutation theory seems implausible, since not only does the mutation frequency have to be very high, but also the mutations have to occur initially only in nonessential genes. One

way out of this difficulty is to argue, as Medvedev (12) has done, that essential genes are in multiple copies which are randomly inactivated with time. In a sense this suggestion attempts to reconcile mutation and clock theories, as the life-span would be a function of the number of repeated genes.

The other type of error theory depends on the accumulation of defects in protein synthesis. It was originally suggested that errors should accumulate exponentially, leading (in the absence of cellular selection) to an irreversible and lethal error catastrophe in protein synthesis (14). A later amendment made it clear that under certain conditions the error level would simply reach a steady state (15).

If errors do accumulate during cell growth, the difference between diploid and transformed cells could lie not only in the probability of errors, but also in the kinetics of the development of a lethal error catastrophe. This can be explained in terms of a simple model, derived from the experimental studies of clonal senescence in the fungus *Podospora* (11, 23). In this organism it has been clearly shown that the cells move from a nonsenescent state with a given probability to a senescent state, where growth rate remains constant but the growth potential of the cells progressively declines. In different populations grown under the same conditions the incubation period from the initiation of the senescent state until death is fairly constant. Applying this to fibroblasts, the model states that normal or uncommitted cells have a steady-state level of protein errors, but there is a given probability, P, that one or more "critical errors" will move the cell into an irreversible or committed state, in which the level of errors gradually increases and finally develops into a lethal error catastrophe. These "critical errors" might, for instance, be in crucial enzyme molecules involved in information transfer, such as RNA polymerase.

At first sight, it would seem that the population of fibroblasts would die out only if P is at least 0.5, but this is not so if the incubation period (the number of cell divisions from commitment to cell death) is very long. The reason for this is that uncommitted cells give rise to committed ones, but the reverse does not happen. If we assume that the two types of cell grow at the same rate, at least until the final stage of the error catastrophe, then the proportion of uncommitted cells is progressively reduced and will eventually

reach a very low frequency in the population. The population sizes routinely used for in vitro aging studies are in the range of $10^5–10^7$ cells. The crucial question is the length of the incubation period that is necessary to dilute out all uncommitted cells from these populations, because once this has happened the population is no longer immortal. Starting with a population of uncommitted cells, Fig. 3 shows the number of cell generations which are necessary to reduce the proportion of uncommitted cells to 10^{-5} or 10^{-7} for various values of P. These results were obtained by T. B. L. Kirkwood, who will publish the mathematical details of the model elsewhere. To account for the observed in vitro life-spans the P value could not be lower than 0.1, but it could be between 0.1 and 0.2 if we take into account the cell generations prior to and during phase I, as well as phase II and III.

For values of P lower than 0.5 the population will be immortal if it is of unlimited size. At the end of the incubation period, whatever its length, committed cells are removed by cell death and the effect will be to counteract the dilution out of uncommitted cells. It can be shown that a steady state will eventually be reached, with a constant proportion of committed, uncommitted, and dead cells.

We can see that changing one of three parameters would convert a population of finite life-span to one with an infinite life-span: a reduction in the value of P, an increase in population size, or a decrease in the incubation time. In the case of transformed cells, therefore, the initial error frequency could be the same as in diploid cells, but the rate at which the errors build up could be faster, leading more quickly to an error catastrophe. The paradox is that this

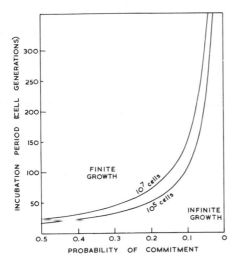

Figure 3. The relationship between the probability of an uncommitted cell giving rise to a committed one, the incubation period before cell death, and the population size (see text). The curves show the incubation periods that are necessary to dilute out all uncommitted cells from populations of 10^5 or 10^7 fibroblasts. With shorter incubation periods, or if the population is of infinite size, growth potential is unlimited.

change will make the population immortal, because the uncommitted cells never get diluted out.

If the model is correct, then it follows that diploid cells per se do not necessarily have a limited growth potential, since if uncommitted cells could be separated from committed ones, the population could be kept going indefinitely. It also follows that in a population of finite life-span, the viable cells will have a wide range of growth potentials, as observed by Smith and Hayflick (22). The exact distribution of clone sizes from individual cells will depend on several factors, but especially on the growth rate of cells nearing the end of their life-span.

Finally, it should be emphasized that the model does not depend on the incubation period being a build-up of protein errors. The same arguments and conclusions would apply if it was initiated, for instance, by the formation of a defective mitochondrion replicating a little more rapidly than normal and eventually killing the cell by diluting out all normal mitochondria.

CELLULAR SELECTION

So far I have not considered the question of cellular selection. The difficulty about both types of error theory is that one would expect cells that have accumulated a given number of mutations or a given proportion of altered proteins to grow more slowly. In this case they should be continually selected against, leaving the cells with the fewest errors and shortest division time to make a correspondingly greater contribution to subsequent generations. This is in itself an argument in favour of clock theories.

The multiple mutation theory is only feasible if many mutations can be present without any effect on growth rate, and the same applies to the initial accumulation of defective proteins. For the protein error theory to be tenable, cells containing an incipient error catastrophe would have to grow at the same rate as uncommitted cells with the basal steady-state level of errors. As has been explained, once all the diploid cells had entered this irreversible condition, the population would die out, irrespective of cellular selection.

This provides the basis for another possible explanation of the difference in growth potential between diploid and heteroploid cells. It is not unreasonable to suppose that diploid cells control cell division in such a way that the rate is not limited by the total amount or activity of any single protein or enzyme. Even simple regulatory controls such as end product feedback inhibition could account for this. A few percent drop in activity of all enzymes as a result of an increase in errors can be compensated for and not affect complex cellular processes such as cell division. On the other hand, the transformed cell has clearly lost a number of cellular controls, and it may well be that its rate of growth *is* dependent on the limiting amount of a single enzyme or protein. If so, a small reduction in the activity of this enzyme, from infidelity in protein synthesis, will reduce growth rate. It makes no difference whether a transformed cell grows slower or faster— as is usually the case—than the diploid one. To achieve immortality all that is required is for cells containing a low frequency of errors to be continually selected against. This theory predicts that transformed cells should be more sensitive than diploid ones to the effect of agents that act by introducing defects into proteins. Experiments to test this prediction are in progress.

IMMORTALITY OF THE GERM LINE

A related problem in higher organisms concerns the immortality of the germ line in comparison to the mortal somatic cells. This is of course most easily explicable on the basis of a program for aging. A developmental or aging clock would run only in somatic cells, but would not be switched on in the germ line. However, as in the case of transformed fibroblasts, it is not impossible to reconcile error theories with the stability of the germ line, provided there is selection against abnormal cells. In protozoa and fungi it is known that the visible signs of clonal senescence are almost always preceded by sterility (11, 21), and it may well be that cells in higher organisms containing minor defects behave in the same way and cannot enter or complete meiotic division. More specifically, it is possible that meiotic cells have a special molecular device for ensuring that the defective gametes are not contributed to the next generation. Suppose these cells synthesize a large amount of a protein which has no function in its normal form. Introduction by mistranslation of one of several errors may convert the innocuous molecule into a lethal "suicide protein." Such a protein might bind irreversibly to the operator of an indispensable structural gene. Alternatively it could kill the cell in the same way as a single colicin molecule kills a bacterium. A cell containing one or a few such molecules "by mistake" would then be removed from the pool of germ cells. If the cell makes 10^6 molecules each of 10^3 amino acids, then according to the best estimates available (8, 9), at least 10^5 of these would contain at least one incorrect amino acid. We can see that the chance of introducing a lethal mistake could be quite small, perhaps the need to introduce a cysteine

residue in a particular region, which would drastically change the structure of the molecule by forming an internal -S-S- bridge with an -SH group normally present. Moreover, if the protein was a dimer or a tetramer and the suicide form had to be made up entirely of altered molecules, then the probability of a cell containing one such molecule would increase as the square or the fourth power of the error frequency. This would provide very sensitive discrimination against cells with only a relatively slight increase in errors above the background level.

SUMMARY AND CONCLUSIONS

Three possible explanations have been considered for the difference in growth potential between diploid fibroblasts and transformed permanent lines. First, that only the former have a genetic program of aging, which is bypassed or inactivated in the latter. Second, that the buildup of errors or defects in macromolecules is much slower in diploids than in transformed cells and leads eventually to the dilution out of diploid cells containing a low steady state level of errors. Third, that cellular selection operates more efficiently against transformed cells that have just begun the aging process than it does against diploid ones.

Several lines of evidence suggest that the aging of diploid cells is more likely to be due to the accumulation of defects than to a genetic program. Populations of fibroblasts are extremely heterogeneous in their growth potential, and environmental agents strongly affect life-span. In addition, there is evidence that altered protein molecules accumulate rapidly during the last few population doublings (6, 7). On the other hand, one of the main predictions of the protein error theory has not so far been fulfilled: viruses grown in senescent cells do not seem to contain defective proteins or have an increased frequency of mutations (5).

One way of distinguishing between different theories of cellular aging may be to answer the crucial questions about the origin and growth potential of heteroploid cells. Can diploids give rise to these cells with equal frequency at all phases of growth? What proportion of the heteroploid cells which arise produce a permanent immortal line, and how many still show senescence and aging? We should not be sidetracked by the semantic problem of whether heteroploid strains of defined life-span are or are not truly transformed. If we are to understand the different growth potentials of diploid strains and heteroploid lines, it will undoubtedly be essential to study cells with some of the phenotypic characteristics of each.

I am grateful to Dr. L. E. Orgel for many stimulating discussions; Mr. T. B. L. Kirkwood for devising the computer program that gave the results in Fig. 3, and Mrs. G. M. Tarrant for carrying out the experiments with 5-fluorouracil.

REFERENCES

1. CRISTOFALO, V. J., AND B. B. SCARF. *Exptl. Cell Res.* 76: 419, 1973.
2. GLUCKSMAN, A. *Biol. Rev. Cambridge Phil. Soc.* 26: 59, 1951.
3. HAYFLICK, L. *Exptl. Cell Res.* 37: 614, 1965.
4. HAYFLICK, L., AND P. S. MOORHEAD. *Exptl. Cell Res.* 25: 585, 1961.
5. HOLLAND, S. S., D. KOHNE AND M. V. DOYLE. *Nature* 245: 318, 1973.
5a. HOLLIDAY, R., AND J. E. PUGH. *Science* In press.
6. HOLLIDAY, R., AND G. M. TARRANT. *Nature* 238: 26, 1972.
7. LEWIS, C. M., AND G. M. TARRANT. *Nature* 239: 316, 1972.
8. LOFTFIELD, R. B. *Biochem. J.* 89: 82, 1963.
9. LOFTFIELD, R. B., AND D. VANDERJAGT. *Biochem. J.* 128: 1353, 1972.
10. MANDEL, H. G. *Progr. Mol. Subcellular Biol.* 1: 82, 1969.
11. MARCOU, D. *Ann. Sci. Nat. Botan. Biol. Vegetale* 12: 653, 1961.
12. MEDVEDEV, ZH. A. *Exptl. Gerontol.* 1: 227, 1972.
13. OLOVNIKOV, A. M. *Dokl. Akad. Nauk USSR* 201: 1796, 1971.
14. ORGEL, L. E. *Proc. Natl. Acad. Sci. U.S.* 49: 517, 1963.
15. ORGEL, L. E. *Proc. Natl. Acad. Sci. U.S.* 67: 1476, 1970.
16. ORGEL, L. E. *Nature* 243: 441, 1973.
17. PONTEN, J. In: *Symposium on Molecular and Cellular Mechanisms of Aging*, Paris: Inst. Natl. Sante Recherche Med. 27: 53, 1973.
18. RABINOVITZ, Z., AND L. SACHS. *Intern. J. Cancer* 6: 388, 1970.
19. SAUNDERS, J. W. *Science* 154: 604, 1966.
20. SCARANO, E. In: *Advances in Cytopharmacology*, edited by F. Clementi and B. Ceccarelli. New York: Raven, 1971, p. 1.
21. SIEGEL, R. W. *Symp. Soc. Exptl. Biol.* 21: 127, 1967.
22. SMITH, J. R., AND L. HAYFLICK. *J. Cell Biol.* 62: 48, 1974.
23. SMITH, J. R., AND I. RUBINSTEIN. *J. Gen. Microbiol.* 76: 283, 1973.
24. THOMPSON, K. V. A., AND R. HOLLIDAY. *Exptl. Cell Res.* 80: 354, 1973.
25. WATSON, J. D. *Nature New Biol.* 239: 197, 1972.
26. WESTERMARK, B. *Acta Univ. Upsal.* 164: 1973.

Pathological implications of cell aging in vitro[1,2]

S. GOLDSTEIN, S. NIEWIAROWSKI AND D. P. SINGAL

Departments of Medicine and Pathology

McMaster University Medical Centre

Hamilton, Ontario, Canada, L8S 4J9 and

Specialized Center for Thrombosis Research

Temple University Health Sciences Center

Philadelphia, Pennsylvania 19122

ABSTRACT

The replicative capacity of cultured human fibroblasts is discussed in relation to three areas, diabetes mellitus, expression of HL-A antigens, and interactions with polymerizing fibrin. The replicative capacity of cells is diminished in diabetes mellitus and certain related disorders such as progeria and Werner's syndrome, all of which feature accelerated aging. Expression of HL-A antigens is reduced in progeria fibroblasts compared to normal cultures at corresponding stages of passage. Normal cells show more subtle alteration during aging in vitro probably related to clonal heterogeneity and/or selection within mass cultures. Early-passage fibroblasts interact rapidly with polymerizing fibrin to form a mature clot which is then retracted by a process dependent on cellular integrity and active metabolism. Late-passage cultures are less active in both parameters as are fibroblasts from a subject with progeria. These observations, in total, may relate to altered self-recognition and certain autoimmune concomitants of aging in vivo. They may also help to explain impaired wound healing and increased predisposition to atherothrombosis in aging and diabetic individuals. This system of cultured human fibroblasts should serve as an excellent model to investigate the cellular and molecular basis of diabetes mellitus, aging and related pathology.—GOLDSTEIN, S., S. NIEWIAROWSKI AND D. P. SINGAL. Pathological implications of cell aging in vitro. *Federation Proc.* 34: 56–63, 1975.

[1] From Session III, *Finite versus infinite proliferative and functional capacities of cells*, of the FASEB Conference on *Biology of Development and Aging*, presented at the 58th Annual Meeting of the Federation of American Societies for Experimental Biology, Atlantic City, N. J., April 10, 1974.

[2] Supported by grants from the Medical Research Council of Canada, the Canadian Diabetic Association Foundation Fund, and Hoechst Pharmaceuticals Limited of Canada and the U.S. during the tenure of a Medical Research Council Scholarship (S.G.).

Abbreviation: MPD = mean population doublings.

While the finite replicative life-span of diploid human fibroblasts has been well documented for hundreds of cell strains in several laboratories (20, 21, 27, 34, 56), the molecular basis of this phenomenon remains obscure. The present status of inquiry indicates that as cells approach the end of their replicative life-span, they accumulate an increasing proportion of abnormal gene products (28, 31). Thus, the heat-labile fraction of glucose-6-phosphate dehydrogenase and 6-phosphogluconate dehydrogenase, two enzymes involved in carbohydrate metabolism, increases in late-passage fibroblasts (28). It has also been shown for a third enzyme of carbohydrate metabolism, lactate dehydrogenase (31), that while the amount of enzyme reactive with specific antiserum remains unchanged during aging in vitro, its specific activity is decreased. More recently, we have demonstrated that hypoxanthine-guanine phosphoribosyltransferase, an enzyme involved in purine metabolism, develops an increasingly heat-labile fraction during serial culture (S. Goldstein and E. J. Moerman, in preparation). Furthermore, the proportion of heat-labile glucose-6-phosphate dehydrogenase, 6-phosphogluconate dehydrogenase and hypoxanthine-guanine phosphoribosyltransferase is greater in extent in fibroblasts derived from subjects with two syndromes of premature aging, progeria and Werner's syndrome (Goldstein and Moerman, in preparation). Additionally, while the HL-A system of surface antigens may undergo subtle alterations during aging of normal cells in vitro (see below), there is clearly altered expression in progeria (54) and Werner's syndrome (23a). In total, these data suggest that conformational changes occur in a variety of proteins during cellular aging, perhaps on the basis of the missense incorporation of amino acids (28, 31). It is noteworthy that these proteins include intracellular enzymes catalyzing diverse metabolic reactions and the surface membrane-related HL-A antigens, which are coded at assorted autosomal and X-linked genetic loci.

In the present report we will attempt to correlate cell aging in vitro with three pathological concomitants of aging in vivo. First, we will develop the concept that impaired growth capacity of cultured cells is frequently associated with the propensity to develop diabetes mellitus. Second, the expression of HL-A antigens in cultured fibroblasts will be discussed vis-à-vis the possibility of age-dependent immunopathology. Last, we will present data on the interaction of cultured fibroblasts with polymerizing fibrin and discuss how disturbances in these processes may relate simultaneously to diminished wound healing and the increased tendency to atherothrombosis seen in aging populations.

CELLULAR AGING AND DIABETES MELLITUS

Hayflick first reported (27) that the replicative life-span of cultured fibroblasts was determined by the chronologic age of the donor. Thus, 13 cultures derived from fetuses of 3–4 months gestation were able to undergo 48 mean population doublings (MPD) (range 35–63) while cells derived from postnatal donors, aged 26–87 years, were only able to undergo 20 MPD (range 14–29) prior to total cessation of growth. However, in these studies the expected inverse correlation between the age of the donor and the MPD prior to phase-out was not seen. It must be emphasized that the genetic identities of these donors were unknown. Moreover, all explant material was obtained after variable intervals post-mortem, introducing the possibility that various degrees of autolysis and other tissue damage could have occurred prior to initiating cultures. Additionally, the majority of adults in this series apparently had protracted cardiopulmonary diseases which may have compromised the viability of the lung tissue used to develop the cultures.

Epidemiologically, a strong positive correlation exists between aging and diabetes mellitus (3). That is, as human populations age, there is a rising prevalence of diabetes, a disease manifest predominantly as an aberration of carbohydrate metabolism, although the other major metabolic areas of lipids and proteins are also adversely affected (47). Therefore, in

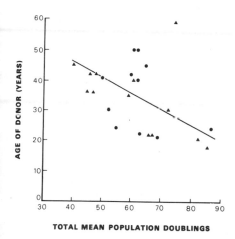

TOTAL MEAN POPULATION DOUBLINGS

Figure 1. Relation between age of donor and mean population doublings achieved prior to cessation of growth. All subcultures were carried out at 1·8 splits counting 3 MPD each time (20, 27, 34). Values include an estimate of 10 MPD occurring within the primary explant before harvest of the first confluent monolayer. Excluding the 60-year-old prediabetic there is an inverse correlation between the age of the donor and the total MPD of cultures ($P < 0.01$). Prediabetic: ▲; Normal: •. Redrawn from ref (20).

an earlier study (20), we explored the possibility that the diabetic genotype had an adverse effect on the life-span of cultured cells. All tissue was obtained from skin of the anterior forearm of living donors and explanted within 1–2 hours. Donors were selected according to stringent criteria and fell into two groups: normals had a negative family history of diabetes mellitus and consistently negative glucose tolerance tests; prediabetics were genetically predisposed to diabetes mellitus because both parents had developed the overt disease, but were not yet affected themselves. In addition, prediabetics were clinically free of other genetic and metabolic diseases to minimize the possibility that secondary endocrine-metabolic phenomena would influence the viability of cultures adversely. Although no significant difference was found between normals and prediabetics (Fig. 1), when data from the two groups were pooled, an inverse correlation was found. In other words the older the donor the fewer MPD occurred in cultured fibroblasts.

Since cell interaction is known to occur within crowded cultures so that hardy cells could assist weaker cells in various ways (20), low density plating experiments were performed (Fig. 2). In these studies prediabetic cultures scored lower than normals at three successive intervals of the in vitro life-span. In addition, the plating efficiency of normal cultures declined as a function of in vitro age while prediabetic cultures plated at a lower level initially. This suggests that prediabetic cultures were prematurely aged within the explant and contained fewer cells capable of growth. Indeed, in a more recent, expanded series of skin cultures from 30 subjects with prediabetes, 26 overt diabetics and 25 normal controls, this notion of premature senescence is supported (21). On monitoring cellular outgrowth from skin fragments starting immediately after explantation, fibroblasts of prediabetic and diabetic donors emerged from explants later, grew more slowly, and with less intensity. Following harvest, they required longer intervals between subculture, and finally, their cumulative MPD were reduced: normals (N) 52.9 ± 2.1 (mean ± SEM); prediabetics (P) 47.7 ± 1.9; diabetics (D) 47.5 ± 2.1, N vs P and D, 0.05 < P < 0.1). In total, these observations indicate that the diabetic genotype decreases the replicative potential of cultured fibroblasts, perhaps as a consequence of premature aging in vivo. Further support for this concept has recently been reported in the laboratory of Vracko and Benditt (62, 63).

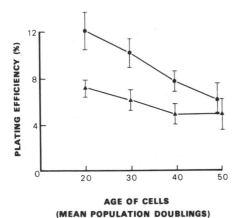

Figure 2. Average plating efficiency of fibroblasts from prediabetic subjects and normal controls during aging in vitro. Cells were removed from mass culture at deciles of MPD and 500 cells were inoculated into each of 4 petri dishes. Cells were refed with fresh medium twice weekly and stained with Giemsa after 2 weeks. Each point represents the mean ± SEM. Experiments were discontinued beyond 50 MPD when several cultures had ceased growth (see Fig. 1). Redrawn from ref (20).

GENETIC HETEROGENEITY IN DIABETES MELLITUS

While the molecular basis of diabetes mellitus is as obscure as that of biological aging, it appears that a number of distinct genetic disorders are frequently associated (Table 1). Indeed, several of these disorders also feature stunting of somatic growth as well as premature aging, especially progeria and Werner's syndrome. It seems clear by our present criteria that diabetes is a disorder of enormous genetic heterogeneity. Moreover, one would predict that more syndromes will be added to the list as further testing is done. Some of these disorders have recently been examined in vitro by looking at the replicative capacity of cultured skin fibroblasts, and the data reveal a decreased replicative capacity compared to normal controls (Table 1). It appears, therefore, that a wide variety of genetic disorders, affecting many metabolic pathways, can simultaneously impair glucose tolerance and the life-span in vivo, as well as the replicative life-span of cultured fibroblasts in vitro (17). The obvious corollary is that any studies which seek to explore the correlation between the age of a given donor and the replicative potential of his fibroblasts must take into account his genetic identity, and especially his predisposition to diabetes. This system should be useful to explore the inheritance and molecular basis of the various forms of diabetes as well as the development of glucose intolerance, insulin resistance, and associated pathology.

EXPRESSION OF HL-A ANTIGENS DURING CELLULAR AGING

Normal mass cultures

While a decreased growth potential during cell aging in vitro may help

TABLE 1. Genetic disorders associated with glucose intolerance and/or insulin resistance

Familial	Familial (Continued)
Alström's syndrome	Optic atrophy and diabetes
Ataxia telangiectasia	Optic atrophy, diabetes insipidus, and
Cockayne's syndrome	diabetes mellitus
Cystic fibrosis	Hereditary relapsing pancreatitis
Friedreich's ataxia	Photomyoclonus, diabetes, deafness,
Glucose-6-phosphate dehydrogenase	nephropathy, and cerebral dysfunction
deficiency	Pineal hyperplasia and diabetes
Type I glycogen storage disease	Acute intermittent porphyria
Gout	Pheochromocytoma
Hemochromatosis	Prader-Willi syndrome
Huntington's disease (36)	Retinitis pigmentosa, neuropathy, ataxia, and
Hutchinson-Gilford (progeria) syndrome	diabetes
(11,16,34,54)	Schmidt's syndrome
Hyperlipemia, diabetes, hypogonadism, and	Werner's syndrome (29,34,57)
short stature syndrome	
Hyperlipoproteinemia III, IV, and V	*Nonfamilial (chromosomal)*
Isolated growth hormone deficiency	
Laurence-Moon-Biedl syndrome	Down's syndrome[a] (51,52)
Lipoatrophic diabetes	Klinefelter's syndrome
Muscular dystrophy	Turner's syndrome
Myotonic dystrophy	
Ocular hypertension induced by	
dexamethasone	

For further details on these disorders see refs (17,35,48). For Huntington's disease see ref (44). Numbers in parentheses refer to published reports of decreased replicative ability in cultured skin fibroblasts.   [a] A small percentage of cases, e.g., balanced translocation, is familial.

to explain certain features of aging in vivo, such as atrophy of tissues and the profound stunting of growth seen in progeria and to a lesser degree in Werner's syndrome, it does not explain some of the other pathology that is frequently present. The HL-A system of histocompatibility of transplantation antigens is found on the surface of all nucleated cells and is the major determinant of immune self-recognition (53). It seems clear, therefore, that any alteration of HL-A antigens with age could predispose the organism to aberrations of self-recognition and hence, to certain forms of pathology that could result from autoimmune tissue injury (17, 18, 64, 65). Genetically, the HL-A system is highly polymorphic and represented at two distinct but closely linked loci (53). Expression of these genes is codominant so that individuals who are homozygous at both loci will have a two-antigen phenotype. Those who are heterozygous at both loci will have four antigens, and intermediate combinations will produce a three-antigen phenotype. Although the structure of HL-A antigens is not yet clearly defined it seems probable that these antigens are derived mainly if not entirely from protein (46) with perhaps a small percentage of carbohydrate (33, 49). Most important in the present context is recent evidence suggesting that the carbohydrate portion is not involved in antigenicity, at least under normal conditions (14). In any case, the HL-A phenotype is determined by suitably characterized, monospecific antisera that also serve as a powerful tool to ascertain whether these surface-associated gene products maintain normal expression during aging in vitro.

HL-A phenotypes are determined routinely on freshly prepared circulating lymphocytes by a standard microdroplet cytotoxicity test (38) directing three or more antisera against each known HL-A specificity. Subsequently, studies can be done on cultured fibroblasts from a given individual of known HL-A identity. In general, our findings on cultures from normal individuals have shown (22, 23, 54), as in other studies (7, 8, 37, 50, 59), a complete concordance of HL-A phenotype be-

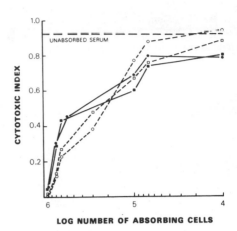

Figure 4. HL-A9 expression in normal mass cultures at early and late passage. Procedure and symbols as in Fig. 3.

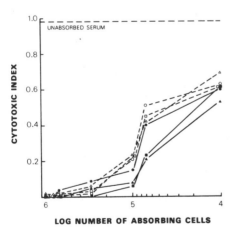

Figure 3. HL-A 2 expression in normal mass cultures at early and late passage by quantitative absorption assay. Early-passage cells were studied 3–5 subcultures after harvesting primary cultures while late-passage cultures were within 1–2 subcultures of termination. D.S.: ▲—▲; J.C.: ●—●; M.S.: ■—■ (all at early passage). Corresponding open symbols and dashed lines: same strains at late passage. The total MPD achieved by each culture were DS: 72; JC: 58; MS: 61.

tween the lymphocytes and cultured fibroblasts of a given donor. In particular, when normal fibroblasts were examined at early passage there is no question about the faithful expression of HL-A antigens. However, as the culture approaches its terminal stages, the cytotoxicity method, which serves only as a screening test, becomes less reliable; cells are devitalized and scoring is done in a background of increasingly dying or dead cells. A more definitive assay is the quantitative absorption technique (30) where fibroblasts are liberated by gentle trypsinization (or a rubber policeman) from the monolayer and suspended in specific antisera for incubation. Antibodies specific to the antigen in question are then absorbed in proportion to the number of antigens expressed so that there are variable degrees of residual cytotoxicity on subsequent testing of the supernatant against appropriate target lymphocytes. In this way, surface antigens can be quantitated and one cell strain can be compared to another

(30, 54, 55). Accordingly, the quantitative expression of HL-A2 in mass cultures of normal fibroblasts, including one strain derived from a 76-year-old normal female (M.S.), may have decreased slightly from early to late passage (Fig. 3). However, this effect was not apparent for HL-A9 (Fig. 4). Our results, therefore, are in general agreement with those of Brautbar et al. (8), who found essentially no change in expression of HL-A antigens during the in vitro life-span of 2 embryonic and 10 adult strains using a virtually identical assay. The different shapes of the curves in Figs. 3 and 4 are worthy of comment and represent a typical day-to-day variation probably related to different batches of antisera, complement and target lymphocytes. Thus, a valid comparison between various cell strains can only be made if they are scored on the same day with identical batches of antiserum, complement and target lymphocytes. While this introduces logistic problems that limit the number of comparisons possible, it underscores the need for cautious evaluation of the exact techniques employed and any data obtained thereby.

Normal clonal cultures

Nevertheless, there appear to be remarkable clonal differences within normal mass cultures (Fig. 5). In the limited sample of four clones examined, two had significantly reduced antigen expression, while the others were similar to the parent mass culture. It is not known whether these results represent quantitative differences between the various cells within the skin dermis that may be the precursor cells of the culture strain, e.g., endothelial, smooth muscle cells, and genuine connective tissue fibroblasts. On the other hand, the variable antigen expression between clones may be a manifestation

of variants that accumulate during cellular aging (22), or alternately, a low frequency of spontaneous variants occurring in cells still capable of vigorous growth (1). In any case, these observations suggest that clonal differences in HL-A expression are obscured by a summation effect in mass cultures, probably because clones with normal antigen expression are selected during growth (22). Studies are now in progress to see whether in several clones isolated at very early passage from a long-lived strain there is sequential alteration of antigen expression as the culture proceeds into senescence.

Progeria cultures

In striking contrast to these relatively subtle events in mass cultures from normal subjects, there was a definite alteration in surface antigens of two

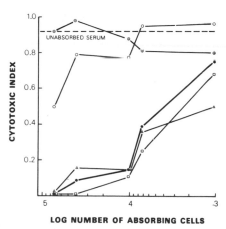

Figure 5. HL-A2 expression in normal mass cultures and 4 subclones of EM. Clones were isolated after low density plating of the mass culture (22) and when grown to requisite numbers were assayed simultaneously (after 40–45 MPD out of a maximum of 52 MPD). Open symbols: 4 clones; closed symbol: parent mass culture.

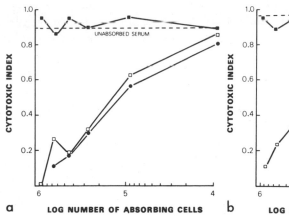
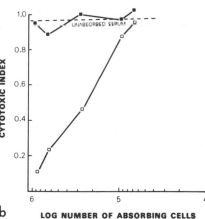

Figure 6. HL-A2 expression in mass cultures of progeria A.K. and normal controls E.M. and J.C. *a*) at early passage and *b*) at late passage. A.K. achieved 46 MPD and controls as before. A.K.: ■ — ■; E.M.: □ — □; J.C.: ● — ●.

progeria strains (Table 2). Thus, we were unable to detect any antigens, albeit by the cytotoxicity test, at early stages of culture, immediately after harvesting the explants and well before the final phaseout of the replicative capacity (54). Indeed, in one culture (A.K.) no antigens could be detected after augmenting the amounts of antiserum and complement five fold, using several additional antisera for all the specificities, and, also, doubling the incubation time (54).

Quantitative absorption studies on A.K. have revealed a variable expres-

TABLE 2. HL-A phenotypes of cells from normal controls and subjects with progeria

Subjects	Age	HL-A phenotype	
		Circulating lymphocytes	Cultured fibroblasts
Normal			
B.G.	17	HL-A3, 7, 17	HL-A3, 7, 17
J.C.	27	HL-A2, 3, 14, W15	HL-A2, 3, 14, W15
T.M.	28	HL-A3, 7, 27	HL-A3, 7, 27
E.M.	30	HL-A2, 9, 5, 7	HL-A2, 9, 5, 7
S.G.	34	HL-A2, 14, W18	HL-A2, 14, W18
D.S.	35	HL-A2, 9, 7, 12	HL-A, 9, 7, 12
M.S.	76	HL-A2, 5, 17	HL-A2, 5, 17
Progeria			
A.K.	9	HL-A2, 9, 14, ±W5	Not detectable
K.H.	14	HL-A11, 28, W15	Not detectable

Assays were performed by standard microdroplet cytotoxicity testing on lymphocytes (38) slightly modified for fibroblasts (22,54).

sion for each antigen. That is, HL-A2 was not detectable at any time in the culture life-span (Fig. 6). In contrast, HL-A9 was somewhat reduced compared to normal control cultures but no significant progression occurred toward terminal stages (Fig. 7). Expression of HL-A14 was also reduced in A.K. fibroblasts at early passage compared to the control (Fig. 8). Because of the possibility that certain substances were masking

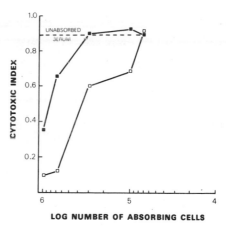

Figure 8. HL-A14 expression in progeria A.K. and normal control S.G. at early passage. S.G. attained a total of 64 MPD. A.K.: ■ — ■; S.G.: □ — □.

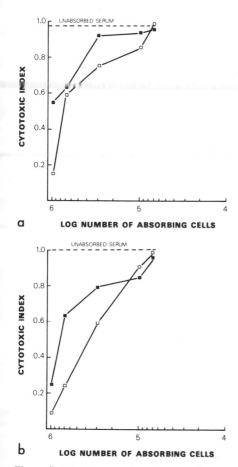

Figure 7. HL-A9 expression in mass cultures of progeria A.K. and normal control E.M. *a*) at early passage and *b*) at late passage. Symbols as in Fig. 6.

the antigens, and thereby interfering with their ability to absorb specific antibody, some cells were first treated with collagenase and neuraminidase to digest putatively masking collagen or excess sialation, respectively. Figure 9 reveals that these treatments did not even partially restore expression of HL-A2. In total, therefore, the variable expression of each of the three HL-A antigens (HL-A2, 9, 14), plus the inability of enzyme pretreatment to increase the reactivity of HL-A2, suggests that cellular aging is associated with a defect in genetic expression. Indeed, similar results are now being found in a culture from a subject with Werner's syndrome (23a), where cultured fibroblasts have a sharply curtailed replicative life-span (29, 34, 57).

However, it is recognized that alternative possibilities exist. Thus, many chemical-masking substances, other than those looked at here, could still be present. Additionally, nothing is known about the topographic distribution of HL-A antigens in normal, progeric or Werner's fibroblasts. Indeed, it is possible that a disturbance of the process normally triggered in lymphocytes after antibody fixation, that of clustering in caps or patches (2, 6, 10, 39) may somehow be restricting antibody binding in aged fibroblasts. Furthermore, the results underscore our relative ignorance about the relation between quantitative antigen expression and complement-mediated cytotoxicity. In the case of HL-A2 in A.K., for example, the drastically reduced expression of antigen readily explains the absence of cytotoxicity. However, in the case of HL-A9 and 14 it appears that a more subtle decrease in antigen expression is able to completely abrogate complement-mediated cell killing.

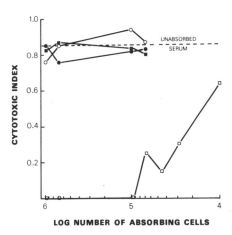

Figure 9. Effect of enzyme pretreatment on HL-A2 expression in progeria A.K. and normal control E.M. Fibroblast suspensions were treated with 50 U/ml of neuraminidase or 100 U/ml of collagenase in CBS buffer (25), or buffer alone for 30 min. Cells were rinsed, recounted and then assayed by quantitative absorption assay. Control cells were pretreated with buffer: □ — □. A.K. plus buffer: ■ — ■; plus neuraminidase ● — ●; plus collagenase: o — o.

INTERACTIONS OF CULTURED FIBROBLASTS WITH FIBRIN

It is now appreciated that the normal processes of tissue repair and hemostasis require extensive interaction between circulating elements, for example, blood platelets and fibrinogen, with fixed tissue cells such as vascular endothelium and connective tissue fibroblasts (4, 41, 43). Previous studies have shown (42) that fibrinogen that is stimulated to undergo polymerization to fibrin can interact with the permanent line of mouse L cells and form a clot. The rationale of our studies, therefore, was first to characterize the interaction with fibrin of human diploid fibroblasts at early passage, and second, to compare senescent fibroblasts and other fibroblasts from disease states known to have increased bleeding or clotting problems (40).

The interaction of fibroblasts with polymerizing fibrin is monitored in an aggregometer wherein light is directed through a cuvette containing a continuously stirred suspension of cells. Fibrin is then added and as interaction occurs, fibroblasts form sedimenting aggregates which clear the turbidity and allow increased light transmission. The interaction was rapid following the addition of polymerizing fibrin to suspensions of early-passage cells from a normal adult (Fig. 10a). Early-passage fibroblasts from a fetus, two normal adult females (one pre- and one postmenopausal) and a boy with Ehlers-Danlos syndrome had similar patterns of interaction. The latter is an inherited disease associated with hyperelastic skin and joints and a severe tendency to bruising, bleeding and impaired wound healing (35). In contrast, late-passage normal fibroblasts had a much slower rate of interaction (Fig. 10b), which was confirmed by finding a smaller amount of [125]I-

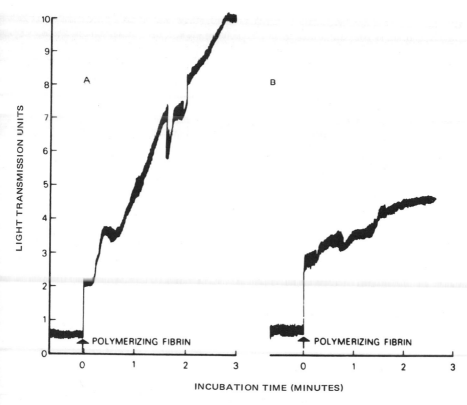

Figure 10. Light transmission in arbitrary units through suspensions of normal fibroblasts (2 × 10⁶ cells/ml) during exposure to polymerizing fibrin *A*) at early passage and *B*) at late passage. Irregularity of curves probably relates to formation of fibrin-fibroblast aggregates which sediment unevenly. Redrawn from ref (40).

fibrin in the cellular sediment (Table 3). Following interaction of the cells and fibrin, a mature gelatinous clot is formed, but after 30–60 min in normal cells at early passage, retraction occurs so that the original volume is reduced by more than 50% (Table 4). Cyclic AMP may be involved in the mediation of retraction because prostaglandin E_1, known to increase cyclic AMP levels in cultured human fibroblasts (19, 32), and dibutyryl-cyclic AMP both inhibited retraction significantly, just as they do in platelet systems (41, 43). Cytochalasin B, which interferes with the function of the cytoskeleton and thus inhibits cytokinesis, cell motility, platelet aggregation and platelet-induced clot retraction, completely inhibited retraction induced by fibroblasts. Retraction also appeared to be energy dependent because it was blocked by the respiratory poison antimycin (not shown); it also depended on cellular integrity because disruption of cells by sonication destroyed the ability to retract fibrin. In any event, late-passage fibroblasts produced markedly less fibrin retraction compared to cells at early passage (Table 4, Fig. 11). Additionally, progeria fibroblasts, with a significant part of the culture life-span still remaining, also promoted less fibrin retraction than early-passage normal fibroblasts (Fig. 11).

In more recent experiments, we have found that both late-passage normal fibroblasts and those from progeria have increased procoagulant activity compared to normal cells at early passage (S. Niewiarowski and S. Goldstein, unpublished observations). That is, these cells have increased amounts of a clot-promoting substance or substances that short-circuit the "intrinsic" clotting mechanism via the "extrinsic" system (66, 67). Normal human fibroblasts also contain potent fibrinolytic activity so that the retracted clot is eventually lysed by one or more proteolytic enzymes (40). Although this activity is inhibited by soy bean trypsin inhibitor (40), it is clearly not related to the trypsin routinely used in tissue culture, because cells harvested with a rubber policeman show the identical activity. It is noteworthy that

TABLE 4. Factors influencing the retraction of fibrin induced by normal human fibroblasts

| Stage of passage | Additive | Fibrin volume,[a] per cent of initial | |
		Mean	SD
Early	None	44.1	± 19.7
Late	None	85.9	± 6.7
Early	PGE$_1$ (10^{-5} M)	94.5	± 8.1
Early	Dibutyryl cylic AMP (10^{-3} M)	84.4	± 5.7
Early	Cytochalasin B (10 μg/ml)	100.0	—

[a] Fibrin volume measured after 120 min incubation at 37 C. All are significantly different from 44.1%, $0.001 < P < 0.005$. Data from ref (40).

mouse L cells are completely devoid of fibrinolytic activity (42), as if during their establishment into a permanent line or during subsequent cultivation, they have lost this capability which persists in the genetically-stable human fibroblast. It will now be of interest to see if procoagulant and fibrinolytic activities are altered during aging of normal cells in vitro, in cultures from subjects with progeria and Werner's syndrome and other disease states associated with a abnormal tendency to atherothrombotic vascular disease.

CONCLUSION

The data suggest that cellular aging is in some way related to the triad of diabetes mellitus, altered expression of HL-A antigens, and reduced interactions with polymerizing fibrin. Indeed, the two latter phenomena may provide insight into the occurrence in many diabetics of insulin insensitivity. HL-A antigens are clearly membrane receptors for the immune system (10, 53, 65), while fibrin interaction probably requires

TABLE 3. Interaction of normal human fibroblasts with polymerizing fibrin

| Stage of passage | ^{125}I associated with cells (% of total) | |
	Mean	SD
Early	31.4	± 7.6
Late	14.9	± 11.5

The interaction of cells (from a young adult male) with polymerizing fibrin prepared from ^{125}I-fibrinogen is expressed as the percentage of the total radioactivity associated with the cell sediment. This is calculated by subtracting the percentage of radioactivity found in the sediment of the control solution (containing no cells) from the percentage of radioactivity found in the cellular sediment. Early versus late $0.001 < P < 0.005$. Data from ref (40).

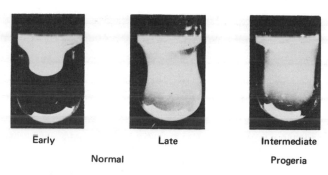

Early   Late   Intermediate

Normal   Progeria

Figure 11. Fibrin retraction induced by cells 2 hours after incubation at 37 C. Progeria fibroblasts A.K. were halfway through their replicative life-span. The opaque fibrin clot (white zone) originally occupied entire volume from meniscus to bottom of test tube which shows light reflection.

its own surface receptors (11, 13) or one for thrombin, a critical enzyme in the clotting mechanism (13). Thus, it may be that the surface receptor for insulin (15) undergoes alteration in its genetic expression during cellular aging and will prove to be the underlying factor in certain forms of insulin resistance, particularly as found in maturity-onset diabetes (2) and in progeria (61) and Werner's syndrome (12).

The cardinal pathological feature of progeria and Werner's syndrome, and indeed of diabetes mellitus generally, is the predisposition to severe and accelerated atherothrombotic disease in large blood vessels (5, 12, 26, 45). It is of great interest that individuals who receive kidney and heart transplants with imperfect histocompatibility and then survive for several months without acute rejection are found to have severe atherosclerosis of the renal and coronary arteries (24, 58), apparently autoimmune in nature (58). We speculate, therefore, that an immune component may be operating along a clonal or patchy distribution during normal cellular aging (17, 18, 22, 60, 64, 65). In this way, immune damage to cells lining the arterial wall could increase cell turnover, accelerate cellular aging (23), and hasten the development of atherosclerosis. This process would be a more universal phenomenon in the vascular tree of individuals with progeria and Werner's syndrome, with perhaps various intermediate degrees of severity in more common forms of diabetes mellitus (17, 60). Clearly an explanation will still be needed for the accumulation of lipids like cholesterol ester in atheromatous foci, but recent studies suggest (9) that a tissue culture approach will be helpful. This system of cultured human fibroblasts holds great promise in exploring the fundamental nature of aging and age-dependent pathology.

REFERENCES

1. ADMAN, R., AND D. A. PIOUS. Isoantigenic variants: isolation from human diploid cells in culture. *Science* 168: 370, 1970.
2. AMOS, D. B., I. COHEN AND W. J. KLEIN. Mechanisms of immunologic enhancement. *Transplantation Proc.* 2: 68, 1970.
3. ANDRES, R., T. POZEFSKY, S. SWERDLOFF, et al. Effect of aging on carbo-

hydrate metabolism, early diabetes. In: *Advances in Metabolic Disorders*, Suppl. 1, edited by R. A. Camerini-Davalos and H. S. Cole. New York: Academic, 1970, p. 349.

4. ASTRUP, T. Blood coagulation and fibrinolysis in tissue culture and tissue repair. *Biochem. Pharmacol.* Suppl. 241, 1968.

5. ATKINS, L. Progeria: report of a case with post-mortem findings. *New Engl. J. Med.* 250: 1065, 1954.

6. BERNOCO, D., S. CULLEN, G. SCUDELLER, G. TRINCHIERI AND R. CEPPELLINI. HL-A molecules at the cell surface. In: *Histocompatibility Testing*, edited by J. Dausset and J. Colombani. Copenhagen: Munksgaard, 1972, p. 527.

7. BRAUTBAR, C., R. PAYNE AND L. HAYFLICK. Fate of HL-A antigens in aging cultured human diploid cell strains. *Exptl. Cell Res.* 75: 31, 1972.

8. BRAUTBAR, C., M. A. PELLEGRINO, S. FERRONE, R. A. REISFELD, R. PAYNE AND L. HAYFLICK. Fate of HL-A antigens in aging cultured human diploid cell strains. *Exptl. Cell Res.* 78: 367, 1973.

9. COOPER, J. T., AND S. GOLDSTEIN. De novo synthesis of lipids and incorporation of oleic acid into cultured human fibroblasts from diabetics and normals. *Atherosclerosis* 20: 41, 1974.

10. CULLEN, S. E., D. BERNOCO, A. O. CARBONARA, H. JAEOT-GUILLARMOD, G. TRINCHIERI AND R. CEPPELLINI. Fate of HL-A antigens and antibodies at the lymphocyte surface. *Transplantation Proc.* 5: 1835, 1973.

11. DANES, B. S. Progeria: a cell culture study on aging. *J. Clin. Intest.* 50: 2000, 1971.

12. EPSTEIN, C. J., G. M. MARTIN, A. S. SCHULTZ AND A. G. MOTULSKY. Werner's syndrome. A review of its symptomatology, natural history, pathology features, genetics and relationship to the aging process. *Medicine* 45: 177, 1966.

13. GANGULY, P. Binding of thrombin to human platelets. *Nature* 247: 306, 1974.

14. GAULDIE, J., S. C. BHANDARI AND D. P. SINGAL. Non-involvement of carbohydrate in the HL-A antigenic site. *Federation Proc.* 33: 719, 1974.

15. GAVIN, J. R., JR., J. ROTH, D. M. NEVILLE, JR., P. DE MEYTS AND D. N. BUELL. Insulin-dependent regulation of insulin receptors concentrations: a direct demonstration in cell culture. *Proc. Natl. Acad. Sci. U.S.* 71: 84, 1974.

16. GOLDSTEIN, S. Lifespan of cultured cells in progeria. *Lancet* 1: 424, 1969.

17. GOLDSTEIN, S. On the pathogenesis of diabetes mellitus and its relationship to biological aging. *Humangenetik* 12: 83, 1971.

18. GOLDSTEIN, S. The biology of aging. *New Engl. J. Med.* 285: 1120, 1971.

19. GOLDSTEIN, S., AND R. HASLAM. Cyclic AMP levels in young and senescent fibroblasts: effects of epinephrine and prostaglandin E_1. *J. Clin. Invest.* 52: 35a, 1973.

20. GOLDSTEIN, S., J. W. LITTLEFIELD AND J. S. SOELDNER. Diabetes mellitus and aging: diminished plating efficiency of cultured human fibroblasts. *Proc. Natl. Acad. Sci. U.S.* 64: 155, 1969.

21. GOLDSTEIN, S., E. J. MOERMAN, J. S. SOELDNER, R. E. GLEASON AND D. M. BARNETT. Diabetes mellitus and prediabetes: decreased replicative capacity of cultured fibroblasts. J. Clin. Invest. 53: 27a, 1974.

22. GOLDSTEIN, S., AND D. P. SINGAL. Loss of reactivity of HL-A antigens in clonal populations of cultured human fibroblasts during aging in vitro. *Exptl. Cell Res.* 75: 278, 1972.

23. GOLDSTEIN, S., AND D. P. SINGAL. Senescence of cultured human fibroblasts: mitotic versus metabolic time. *Exptl. Cell Res.* In press.

23a GOLDSTEIN, S., AND D. P. SINGAL. Alteration of fibroblast gene products in vitro from a subject with Werner's syndrome. *Nature* in press.

24. GRAHAM, A. F., J. S. SCHROEDER, R. B. GRIEPP, E. B. STINSON AND D. C. HARRISON. Does cardiac transplantation significantly prolong life and improve its quality? *Circulation* 48: Suppl. III, 116, 1973.

25. GROTHAUS, E. A., M. W. FLYE, E. YUNIS AND D. B. AMOS. Human lymphocyte antigen reactivity modified by neuraminidase. *Science* 173: 542, 1971.

26. HAIMOVICI, H. Peripheral arterial disease in diabetes mellitus. In: *Diabetes Mellitus: Theory and Practice*, edited by M. Ellenberg and H. Rifkin. New York: McGraw-Hill, 1970.

27. HAYFLICK, L. The limited in vitro lifetime of human diploid cell strains. *Exptl. Cell Res.* 37: 614, 1965.

28. HOLLIDAY, R., AND G. M. TARRANT. Altered enzymes in aging human fibroblasts. *Nature* 238: 26, 1972.

29. HOLLIDAY, R., J. S. PORTERFIELD AND D. D. GIBBS. Werner's syndrome: premature aging in vivo and in vitro. 248: 762, 1974.

30. KLEIN, G., S. FRIBERG, JR. AND H. HARRIS. Two kinds of antigen suppression in tumor cells revealed by cell fusion. *J. Exptl. Med.* 135: 839, 1972.

31. LEWIS, C. M., AND G. M. TARRANT. Error theory and ageing in human diploid fibroblasts. *Nature* 239: 316, 1972.

32. MANGANIELLO, V., J. BRESLOW AND M. VAUGHAN. An effect of dexamethasone on the cyclic AMP content of human fibroblasts stimulated by catecholamines and prostaglandin E_1. *J. Clin. Invest.* 51: 60a, 1972.

33. MANN, D. L., G. N. ROGENTINE, J. L. FAHEY AND S. G. NATHENSON. Solubilization of human leukocyte membrane isoantigens. *Nature* 217: 1180, 1968.

34. MARTIN, G. M., C. A. SPRAGUE AND C. J. EPSTEIN. Replicative lifespan of cultivated human cells. Effects of donor's age, tissue, and genotype. *Lab. Invest.* 23: 86, 1970.

35. MCKUSICK, V. A. *Mendelian Inheritance in Man.* Baltimore: Johns Hopkins Press, 1968.

36. MENKES, J. H., AND N. STEIN. Fibroblast cultures in Huntington's disease. *New Engl. J. Med.* 288: 856, 1973.

37. MIGGIANO, V. C., M. NABHOLZ AND W. F. BODMER. Detection of HL-A and other antigens on fibroblast micro monolayers using a fluorochromatic cytotoxicity assay. In: *Histocompatibility Testing*, edited by P. I. Terasaki. Copenhagen: Munksgaard. 1970, p. 623.

38. MITTAL, K. K., M. R. MICKEY, D. P. SINGAL AND P. I. TERASAKI. Serotyping for homotransplantation XVIII. Refinement of microdroplet lymphocyte cytotoxicity test. *Transplantation* 6: 913, 1968.

39. MIYAJIMA, T., A. A. HIRATA AND P. I. TERASAKI. Escape from sensitization to HL-A antibodies. *Tissue Antigens* 2: 64, 1972.

40. NIEWIAROWSKI, S., AND S. GOLDSTEIN. Interaction of cultured human fibroblasts with fibrin: modification by drugs and aging in vitro. *J. Lab. Clin. Med.* 82: 605, 1973.

41. NIEWIAROWSKI, S., E. REGOECZI AND J. F. MUSTARD. Platelet interaction with fibrinogen and fibrin: comparison of the interaction of platelets with that of fibroblasts, leukocytes, and erythrocytes. *Ann. N.Y. Acad. Sci.* 201: 72, 1972.

42. NIEWIAROWSKI, S., E. REGOECZI AND J. F. MUSTARD. Adhesion of fibroblasts to polymerizing fibrin and retraction of fibrin induced by fibroblasts. *Proc. Soc. Exptl. Biol. Med.* 140; 199, 1972.

43. NIEWIAROWSKI, S., E. REGOECZI, G. J. STEWART et al. Platelet interaction with polymerizing fibrin. *J. Clin. Invest.* 51: 685, 1972.

44. PODOLSKY, S., N. A. LEOPOLD AND D. S. SAX. Increased frequency of diabetes mellitus in patients with Huntington's chorea *Lancet* 1, 1356, 1972.

45. REICHEL, W., AND R. GARCIA-BUNUEL. Pathologic findings in progeria: myocardial fibrosis and lipofuscin pigment. *Am. J. Clin. Pathol.* 53: 243, 1970.

46. REISFELD, R. A., M. A. PELLEGRINO, S. FERRONE AND B. D. KAHAU. Chemical and molecular nature of HL-A antigens. *Transplantation Proc.* 5: 447, 1973.

47. RENOLD, A. D., W. STAUFFACHER AND G. F. CAHILL. Diabetes mellitus. In: *The Metabolic Basis of Inherited Disease*, edited by J. B. Stanbury, J. B. Wyngaarden and D. S. Fredrickson. New York: McGraw-Hill, 1972, p. 83.

48. RIMOIN, D. L., AND N. SCHIMKE. *Genetic Disorders of the Endocrine Glands.* St. Louis: Mosby, 1971, p. 163.

49. SANDERSON, A. R. HL-A substances from human spleens. *Nature* 220: 192, 1968.

50. SASPORTES, M., C. DEHAY AND M. FELLOUS. Variations of the expression of HL-A antigens on human diploid fibroblasts in vitro. *Nature* 233: 332, 1971.

51. SCHNEIDER, E. L., AND C. J. EPSTEIN. Replication rate and lifespan of cultured fibroblasts in Down's syndrome. *Proc. Soc. Exptl. Biol. Med.* 141: 1092, 1972.

52. SEGAL, D. J., AND E. E. MCCOY. Studies on Down's syndrome in tissue culture. I. Growth rate and protein contents of fibroblast cultures. *J. Cellular Physiol.* 83: 85, 1974.

53. SINGAL, D. P. Tissue typing and organ transplantation. *Can. J. Surg.* 15: 295, 1972.

54. SINGAL, D. P., AND S. GOLDSTEIN. Absence of detectable HL-A antigens on cultured fibroblasts in progeria. *J. Clin. Invest.* 52: 2259, 1973.

55. SINGAL, D. P., V. R. VILLANUEVA AND N. NAIPAUL. Effect of phytohemagglutinin on expression of human histocompatibility antigens. *J. Immunol.* 112: 852, 1974.

56. SWIM, H. E., AND R. F. PARKER. Culture characteristics of human fibroblasts propagated serially. *Am. J. Hyg.* 66: 235, 1957.

57. TAO, L. C., E. STECKER AND H. A. GARDNER. Werner's syndrome and acute myeloid leukemia. *Can. Med. Assoc. J.* 105: 951, 1971.

58. TAYLOR, H. E. Pathology of organ transplantation in man. *Pathology Annual* 7: 1973, 1972.

59. THORSBY, E., AND S. LIE. Antigens on human fibroblasts demonstrated with HL-A antisera and anti-human lymphocytic sera. *Vox Sanguinis* 15: 44, 1968.

60. UNGAR, B., A. E. STOCKS, F. I. R. MARTIN, S. WHITTINGHAM AND I. R. MACKAY. Intrinsic factor antibody, parietal-cell antibody, and latent pernicious anemia in diabetes mellitus. *Lancet* 2: 415, 1968.

61. VILLEE, D. B., G. NICHOLS, JR. AND N. B. TALBOT. Metabolic studies in two boys with classical progeria. *Pediatrics* 43: 207, 1969.

62. VRACKO, R. Basal lamina layering in diabetes mellitus. Evidence for accelerated rate of cell death and cell regeneration. *Diabetes* 23: 94, 1974.

63. VRACKO, R., AND E. P. BENDITT. Replicative life-span of diabetic fibroblasts. *Federation Proc.* 33: 607, 1974.

64. WALFORD, R. L. *The Immunologic Theory of Aging.* Copenhagen: Munksgaard, 1969.

65. WALFORD, R. L. Immunologic theory of aging: current status. *Federation Proc.* 33: 2020, 1974.

66. ZACHARKSI, L. R., AND O. R. McINTYRE Membrane-mediated synthesis of tissue factor (thromboplastin in cultured fibroblasts. *Blood* 41: 679, 1973.

67. ZACHARSKI, L. R., AND O. R. McINTYRE Tisue factor (thromboplastin, Factor-III) synthesis by cultured cells. *J. Med. Exptl. Clin.* 4: 118, 1973.

Unlimited division potential of precancerous mouse mammary cells after spontaneous or carcinogen-induced transformation[1,2]

C. W. DANIEL, B. D. AIDELLS
D. MEDINA[3] AND L. J. FAULKIN, JR.[4]
*Division of Natural Sciences, University of California
Santa Cruz, California 95064*

ABSTRACT

Serial transplantation of normal mouse mammary gland in young, isogenic hosts results in progressive loss of division potential, and the transplant line is eventually lost. This is interpreted as an expression of senescence at the cell and tissue level, and it inevitably occurs even though experimental conditions for growth are judged to be optimal. An indefinite extension of mammary growth span can be accomplished by transformation of these normal cells into precancerous cell types, which grow as a benign tissue but which may, however, occasionally undergo a second transformation into a malignant carcinoma. All precancerous tissues tested displayed unlimited growth potential, regardless of whether they occurred spontaneously, or were induced by oncogenic viruses or by administration of chemical carcinogens. Precancerous tissues of both ductal and lobuloalveolar morphology grew continuously. These results indicate that release from cell aging, as measured by the acquisition of unlimited growth potential, is associated with the precancerous state per se, and occurs as an early event in the transition from normal to malignant mammary cells.— DANIEL, C. W., B. D. AIDELLS, D. MEDINA AND L. J. FAULKIN, JR. Unlimited division potential of precancerous mouse mammary cells after spontaneous or carcinogen-induced transformation. *Federation Proc.* 34: 64–67, 1975.

[1] From Session III, *Finite versus infinite proliferative and functional capacities of cells*, of the FASEB Conference on *Biology of Development and Aging*, presented at the 58th Annual Meeting of the Federation of American Societies for Experimental Biology, Atlantic City, N. J., April 10, 1974.

[2] These investigations were supported by Public Health Service Grants HD 04164 from the National Institute of Child Health and Human Development, and by CA 11944 from the National Cancer Institute.

[3] Address: Baylor College of Medicine, Department of Anatomy, Houston, TX 77025.

[4] Address: Department of Anatomy, University of California, Davis, CA 95616.

Abbreviation: MTV = mouse mammary tumor virus; NIV = nodule inducing virus.

123

A striking relationship exists between cellular growth span and neoplasia. Most normal, nontransformed cells display a limited ability to proliferate when serially propagated either in vitro or in vivo (2, 9). This finite proliferative capacity of somatic cells has been demonstrated in many laboratories, and it is widely considered to be an expression of senescence at the cellular level. Although improvements in the conditions of culture or of serial transplantation may slightly extend the growth span, a limit is ultimately reached beyond which proliferation does not occur. In contrast, transformed cells, which generally display either malignant or premalignant characteristics, are able to grow without apparent limit under identical conditions of serial culture or transplantation. This correlation between transformation and unlimited growth potential suggests that common or shared mechanisms may be involved in these apparently different processes, and if so this becomes a matter of potential importance to both aging and to the problem of cancer (9).

The studies reported in this paper were designed to explore this interrelationship with the ultimate aim of discovering whether the apparently obligatory coincidence of neoplasia and infinite growth is causal or merely casual. More particularly, we have been concerned with the growth potential of precancerous cell types— intermediate cells that do not display malignant growth habits, but which may develop into frankly malignant cells.

FINITE GROWTH SPAN OF NORMAL CELLS IN VIVO

In vivo experiments that measure division potential require the repeated transfer of cells or tissues between animals in such a manner that at each passage conditions are optimal for survival, growth, and function. The number of suitable transplant systems is limited, due principally to difficulties in the identification of transplanted cells. An example is found in a series of very long-term experiments in which Krohn (10, 11) studied the life-span of mouse skin by serially grafting small explants. These grafts could be carried for long periods, with the oldest surviving for 10.25 years—far longer than the life-span of the laboratory mouse (Krohn, unpublished data). The grafts became smaller and more difficult to transplant with each passage, however, and a finite life-span for skin is indicated. A difficulty in interpreting these results arises because of the possibility that grafts were invaded with host cells, making it difficult to accurately determine the true age of the graft.

The problem of identification of transplanted cells was avoided by passaging hemopoietic cells in mice that had been heavily irradiated. The ability of transplanted cells to repopulate hosts declined markedly during serial passage, and the ability of transplants to promote survival of the hosts similarly declined (17, 18). Harrison avoided the necessity of irradiation by transplanting hemopoietic cells into genetically anemic mice, and found that although mice could be cured by receiving cells that had been functioning for 73 months and four transplant generations, nevertheless there was a trend for cell proliferation, as measured in colony-forming units, to decline with successive transplants. Although these experiments are still in progress, this suggests that these cell lines may not be maintained for an indefinite period (8).

Many of the difficulties associated with the design and interpretation of serial transplant experiments are avoided with the mouse mammary transplant system. In order to perform transplants, host mice 3 weeks of age are prepared to receive implants by surgically excising the small mammary rudiment from each inguinal (no. 4) mammary fat pad. This simple operation prevents host mammary tissue from populating the fatty stroma, and provides in each host two mammary-gland-free fat pads (5). These are a natural site for the transplantation of mammary cells and there is no possibility of confusing transplants with host material. Primary implants characteristically grow to fill the available fat in 2–3 months, when tissue can again be removed for subsequent transplantation (Fig. 1). By maintaining a constant transplant interval, any decline in the proliferative capacity of mammary cells can be identified and expressed in terms of the mean percent fat pad filled at each passage.

Serial transplantation of normal mammary tissues produces a progressive loss of proliferative capacity (3), with the result that older transplants are unable to fill more than a portion of the available fat during the usual transplant interval of 2–3 mo (Fig. 2). This decline in growth rate is approximately linear, and it is estimated that approximately 15% of the primary implant's proliferative potential is lost at each transplant generation (Fig. 3). It has also been shown that this reduction in viability is a result of the number of cell divisions undergone, and cannot be ascribed to the passage of chronological or metabolic time (4). This loss of division potential appears to be an inevitable consequence of serial propagation, and occurs even when careful selection is made for the most vigorously growing line, and when all conditions for growth are judged to be optimal.

SERIAL TRANSPLANTATION OF MAMMARY NODULES

The best studied example of precancerous transformation is found in the mouse mammary tumor system. These preneoplastic lesions (nodules) appear in the mammary glands of old, multiparous mice of certain strains. Their occurrence is usually associated with infection with the mouse mammary tumor virus (MTV),

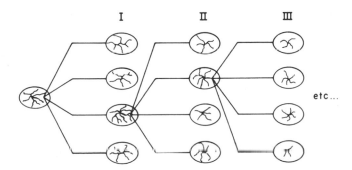

Figure 1. Diagram illustrating serial transplantation of mouse mammary tissues. Primary implants are removed from a single donor gland and transplanted into 10–14 gland-free fat pads, which represent generation I. Subsequent transplants are always taken from the most vigorously growing outgrowth of the preceding generation. Growth rate is expressed as mean percent fat pad filled at each generation.

but they may also be introduced in MTV-free mice by treatment with carcinogenic hydrocarbons (6). Nodules may be distinguished because they retain an alveolar morphology in nonpregnant females. That is, nodules have altered hormonal requirements for maintenance of alveolar cells such that they are maintained under circumstances in which all normal alveoli are regressed, and in which normal mammary tissue exists as a simple network of ducts.

Nodules remain as small, discrete alveolar structures because their growth is completely inhibited by contiguous normal duct tissues (7). If transplanted into gland-free fat pads and removed from the growth-in-hibiting effects of normal gland, however, nodules proliferate and retain their characteristic alveolar morphology. Their growth is limited by the boundaries of the fat pads, as is normal gland, and growth stops when the available fat is occupied.

Like normal mammary tissues, nodules can be serially propagated by repeated transplantation into gland-free fat pads of young, isogenic mice. In a long-term serial transplantation study, the growth spans of normal and preneoplastic mammary tissues were compared (3). Normal gland could be carried for a maximum of 2 years and 8 transplant generations, after which age-associated reduction in growth rate made subsequent propagation impossible.

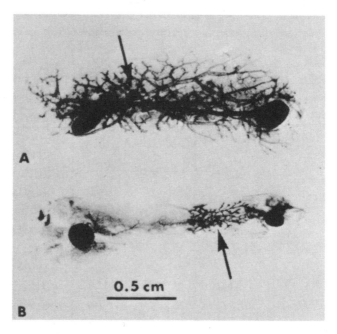

Figure 2. Typical mammary outgrowths arising from serially transplanted mammary tissues, using a transplant interval of 3 mo. Arrows indicate the origin of growth. *A*) Generation I outgrowth which has grown rapidly to fill the available fat. *B*) Generation IV outgrowth which has been propagated for 16 mo. and fills about 25% of the fat pad. Hematoxylin staining. (From Daniel and Young (3).)

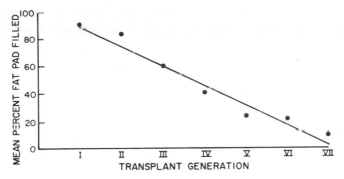

Figure 3. Decline in growth rate of mammary tissue during serial propagation. This plot summarized results of eight transplant lines, and each point represents 80–100 transplants. The regression is approximately linear, and the slope indicates a 15% loss of growth potential at each passage. Line fitted by method of least squares.

In contrast, two MTV-induced nodules grew for longer than 8 years and 30 transplant generations; both lines were proliferating vigorously when the experiment was terminated. These results clearly indicated that unlimited growth potential, in the case of mammary cells, is associated with a preneoplastic transformation.

In these investigations all nodules tested were MTV-induced, and it is known that nodule cells represent a particularly favorable site for virus production. The question arises whether MTV infection and production, rather than other precancerous characteristics of nodule cells, might be responsible for the observed extension of growth span. This was resolved by inducing nodules in mice of the BALB/c/Crgl strain, which is free of both MTV and of the nodule inducing virus, NIV (16). One such line was obtained by administration of 3-methylcholanthrene (for details see ref (6)). The outgrowth line resulting from transplantation of this nodule is characterized by hyperplastic morphology (Fig. 4), which is similar to that of MTV-induced nodule outgrowths. The tissue has

been periodically examined by electron microscopy for the presence of MTV, and has been consistently negative. Its potential for growth, however, appears to be unlimited. The line presently is in its 5th year and 27th serial passage (Fig. 5).

Other nodules were obtained in virus-free mice of the BALB/c strain either by examination of old, retired breeders, or by implanting pituitary isografts (12). In addition, two nodules from the C3Hf/Crgl strain, which lacked MTV but were infected with NIV, were serially transplanted. Details concerning the origin of these tissue lines and evidence for their virus-free nature are available

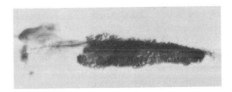

Figure 4. Characteristic dense, lobuloalveolar outgrowth arising from serial transplantation of carcinogen-induced nodule. Transplant generation XXI. Hematoxylin staining. × 3.5.

TABLE 1. Serial transplantation of mouse mammary nodule outgrowth lines

Nodule line	Strain	Virus	Origin	Age of host when HAN noticed, mo[a]	Total time carried, yr	Total generations carried
D1	BALB/c	MTV−, NIV−	retired breeder	18	10	29
D2	BALB/c	MTV−, NIV−	pituitary iso-grafts, 11 mo	18	8.5	26
D2a	BALB/c	MTV−, NIV−	pituitary iso-grafts,11 mo	18	5.5	13
D7	BALB/c	MTV−, NIV−	pituitary iso-grafts, 14 mo	16	5.0	11
D8	BALB/c	M.TV−, NIV−	pituitary iso-grafts, 14 mo	16	3.5	8
F1	C3Hf	MTV−, NIV+	retired breeder	18	4.0	13
F2	C3Hf	MTV−, NIV+	retired breeder	18	3.5	12

(13–15). The data from these experiments are summarized in Table 1, and indicate that in all cases the nodule lines, regardless of source or origin, have a seemingly limitless potential for growth.

GROWTH SPAN OF PRENEO-PLASTIC DUCTS DERIVED FROM HORMONE-DEPENDENT TUMORS

In strain GR mice mammary tumors occur that display properties of hormone dependence. These tumors appear early in pregnancy and grow rapidly until parturition, after which they regress, usually within days. In subsequent pregnancies a tumor arises at the same site, indicating that a small population of preneoplastic cells must persist in the hormonal environment of the nonpregnant mouse. When samples of hormone-dependent tumors were removed from pregnant donors and transplanted into gland-free fat pads of

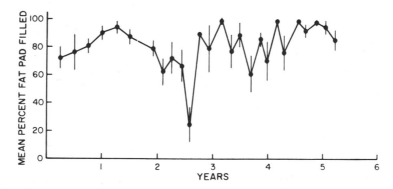

Figure 5. Serial transplantation of outgrowth line 115 originating from a carcinogen-induced nodule in the MTV-free stain BALB/c. Proliferation is vigorous after 5 years of continuous passage. Vertical lines indicate 95% confidence intervals.

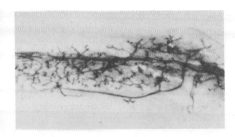

Figure 6. Generation VII outgrowth of pre-cancerous tissue originally derived from a hormone-dependent mammary tumor arising in strain GR mice. The morphology is essentially normal, but its ability to proliferate during serial passage is significantly increased. Hematoxylin staining. × 3.5.

transformed into large, rapidly growing tumors. After parturition the tumor regressed, and residual ducts remained (1).

It was of interest to determine whether this ductal tissue, in spite of its lack of resemblance to nodules, had acquired the ability to grow indefinitely. The results of serial transplantation in nonpregnant hosts are shown in Fig. 7. The outgrowth line was carried for nine transplant generations, and was growing vigorously when it was accidentally lost. Transplants of normal tissue, in contrast, displayed a rapid decay in growth rate and could not be carried beyond generation four.

nonpregnant hosts, outgrowths resulted that were ductal in nature, and in spite of considerable variability, usually resembled normal ducts morphologically (Fig. 6). There was no evidence of hyperplasia in these outgrowths, and in this respect they differed conspicuously from the lobuloalveolar nodules described earlier. The ducts were precursors to neoplasia however, for when the hosts were bred the ductal outgrowths

CONCLUDING REMARKS

In considering the relationship of growth span to neoplasia, it is important to point out that tissue lines derived from either nodules or from hormone-dependent tumors are not themselves tumors. The most important characteristic of malignancy, the continuous and invasive growth of cancer cells in situ, is not a quality of any of the tissue lines. The trans-

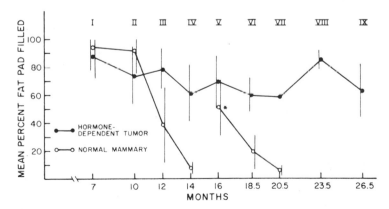

Figure 7. Serial transplantation of hormone-dependent mammary tumor tissue, and normal mammary tissue in virgin hosts. Each point denotes a transplant generation and vertical lines indicate 95% confidence intervals. From Aidells et al. (1). *A second normal mammary tissue line was initiated.

plants grow to fill the available fat, after which normal growth-controlling restraints prevent further cell proliferation; the potential for continued growth can be demonstrated only by transplantation into other gland-free fat pads. Occasionally as the tissues are repeatedly propagated a second transformation occurs, and a carcinoma is found in one of the outgrowths that then proceeds to enlarge at the expense of the host. In several of these lines this is a very rare event however, and the observed phenotype is quite stable.

The studies reviewed and presented here clearly indicate that extended growth spans, perhaps infinitely extended, are associated with transformation from a normal to a precancerous cell type, regardless of the etiologic agents responsible. In these mammary tissues, release from cell aging, as measured by extended division potential, occurs very early on the pathway leading from normality to the frankly cancerous.

REFERENCES

1. AIDELLS, B. D., AND C. W. DANIEL. *J. Natl. Cancer Inst.* 52: 1855, 1974.
2. DANIEL, C. W. *Advan. Gerontol. Res.* 4: 167, 1972.
3. DANIEL, C. W., K. B. DeOME. L. J. T. YOUNG, P. B. BLAIR AND L. J. FAULKIN, JR. *Proc. Natl. Acad. Sci. U.S.* 61: 53, 1968.
4. DANIEL, C. W., AND L. J. T. YOUNG. *Exptl. Cell Res.* 65: 27, 1971.
5. DeOME, K. B., L. J. FAULKIN, JR, H. A. BERN AND P. B. BLAIR. *Cancer Res.* 19: 515, 1959.
6. FAULKIN, L. J., JR. *J. Natl. Cancer Inst.* 36: 289, 1966.
7. FAULKIN, L. J., JR., AND K. B. DeOME. *J. Natl. Cancer Inst.* 24: 953, 1960.
8. HARRISON, D. E. *Proc. Natl. Acad Sci. U.S.* 70: 3184, 1973.
9. HAYFLICK, L. *Exptl. Cell Res.* 37: 614, 1965.
10. KROHN, P. L. *Proc. Roy. Soc. London Ser. B.* 157: 128, 1962.
11. KROHN, P. L. In: *Topics of the Biology of Aging*, edited by P. L. Krohn. New York: Wiley, 1966, p. 125.
12. LOEB, J., AND M. M. KIRTZ. *Am. J. Cancer* 36: 56, 1939.
13. MEDINA, D., AND K. B. DeOME. *J. Natl. Cancer Inst.* 40: 1303, 1968.
14. MEDINA, D., AND K. B. DeOME. *J. Natl. Cancer Inst.* 45: 353, 1970.
15. MEDINA, D., K. B. DeOME, AND D. R. PITELKA. *J. Natl. Cancer Inst.* 46: 1153, 1971.
16. NANDI, S., AND C. M. MCGRATH. *Advan. Cancer Res.* 17: 353, 1973.
17. TILL, J. E., AND E. A. MCCULLOCH. *Radiation Res.* 14: 213, 1961.
18. TILL, J. E., E. A. MCCULLOCH AND L. SIMINOVITCH. *J. Natl. Cancer Inst.* 33: 707, 1964.

Restricted replicative life-span of diabetic fibroblasts in vitro: its relation to microangiopathy[1,2]

RUDOLF VRACKO AND EARL P. BENDITT

Laboratory Service, Veterans Administration Hospital
Seattle, Washington 98108 and
Department of Pathology
University of Washington School of Medicine
Seattle, Washington 98105

ABSTRACT

The finding that diabetic microangiopathy is caused by accumulation of multiple layers of basal lamina and experiments in which similar basal lamina layering is produced when new cell generations repopulate preexisting basal lamina scaffolding (from which previous cell generations have shed) indicate, that the rates of cell death and cell replenishment are accelerated in diabetics. Because the lesions are focal and regional and develop at different ages and in different time sequences, we have proposed that the accelerated cell turnover is probably caused by increased vulnerability of diabetic cells to injury which in turn may represent the expression of a genetically transmitted defect. To test whether this aberration can be detected in vitro, we examined the replicative life-span of skin fibroblasts from three nondiabetics, three age- and sex-matched diabetics and one individual with acquired hyperglycemia due to pancreatitis. Cells of diabetics exhibited about half the number of population doublings as cells from nondiabetics ($0.01 < P < 0.025$). Cells of the individual with pancreatitis generated a normal number of cell doublings. The interpretation that fits best with all data is that decreased replicative life span of diabetic fibroblasts in vitro is also an expression of increased susceptibility of diabetics' cells to injury and dying. — VRACKO, R. AND E. P. BENDITT. Restricted replicative life-span of diabetic fibroblasts in vitro: its relation to microangiopathy. *Federation Proc.* 34: 68–70, 1975.

[1] From Session III, *Finite versus infinite proliferative and functional capacities of cells*, of the FASEB Conference on *Biology of Development and Aging*, presented at the 58th Annual Meeting of the Federation of American Societies for Experimental Biology, Atlantic City, N. J., April 10, 1974.
[2] This study was supported in part by Public Health Service Grants HE-03174 and GM-13543.

131

Microangiopathy, a common and serious manifestation of diabetes mellitus, sets in prior to detectable deficiency of insulin and progresses in spite of careful therapy (4). Capillaries of skeletal muscle, skin, kidney, retina and other organs are involved (7). The typical lesion is caused by excessive deposition of basal lamina[3] as shown in Fig. 1. Characteristically, the basal lamina is not diffusely thickened but the excessive investment is composed of multiple apposing layers (6, 7, 9).

Similar reduplication of basal lamina can be produced in normoglycemic animals by killing cells and letting the injury heal. In these experiments, the newly formed cells repopulate the preexisting basal lamina scaffolds and deposit a new layer of basal lamina in apposition to the old one (8–10). This, and other evidence, suggests a) that accumulation of basal lamina is a quantized phenomenon where each layer of basal lamina represents the residual evidence of one cell generation; and b) that excessive accumulation of basal lamina in diabetics is an indication that cells are dying and are being replenished at an accelerated rate (7, 9, 11).

Because basal lamina accumulation in diabetics is not a uniform process, but occurs regionally and focally within the body (4, 6), we concluded that a pathogenesis of cell death having uniform action such as systemic metabolic, toxic or endocrine events appears unlikely. This, and the fact that microangiopathy and other manifestations of diabetes mellitus appear in diabetics at different ages and in different time sequences (11), fits best with the concept that accelerated turnover is initiated by injurious events that have a greater kill rate among diabetic than nondiabetic cells. This suggests that cells of diabetics are more vulnerable to injury than cells of nondiabetics. Such lowered threshold of diabetic cells for injury could be a manifestation of a genetically-transmitted defect inherent in all cells of the body.

In the search for an expression of this defect in cell culture, we examined the replicative life-span of fibroblasts from three nondiabetics (aged 43, 56 and 69) who had no family history of hyperglycemia and no clinical or postmortem evidence of microangiopathy; from three insulin-dependent diabetics (aged 35, 53 and 68) who had received insulin for 14, 18 and 36 years respectively and had family histories of diabetes mellitus and morphologic evidence of microangiopathy; and from a 49-year-old alcoholic who was on insulin for 12 years following an episode of pancreatitis, who had no family history of diabetes mellitus and who, at time of death, had no evidence of microangiopathy. The methods used were essentially those of Martin et al. (3), except that cells were harvested and counted at weekly intervals.

The data are shown in Fig. 2. The slopes of the regression lines for the controls (−0.33) and diabetics (−0.29) are similar. The regression line for controls is also similar in slope and elevation to that reported originally by Martin et al. (3). The intercepts on the cell-doubling axis are clearly different, the diabetic value (33 doublings) being about two-thirds that of the nondiabetic value (52 doublings). The difference between the two when tested by analysis of covariance (5) is statistically significant ($0.01 < P < 0.025$).[4]

---

[3] The term basal lamina is used synonymously with basement membrane and basement lamina.

[4] Data from Martin et al. (3) and from the patient with hyperglycemia due to pancreatitis were excluded from calculations of the regression lines and analysis of covariance.

The finite characteristic of the replicative life-span of cells in vitro has been interpreted as expression of cell senescence (2). Its inverse relationship to donor age (3) suggests that it is an expression of events that took place in vivo. Since the in vivo rate of cell replenishment in an adult organism is determined by the rate at which cells are dying, a decreased replicative life-span in vitro, as found with diabetic cells, suggests one of three possibilities: *a*) cell senescence is accelerated; *b*) cells are exposed to increased intensity and/or frequency of cell injury; or *c*) cells are unusually susceptible to ordinary levels of injury.

Acceleration of cell senescence by inappropriately set clock mechanism appears to be an unlikely explanation for the decreased in vitro life-span of diabetic cells because reduplication of basal lamina, which we interpret as an expression of accelerated cell turn-over rate in vivo, is not a generalized phenomenon, but occurs in focal and regional distribution.

The second possibility, that diabetics' cells are exposed to increased intensity and/or frequency of injury, also seems unlikely; insulin deficiency

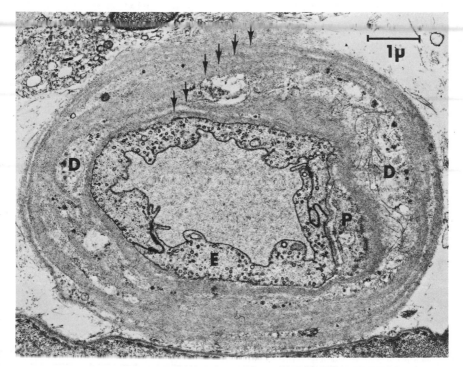

Figure 1. Cross-section of a skeletal muscle capillary from a 70-year-old diabetic who was receiving insulin for 13 years. Although some reduplication of basal lamina normally occurs with advancing age, the capillaries of this individual were surrounded by unusually large number of basal lamina layers (arrows). The layers are frequently separated by cell debris (D), and between endothelial cells (E) and pericytes (P) a single layer of basal lamina is usually present. This suggests that reduplication of basal lamina is not caused by periodic "turning on and off" of basal lamina production.

and associated metabolic aberrations are not the primary injurious events as documented by the following observations: *a*) fibroblasts from prediabetics already exhibit a defect in vitro (1); *b*) excessive accumulation of basal lamina becomes evident in prediabetics (4); *c*) hyperglycemia due to loss of pancreas or hyperfunction of other endocrine organs is not associated with diabetic microangiopathy (4); and *d*) fibroblasts from an individual with acquired insulin deficiency and hyperglycemia from pancreatic destruction 12 years previously show a normal replicative life-span.

The possibility that cells of patients with diabetes mellitus are excessively vulnerable to injury and death appears to best explain all manifestations of diabetes mellitus. According to this concept, any one of a variety of injurious events or insults that normally affect cells, kill a larger number of cells in diabetics than in nondiabetics. Cell loss is

followed by cell replenishment, as in normal circumstances, except that in diabetics, in a given time interval, a larger number of cell divisions is required to maintain the integrity of tissues. The accelerated rate of cell death and cell replenishment in diabetics brings on prematurely and with greater severity certain manifestations that are normally seen as "degenerative" changes associated with aging. Whether diabetic cells are multiplying at faster rates than normal in culture is not yet known. The decreased plating efficiency that occurs even with cells of prediabetics (1) could be the evidence that increased susceptibility of diabetic cells can also be elicited by trauma of culture.

REFERENCES

1. GOLDSTEIN, S., J. W. LITTLEFIELD AND J. S. SOELDNER. Diabetes mellitus and aging: diminished plating efficiency of cultured human fibroblasts. *Proc. Natl. Acad. Sci. U.S.* 64: 155, 1969.
2. HAYFLICK, L. The limited in vitro lifetime of human diploid cell strains. *Exptl. Cell Res.* 37: 614, 1965.
3. MARTIN, G. M., C. A. SPRAGUE AND C. J. EPSTEIN. Replicative life span of cultivated human cells: effects of donor's age, tissue, and genotype. *Lab. Invest* 23: 86, 1970.
4. SIPERSTEIN, M. D., R. H. UNGER AND L. L. MADISON. Studies of muscle capillary basement membrane in normal subjects, diabetic and prediabetic patients. *J. Clin. Invest.* 47: 1973, 1968.
5. SNEDECOR, G. W., AND W. G. COCHRAN. *Statistical Methods,* Sixth ed. Ames, Iowa: Iowa State Univ. Press, 1967.
6. VRACKO, R. Skeletal muscle capillaries in diabetics: quantitative analysis. *Circulation* 41: 271, 1970.
7. VRACKO, R. Basal lamina layering in diabetes mellitus: evidence for accelerated rate of cell death and cell regeneration. *Diabetes* 23: 94, 1974.
8. VRACKO, R. Basal lamina scaffold: anatomy and significance for maintenance of orderly tissue structure. *Am. J. Path.* 77: 314–346, 1974.

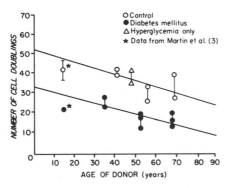

Figure 2. Cumulative number of fibroblast doublings is plotted as function of donor age (each point represents one determination; results from the same donor are connected by a vertical line). Also shown (but not used for calculation of regression lines and analysis of covariance) are the data for a diabetic and four age-matched nondiabetics (mean ± SD) reported by Martin et al. (3).

9. VRACKO, R., AND E. P. BENDITT. Capillary basal lamina thickening: its relationship to endothelial cell death and replacement. *J. Cell Biol.* 47: 281, 1970.

10. VRACKO, R., AND E. P. BENDITT. Basal lamina: the scaffold for orderly cell replacement. *J. Cell Biol.* 55: 496, 1972.

11. VRACKO, R., AND E. P. BENDITT. Manifestations of diabetes mellitus: their possible relationships to an underlying cell defect. *Am. J. Path.* 75: 270, 1974.

Hayflick's hypothesis:
an approach to in vivo testing[1,2]

U. REINCKE, H. BURLINGTON

E. P. CRONKITE AND J. LAISSUE

Medical Research Center, Brookhaven National Laboratory
Upton, Long Island, New York 11973 and
Mount Sinai School of Medicine
City University of New York, New York 10029

ABSTRACT

The experimental evidence relating to the hypothesis of finite cellular life is reviewed. It is emphasized that even if somatic cell production were limited its total potential would have to be vast to provide for extensive cellular regeneration. The actual limit of reproductive cell life would therefore not likely be reached in a normal life-span. It is proposed to test the hypothesis by deliberate exhaustion of stem-cell reserve, and iron-55 cytocide is described as an experimental system that might be applicable.—REINCKE, U., H. BURLINGTON, E. P. CRONKITE AND J. LAISSUE. Hayflick's hypothesis: an approach to in vivo testing. *Federation Proc.* 34: 71–75, 1975.

We will review the existing evidence regarding Hayflick's hypothesis in the light of a theoretical model based on predictable features of stem cells with finite reproductive life, and will then proceed to describe results of our own experiments.

The hypothesis of finite reproductive cell life predicts that the zygote has a restricted capacity to generate somatic cells and that cellular renewal is not unlimited. If true, one profound implication would be a possible life-shortening effect of medical treatment utilizing cytotoxic agents.

Assuming that evolutionary safeguards have developed to protect a limited cell reduplication potential,

one can predict some likely features of stem cells with finite self-reproduction and construct a model of stem-cell regulation. Figure 1 lists three essential features of stem cells with limited reduplication. First, differen-

[1] From Session III, *Finite versus infinite proliferative and functional capacities of cells*, of the FASEB Conference on *Biology of Development and Aging*, presented at the 58th Annual Meeting of the Federation of American Societies for Experimental Biology, Atlantic City, N.J., April 10, 1974.

[2] Research supported by the Atomic Energy Commission, the Leukemia Society of America, Inc., and by National Institutes of Health research grant number HL 15685-02.

LIKELY FEATURES OF STEM CELLS WITH LIMITED SELF RENEWAL

1. Division - Differentiation Sequence : to Protect Potential

2. Resting Pools with Reservoir Function : to Permit Regulation

3. Embryonal Pool : to Secure Life - Time Supply

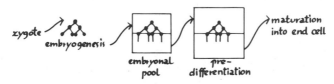

Figure 1. Three hypothetical properties to be expected of stem cells with finite reproductive life-span.

tiated end cells would emerge as off-spring from stem cells whose reproductive potential has been spent. Second, variable periods of rest between divisions would provide the possibility for a regulatory mechanism: resting cells would form reservoirs to be expanded or depleted according to demand. The final condition predicts a finite pool of stem cells that have conserved all or most of their reproductive potential. This "embryonal" pool would contain the supply of stem cells that is to be utilized through life. The following stem-cell model is similar to Kay's concept of "clonal succession."

Figure 2 depicts three pools that symbolize stages of an irreversible sequence of multiplication and rest periods during the hypothetical life history of a hemopoietic stem cell

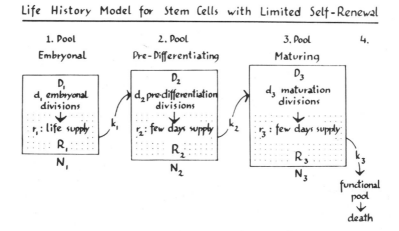

Figure 2. Hypothetical model of stem-cell regulation based on features listed in Fig. 1.

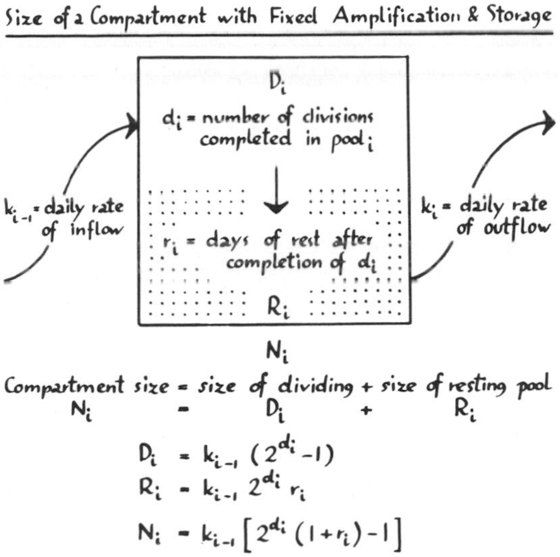

Size of a Compartment with Fixed Amplification & Storage

$$N_i$$

$$\text{Compartment size} = \text{size of dividing} + \text{size of resting pool}$$
$$N_i \quad = \quad D_i \quad + \quad R_i$$

$$D_i = k_{i-1}(2^{d_i}-1)$$
$$R_i = k_{i-1} 2^{d_i} r_i$$
$$N_i = k_{i-1}\left[2^{d_i}(1+r_i)-1\right]$$

Figure 3. Definitions of parameters used in Figs. 2 and 4. The formulas to obtain D_i, R_i and N_i have been used to compute N_1, N_2 and N_3 in Fig. 4.

with limited duplication capacity. Embryonal stem cells form a reservoir that suffices for life. On stimulation an embryonal stem cell enters the predifferentiation multiplicative phase. Differentiation follows as defined by emergence of functional end cells or their recognizable precursors. Few further divisions occur and after a variable delay the finished blood cells are released. A minimum of three stages describes the process. The predifferentiating stage may constitute several sequences of division and rest periods. Demand for extra cells can be satisfied by drawing upon the resting pools.

Figure 3 provides explanation of symbols. Three formulas describe the size of the dividing and resting subpopulation and total pool size for the simplest possible case that all parameters are constant.

A numerical application of the hypothetical model to human hemopoiesis is shown in Fig. 4. Asterisks denote experimentally verified values.

The daily replacement rate of 3.7 $\times 10^{11}$ (Table 1) cells per day is numerically equivalent to the progeny of one cell that has expanded geometrically for about 39 divisions. The integral production over 100 years at the same production rate is 1.35 $\times 10^{16}$ and is numerically equivalent to the progeny of 36,525 cells that have divided 39 times. The minimum of 36,525 embryonal cells required could be the progeny of 1 cell that has undergone about 15 successive mitoses. A total stem-cell production from about 54 duplications can therefore support 100 years of human hemopoiesis. An additional embryonal division doubles the embryonal progeny which might be sufficient to compensate for episodes of necessary regeneration. The embryonal stem-cell population grows to some maximum and thereafter under the assumptions imposed must decrease in size with advancing age. Pool

TABLE 1. Daily replacement of red and white blood cells in 70 kg man

	Cell count		Survival time	Daily replacement
	per μl	in 5 l blood		
Red blood cells	6×10^6	3×10^{13}	120 days	2.5×10^{11}
Granulocytes	6×10^3	3×10^{10}	6 hours	1.2×10^{11}
Total				3.7×10^{11}

Daily replacement of red cells and granulocytic white cells in 5 l blood of a 70 kg man. The obtained value of 3.7×10^{11} cells was used to estimate K_3 in Fig. 4. Total number of bone marrow cells ($N_1 + N_2 + N_3$ in Fig. 4) is consistent with ref (11), proportion of colony-forming stem cells is consistent with ref (23).

sizes are derived from arbitrarily chosen parameters applying the formulas in Fig. 3. The numbers do not illustrate actual conditions but are used only to show that known features of hemopoiesis comply with the model.

Although the present model amounts to an oversimplification, its elements appear essential to a renewal system with finite reduplication potential. Table 2 summarizes hypothetical stem-cell features, their compatibility with finite or infinite self-renewal capacity, and the available supporting experimental evidence. Supportive evidence exists, but conclusive proof is lacking. Hemopoietic stem cells pass an intermediate pre-differentiating stage (3, 10, 27) in which they undergo rapid multiplication (21, 27). This intermediate

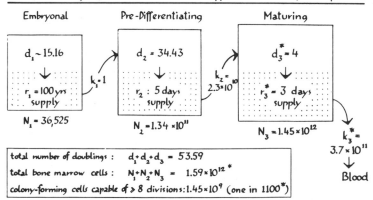

Figure 4. Known parameters of human hemopoiesis (* see Table 1) can be derived using assumed values for the unknown model parameters. This shows that current knowledge about hemopoiesis is compatible with the hypothesis of finite reproductiive cell life. It is not an attempt to describe actual stem-cell regulation.

TABLE 2. Is Hayflick's hypothesis refutable on the grounds of available knowledge?

Hypothetical feature	Reduplication potential		Evidence and reference	Interpretation for H_1
	Finite, H_1	Infinite, H_0		
1) Differentiation schedule				
Stem cell loss at random	No	Yes or no	CFU-content of spleen colonies (28,31,33)	Open
Stem cell loss non-random	Yes	Yes or no		
Series of predifferentiation divisions	Yes	Yes or no	"Committed stem cells" (8,10,21,27)	Compatible
Unequal division potential	Yes	No	Renewal capacity related to cell size (33), lower in spleen-CFU than in bone marrow CFU (18), higher in resting than in cycling CFU (23)	Supportive
2) Supplies of resting stem cells				
with unequal division potential	Yes	Yes or no	Cells in "G_0" (1,20,21)	Compatible
	Yes	No	See above and (26a)	
3) Embryonal stem cell reserve				
Infinite, inexhaustible	No	Yes	Transplanted cells? (11a)	Not supportive
Finite, exhaustible	Yes	No	Diploid cell cultures (7, 12–14, 21a, 22, 29)	Supportive
			Transplanted cells (23,25,26,30)	Supportive
			Interval-dependent decline ? (6,23,32)	Not supportive
			Transplanted tissues (8,19)	Supportive
Regenerative ability exhaustible	Yes	No	Whole-body irradiated mice (2,9)	Compatible
			^{55}Iron cytocide	?

Available evidence relating to Hayflick's hypothesis is examined in comparison to features of stem cells that must be expected if the hypothesis is true. CFU = colony forming units. G_0 = state of rest as opposed to the four phases of the mitotic cycle.

pool could contain stem cells with unequal potential for self-reduplication. Proof of unequal stem-cell reduplication potential would constitute a strong argument for finite reproductive stem-cell life. This has been reported in relation to cell size (33), origin (18), cycle phase (23, p. 99) and was also directly observed in cloned fetal cells (26a).

Random loss of stem cells to the differentiation process appears to be incompatible with life-long maintenance of tissues limited as to their self-renewal capacity. Proof of an existing random mechanism in the selection of stem cells for differentiation could therefore conclusively refute the hypothesis of limited reduplication potential but such proof has not so far been obtained (28, 31, 33).

Existence of a large reservoir of resting hemopoietic stem cells is well established (1, 20, 21). Depending on which hypothesis is true, the embryonal stem-cell reserve will be either finite or unlimited. Evidence supporting the former is strong in cultured (7, 11a, 12–14, 22, 29) and serially transplanted (23, 25, 26, 30) cells, although the interval between passages may be relevant (6, 23, 32). Only one report suggests long continued proliferation of serially transplanted bone marrow (11a). Serially transplanted mouse tissues survive considerably longer than the donor animals (15, 19) but their ultimate decline is well documented (8, 19).

Yet it still is undetermined whether reduplication is limited in cells that were never removed from the body.

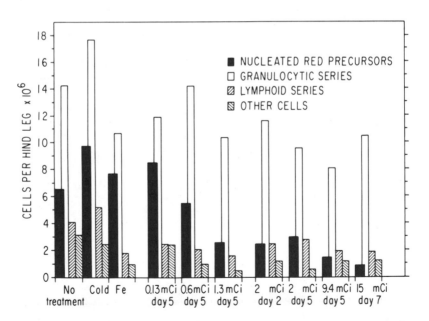

Figure 5. Absolute numbers of erythropoietic granulopoietic, lymphoid, and "other" bone marrow cells per hind leg in seven ^{55}Fe injected mice and three controls. Doses and killing intervals as indicated.

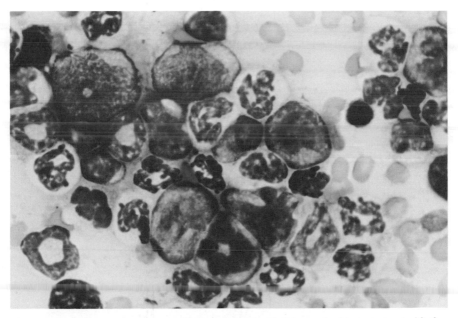

Figure 6. Mouse bone marrow smear 7 days after 15 mCi. Rare erythroblasts contrast with the relative abundance of granulopoiesis. A mitotic figure appears on bottom of picture. ×940.

No significant reduction of hemopoietic stem cells is seen in aging mice (5, 24) although their concentration may decrease (5, 9). This does not contradict exhaustibility of their division potential. The aging mammal still maintains self-renewal of skin, intestine and blood even though at reduced rates (4). Since renewal tissues are endowed with capacity for extensive regeneration it is unlikely that a limited reduplication potential would be exhausted by aging alone. On the other hand, extraordinary demand for regeneration might possibly exhaust a limited potential before an individual's life expectancy is realized. Demonstration of the exhaustibility of the regenerative reserve could therefore prove the hypothesis.

In a deliberate attempt to drain hemopoietic stem cells to possible exhaustion we use ^{55}Fe. The isotope has a half-life of 2.6 years and decays to stable ^{55}Mn by electron capture, releasing low energy Auger electrons and X-rays. Since the greatest electron path length is less than one μm, virtually all of their energy is absorbed in the cell where decay occurs. Iron is predominantly incorporated into the erythropoietic bone marrow, thus ^{55}Fe radiotoxicity should impede red cell formation with only minimal damage to other cells. Depending on the final intracellular ratio of radioactive and stable iron, nucleated red precursors could accumulate a lethal radiation dose before maturation is completed. Such self-destruction may be termed "radioiron cytocide." A pilot experiment in random-bred albino mice demonstrates the feasibility of this approach.

Selective damage to erythroblasts following ^{55}Fe is illustrated in Fig. 5 which shows absolute bone marrow counts of the red and white cell series. A dose-dependent decrease to about 10 percent of normal in red cell precursors is contrasted with a decrease to about 70 percent in each of the other cell series. These mice received a single intravenous dose of high specific activity $^{55}FeCl_3$ (363 mCi/mg Fe). Figure 6 illustrates the relative abundance of white cell precursors in bone marrow 7 days after 15 mCi.

The effect of ^{55}Fe on stem cells was measured by the spleen colony assay.

In Fig. 7, stem cells are represented as colony-forming units (CFU). Mice tested within 3 days after injection showed a reduction of bone marrow CFU to about 10 percent regardless of dose. Colony-forming units in mice tested 3 to 7 days after injection were decreased exponentially in dose-dependent fashion down to 1 percent of the number obtained in iron-loaded controls. This massive effect is unlikely to have arisen from radiation injury. The possible extent of X-ray damage can be extrapolated from

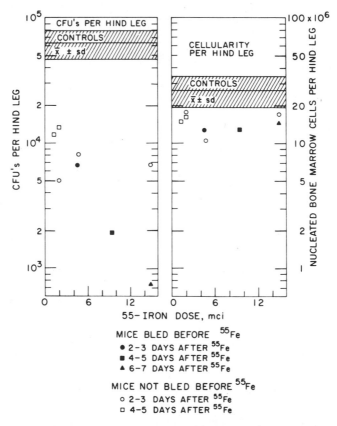

Figure 7. Number of nucleated cells per hind leg (right) and colony forming units per hind leg (left) in eight ^{55}Fe-treated mice, plotted against ^{55}Fe dosage. Pretreatment and interval of killing are indicated in the table. Hatched bands show values and standard deviations of six cold-iron-burdened controls.

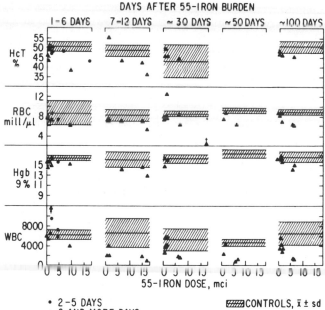

Figure 8. Peripheral blood counts in ^{55}Fe-burdened mice. Each symbol denotes one mouse treated with a single ^{55}FeCl$_3$ dose between 0.5 mCi and 17 mCi. Mean blood counts and standard deviations in 21 cold-iron-burdened controls are shown as hatched bands.

differential cell counts of bone marrow (cf. Fig. 5) and from total marrow cellularity. The latter is plotted on the right of Fig. 7 and shows generalized reduction to 50 percent. Significant radiation damage to other than erythropoietic cells would have been signaled by a dose-dependent decrease in total cellularity, which did not occur.

Since the stem-cell depletion appears unrelated to direct radiation injury it likely reflects stem-cell responses to perturbations in the offspring population. Increased death rate of maturing erythroblasts will be compensated by accelerated stem-cell differentiation into new erythroblasts. The cytocide is perpetuated through reutilization of ^{55}Fe liberated from disintegrated cells. Stem-cell

turnover is enhanced in proportion to the extent of ongoing cytocide which can account for the exponential decrease of CFU's. This implies that stem-cell counts obtained under normal conditions include a substantial reserve that can be diminished rapidly upon demand (3).

Peripheral blood counts (Fig. 8) revealed early reduction in white blood cells which became more significant with time; in addition, moderate anemia began to develop after several weeks. Thus, compensation for erythroblast cytocide appears to have been at least partially effective. The low stem-cell numbers did not impede, but rather were a component of, the regulatory adaptation. It is not clear whether this is mediated by erythropoietin. The early manifestation of stem-cell response before appearance of anemia suggests existence of a direct intramedullary regulatory mechanism.

Approaches to stem-cell exhaustion other than radioiron cytocide are, of course, possible and necessary. No single experiment will decide whether stem cells can continue to divide without limit. But a definitive answer can only be obtained through in vivo studies and, we believe, through maximal challenge of regenerative renewal capacity.

REFERENCES

1. BECKER, A. H., E. A. McCULLOCH, L. SIMINOVITCH AND J. E. TILL. The effect of differing demands for blood cell production on DNA synthesis by hemopoietic colony-forming cells of mice. *Blood* 26: 296, 1965.
2. BOGGS, D. R., J. C. MARSH, P. A. CHERVENICK, G. E. CARTWRIGHT AND M. M. WINTROBE. Factors influencing hematopoietic spleen colony formation in irradiated mice. III. The effect of repetitive irradiation upon proliferative ability of colony-forming cells. *J. Exptl. Med.* 126: 871, 1967.
3. BRUCE, W. R., AND E. A. McCULLOCH. The effect of erythropoietic stimulation on the hemopoietic colony-forming cells of mice. *Blood* 23: 216, 1964.
4. BUETOW, D. E. Cellular content and cellular proliferation changes in the tissues and organs of the aging mammal. In: *Cellular and Molecular Renewal in the Mammalian Body*, edited by Cameron, I. L. and J. D. Thrasher. New York: Academic, 1971, p. 87.
5. CHEN, M. D. Age-related changes in hematopoietic stem cell populations of a long-lived hybrid mouse. *J. Cellular Physiol.* 78: 225, 1971.
6. CUDKOWICZ, G., A. C. UPTON, L. H. SMITH, D. G. GOSSLEE AND W. L. HUGHES. An approach to the characterization of stem cells in mouse bone marrow. *Ann. N.Y. Acad. Sci.* 114: 571, 1964.
7. DANES, B. S. Progeria: a cell culture study on aging. *J. Clin. Invest.* 50: 2000, 1971.
8. DANIEL, C. W., L. J. T. YOUNG, D. MEDINA AND K. B. DeOME. The in-

fluence of mammogenic hormones on serially transplanted mouse mammary gland. *Exptl. Gerontology* 6: 95, 1971.
9. DAVIS, M. L., A. C. UPTON AND L. C. SATTERFIELD. Growth and senescence of the bone marrow stem cell pool in RFM/Un mice. *Proc. Soc. Exptl. Biol. Med.* 137: 1452, 1971.
10. DELMONTE, L. Hemopoietin-initiated changes in differential retransplantability of mouse femoral marrow-derived colony-forming units (CFU). *Proc. Soc. Exptl. Biol. Med.* 141: 227, 1972.
11. DONOHUE, D. M., B. W. GABRIO AND C. A. FINCH. Quantitative measurement of hematopoietic cells of the marrow. *J. Clin. Invest.* 37: 1564, 1958.
11a HARRISON, D. E., Normal production of erythrocytes by mouse bone marrow continuous for 73 months. *Proc. Natl. Acad. Sci. U.S.* 70: 3184, 1973.
12. HAYFLICK, L. The limited in vitro lifetime of human diploid cell strains, *Exptl. Cell Res.* 37: 614, 1965.
13. HAYFLICK, L., AND P. S. MOORHEAD. The serial cultivation of human diploid cell strains. *Exptl. Cell Res.* 25: 585, 1961.
14. HOLEČKOVÁ, E., AND V. J. CRISTOFALO (editors) *Aging in Cell and Tissue Culture.* New York: Plenum, 1970.
15. HOSHINO, K. Indefinite in vivo life span of serially iso-grafted mouse mammary gland. *Experientia* 26: 1393, 1970.
16. KAY, H. G. M. How many cell generations? *Lancet* 2: 418, 1965.
17. KOUKALOVA, B., AND Z. KARPFEL. Proliferative ability of X-irradiated bone marrow from donors of different ages. *Folia Biol., Prague* 12: 283, 1966.
18. KRETCHMAR, A. L., AND W. R. CONOVER. A difference between spleen-derived and bone marrow-derived colony-forming units in ability to protect lethally irradiated mice. *Blood* 36: 772, 1970.
19. KROHN, P. L. Review lecture on senescence: II. Heterochronic transplantation in the study of ageing. *Proc. Roy. Soc. London, Ser. B.* 157: 128, 1963.
20. LAJTHA, L. G., R. OLIVER AND C. W. GURNEY. Kinetic model of a bone marrow stem-cell population. *Brit. J. Haematol.* 8: 442, 1962.
21. LAJTHA, L. G., L. V. POZZI, R. SCHOFIELD AND M. FOX. Kinetic properties of haemopoietic stem cells. *Cell Tissue Kinet.* 2: 39, 1969.
21a LeGUILLY, Y., M. SIMON, P. LENOIR AND M. BOUREL. Long-term culture of human adult liver cells: morphological changes related to in-vitro senescence

and effect of donor's age on growth potential. *Gerontologia* 19: 303, 1973.

22. MARTIN, G. M., C. A. SPRAGUE AND C. J. EPSTEIN. Replicative life-span of cultivated human cells. Effect of donor's age, tissue, and genotype. *Lab. Invest.* 23: 86, 1970.

23. METCALF, D., AND M. A. S. MOORE. *Haemopoietic Cells.* Amsterdam: North-Holland, 1971.

24. PROUKAKIS, C., J. E. COGGLE AND P. J. LINDOP. Effect of age at exposure on the bone-marrow stem-cell population in relation to 30-day mortality in mice. In: *Radiation Biology of the Fetal and Juvenile Mammal,* edited by M. R. Sikov and D. O. Mahlum. U.S. Atomic Energy Commission Div. Tech. Inf. 1969, p. 603.

25. SCHOOLEY, J. C. AND D. H. Y. LIN. Hematopoiesis and the colony-forming unit. In: *Regulation of Erythropoiesis,* edited by A. S. Gordon, M. Condorelli and C. Peschle. Milano: Il Ponte 1972, p. 52.

26. SIMINOVITCH, L., J. E. TILL AND E. A. MCCULLOCH. Decline in colony-forming ability of marrow cells subjected to serial transplantation into irradiated mice. *J. Cellular Comp. Physiol.* 64: 23, 1964.

26a SMITH, J. R. AND L. HAYFLICK. Variation in the life-span of clones derived from human diploid cell strains. *J. Cell Biol.*

62: 48, 1974.

27. STOHLMAN, F., JR., S. EBBE, B. MORSE, D. HOWARD AND J DONOVAN. Regulation of erythropoiesis XX. Kinetics of red cell production. *Ann. N.Y. Acad. Sci.* 149: 156, 1968.

28. TILL, J. E., E. A. MCCULLOCH AND L. SIMINOVITCH. A stochastic model of stem cell proliferation based on the growth of spleen colony-forming cells. *Proc. Natl. Acad. Sci. U.S.* 51: 29, 1964.

29. TODARO, G. J., AND H. GREEN, Serum albumin supplemented medium for long term cultivation of mammalian fibroblast strains. *Proc. Soc. Exptl. Biol. Med.* 116: 688, 1964.

30. VAN BEKKUM, D. W., AND W. W. H. WEYZEN. Serial transfer of isologous hematopoietic cells in irradiated hosts. *Pathol. Biol. Semaine Hop.* 9: 888, 1961.

31. VOGEL, H., M. NIEWISCH AND G. MATIOLI, The self renewal probability of hemopoietic stem cells. *J. Cellular Physiol.* 72: 221, 1968.

32. VOS, O., AND M. J. A. S. DOLMANS. Self-renewal of colony forming units (CFU) in serial bone marrow transplantation experiments. *Cell Tissue Kinet.* 5: 371, 1972.

33. WORTON, R. G., E. A. MCCULLOCH AND J. E. TILL. Physical separation of hemopoietic stem cells differing in their capacity for self-renewal. *J. Exptl. Med.* 130: 91, 1969.

Contributions of cytoplasmic factors to in vitro cellular senescence[1,2]

WOODRING E. WRIGHT AND LEONARD HAYFLICK

Department of Medical Microbiology

Stanford University School of Medicine, Stanford, California 94305

ABSTRACT

Mass populations of normal human lung fibroblasts were enucleated by centrifugation at $\geq 25,000\,g$ in 4 μg/ml cytochalasin B. The 1% of cells that did not enucleate were rendered nonviable by treatment with mitomycin C. Whole cells were poisoned with a 99% lethal dose of the sulfhydryl reagent iodoacetate. The washed cells were then mixed with the anucleate cytoplasms, fused with inactivated Sendai virus, and planted in rotenone for 20 hours. Whereas normal cells are able to survive this rotenone treatment, the 1% surviving iodoacetate-treated cells cannot withstand this additional stress. However, iodoacetate-treated cells that fuse to untreated cytoplasms receive sufficient amounts of active enzymes to allow them to survive. Since this selective system does not rely on using enzymatic mutants, it should permit the selection of hybrids between anucleate cytoplasms and any type of whole cell. Cytoplasmic hybrids were cultured in order to determine their proliferative capacity. The life-spans of cytoplasmic hybrids between young and old cells were compared to those of young/young and old/old controls. Cytoplasmic factors do not appear to control in vitro cellular senescence.—WRIGHT, W. E. AND L. HAYFLICK. Contributions of cytoplasmic factors to in vitro cellular senescence. *Federation Proc.* 34: 76–79, 1975.

We have shown that normal human diploid cells have a limited ability to proliferate in vitro (11). As these cells are serially propagated they exhibit an increased doubling time, accumulation of cellular debris, gradual cessation of mitotic activity, and in the case of embryo donors, the culture degenerates (Phase III) after a total of 50 ± 10 population doublings. These findings have been interpreted as an in vitro expression of cellular aging (8). Sup-

[1] From Session III, *Finite versus infinite proliferative and functional capacities of cells*, of the FASEB Conference on *Biology of Development and Aging*, presented at the 58th Annual Meeting of the Federation of American Societies for Experimental Biology, Atlantic City, N.J., April 10, 1974.

[2] This study was supported, in part, by research grant IID 04004 from the National Institute of Child Health and Human Development, by contract NIH 69-2053 within the Virus Cancer Program of the National Cancer Institute, and by Medical Scientist Training Grant No. GM 1922 from the National Institute of General Medical Sciences.

port for this hypothesis has come from many different studies demonstrating such phenomena as *1*) an inverse correlation between population doubling potential of cultured cells in vitro and donor age (5, 8, 16), *2*) a direct correlation between mean maximum species life-span (9, 10) and in vitro proliferative capacity (5, 7, 20, 22, 27) and *3*) studies showing a limited proliferative capacity for cells serially transplanted in vivo in syngeneic hosts (3, 14, 21).

Two classes of hypotheses have been offered to explain these phenomena. One interprets cellular aging as an expression of specific genetic events, such as "aging genes" or the exhaustion of genetic information. The other relies on a progressive deterioration owing to the accumulation of damage caused by either the internal or the external environment. Many of the theories in the latter class imply that a significant contribution to cellular aging is made by cytoplasmic events (12, 18, 19). Many cytoplasmic functions have been found to change as a function of the in vitro age of cultured cells (2), and in lower organisms such as the fungi (13, 23), amoebas (17) and paramecia (24, 25), cytoplasmic senescence factors have been identified.

Recent experiments in which young and old whole cells have been fused indicate that senescence may be dominant, since the hybrids failed to multiply (15). However, such experiments do not distinguish between nuclear and cytoplasmic contributions to in vitro cellular senescence. The ability to enucleate mass populations of human cells (28–30), and to fuse the anucleate cytoplasms ("cytoplasts")[3] to whole cells of a different in vitro age provides a method of performing what amounts to cytoplasmic transplants between young and old cells. The present study was undertaken to test the aforemen-

tioned theories of aging by determining the proliferative capacity of such cytoplasmic hybrids, and thus to discover if cytoplasmic factors play a causal role in the senescence of cultured normal human cells.

MATERIALS AND METHODS

The normal human diploid fetal lung fibroblast strain WI-38 (8) was enucleated by a method previously described (28, 29) which depends on the ability of the mold metabolite cytochalasin B to cause occasional cells to extrude their nuclei (1). This process is greatly facilitated by subjecting the cells to forces of $\geq 25,000\,g$. The nucleus then migrates through the cytoplasm to one end of the cell, where the cytochalasin B acts to permit its exit from the cell (30). Approximately 99% of the cells become anucleate under these conditions. The few cells that fail to enucleate are rendered incapable of further multiplication by treatment with mitomycin C (26). The cytoplasts are then fused to whole cells using β-propio-lactone-inactivated Sendai virus (6).

Cells with hybrid cytoplasms were isolated by a method described in detail elsewhere (submitted for publication). Briefly, a wide variety of enzymes in the whole cells were inactivated by a near lethal treatment with iodoacetate, an agent that irreversibly alkylates sulfhydryl groups. Whereas untreated cells can easily survive for 24 hours in the presence of rotenone, an inhibitor of oxidative metabolism, iodoacetate-treated cells cannot. However, such cells can survive this treatment if they are first fused to anucleate cytoplasms containing active enzymes (Figs. 1, 2).

---

[3] Anucleate cytoplasms will be referred to as "cytoplasts" following the suggestion of D. Prescott (personal communication).

Thus, only cells with hybrid cytoplasms survive. These cells were then subcultivated in rotenone-free medium until they reached Phase III in order to determine their total proliferative capacity. In each experiment a control consisting of an aliquot of approximately 10^7 iodoacetate-treated cells was cultivated alone for 24 hours in rotenone in order to verify an adequate killing (whole cell control). Any experiments where more than two of the cells in this aliquot survived were discarded to

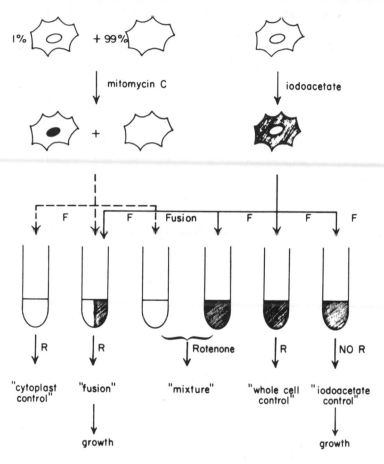

Figure 1. Experimental protocol. The cytoplast control defines the background survival of cells that failed to enucleate, and verifies that they have been rendered unable to divide by treatment with mitomycin C. The whole cell control verifies adequate killing of the whole cells by iodoacetate. The iodoacetate control shows the behavior of cells subjected to all the experimental manipulations except the final killing by rotenone. The "mixture" is treated with Sendai virus in order to make the total stress experienced by these cells equivalent to that in the "fusion." Washing the cytoplasts and cells free of virus before mixing them is effective in preventing cytoplasmic hybridization in the "mixture." The difference in cell density and subsequent growth between the "fusion" and the "mixture" are the criteria for identifying rescue of treated cells by untreated cytoplasts.

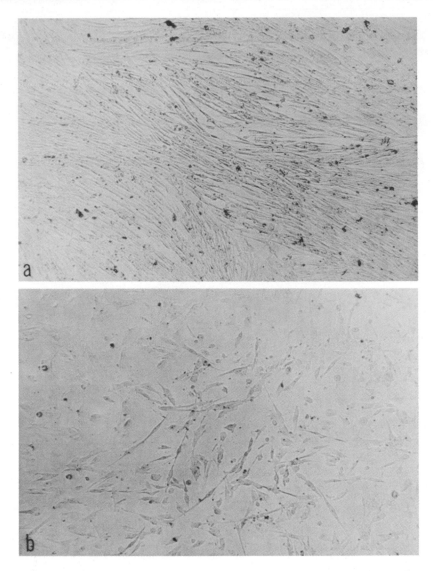

Figure 2. Rescue of iodoacetate-rotenone treated cells by fusion to cytoplasts. Whole cells were treated with 9×10^{-4}M iodoacetate for 30 min at 0–5 C. *a*) "fusion," *b*) "mixture," *c*) whole cell control, *d*) iodoacetate control, and *e*) cytoplast control. See Fig. 1 for the definition of these terms. × 75. Line indicates 200 μ.

avoid the possibility of nonhybridized young cells multiplying and overgrowing the culture. In some experiments, an equal aliquot of treated cells was also cultivated in the absence of rotenone, thus permitting the cells to survive (iodoacetate control). These cells were then subcultivated

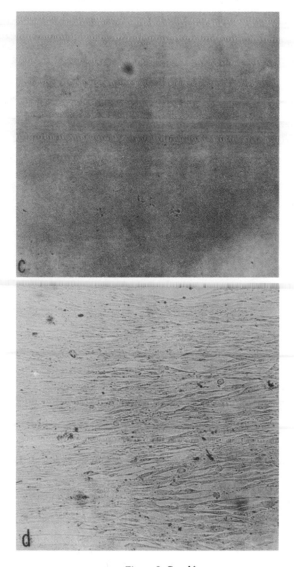

Figure 2. Cont'd.

until Phase III in order to assess the effect of the iodoacetate treatment alone on total proliferative capacity. In these experiments, "young" refers to cells of population-doubling level 20–26 and "old" to cells of population-doubling level 49–60.

RESULTS

Figure 3 summarizes the results of these experiments. Eight of 12 (67%) "iodoacetate control" cultures divided significantly following these manipulations. The failure of four cultures

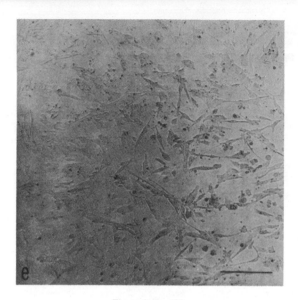

Figure 2. Cont'd.

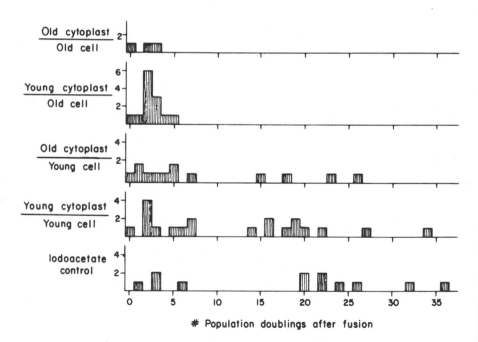

Population doublings after fusion

Figure 3. Population doubling levels following cytoplasmic hybridization. Each square represents one experiment. "Young" = population doubling level 20–26. "Old" = population doubling level 49–60. The iodoacetate control consists of young cells treated with iodoacetate but not rotenone, thus permitting cell survival.

is not surprising in view of the number of traumatic procedures to which these cells were subjected. Of the eight cultures that did reenter the log phase of growth, the average number of subsequent population doublings was 25, which is 4 less than untreated parallel cultures. This is the baseline with which to compare the behavior of cells with hybrid cytoplasms. Ten of 20 (50%) young cytoplast/young cell hybrid cultures yielded more than 7 population doublings. Of these, the average subsequent population doublings was 20. This is grossly comparable to the behavior of the "iodoacetate controls." Four of 13 (31%) old cytoplast/young cell cultures yielded more than 7 population doublings, and their average number of subsequent population doublings was also 20. The differences between the young cytoplast/young cell hybrids and the old cytoplast/young cell hybrids are not statistically significant ($P \geqslant 0.05$). None of the young cytoplast/old cell or old cytoplast/old cell cultures ever yielded more than 5 population doublings following hybridization.

DISCUSSION

Because of the wide variation in proliferative capacity following cytoplasmic hybridization, only the most gross changes could be observed in these experiments. Within this limitation, the following conclusions can be drawn: In no case were young cytoplasts able to rejuvenate old cells. This implies that cellular senescence is not a result of the selective depletion of any cytoplasmic component over time. Alternatively, since old cells are probably more subject to stress than young cells, they could simply have sustained so much damage from the experimental manipulations that even young cytoplasm could not restore their proliferative capacity.

Old cytoplast/young cell hybrid cultures had as great a proliferative capacity as young cytoplast/young cell controls. This suggests that old cytoplasm is not able to age young cells. These interpretations imply that the control of cellular senescence is intranuclear rather than intracytoplasmic. However, it is necessary to add several important qualifications. First, since the evidence for the isolation of hybrids is only indirect (growth of the "fusion" and not the "mixture", see Figure 1), there is a possibility of artifacts affecting the results. For example, agglutination of cytoplasts and iodoacetate-treated cells by Sendai virus might have permitted metabolic rescue of some cells in the absence of actual fusion. Thus, it is possible that old cytoplast/young cell cultures contained some nonhybridized young cells that eventually overgrew the cultures. However, since there was ample opportunity for cytoplast/cell contact in the "mixture" control, the fact that the "mixture" failed to divide argues against this possibility.[4] Second, since only the most gross changes would have been observed, these results do not rule out important but more subtle cytoplasmic contributions to cellular senescence. In addition, the amount of cytoplasm necessary to just rescue an iodoacetate-treated cell might be less than that needed to allow the expression of cytoplasmic senescence factors. Although the present evidence is sufficiently ambiguous to prevent a definitive conclusion at this time, the results nonetheless suggest that nuclear factors and not cytoplasmic factors limit the proliferative

---

[4] A more thorough discussion of the possible sources of artifact in using iodoacetate for the isolation of cytoplasmic hybrids is discussed in two subsequent publications (submitted for publication).

capacity of cultured normal human cells. As experience accumulates in the use of iodoacetate for the isolation of cytoplasmic hybrids, it should be possible to verify or refute this interpretation by more accurately defining the role of cytoplasmic factors in the control of in vitro cellular senescence.

REFERENCES

1. CARTER, S. B. Effects of cytochalasins on mammalian cells. *Nature* 213: 261, 1967.
2. CRISTOFALO, V. J. Animal cell cultures as a model system for the study of ageing. *Advan. Gerontol. Res.* 4: 45, 1972.
3. DANIEL, C. W., K. B. DE OME, L. J. T. YOUNG, P. B. BLAIR AND L. J. FAULKIN, JR. The in vivo life span of normal and preoplastic mouse mammary glands: a serial transplantation study. *Proc. Natl. Acad. Sci. U.S.* 61: 53, 1968.
4. GOLDSTEIN, S. Aging in vitro-Growth of cultured cells from the Galapagos tortoise. *Exptl. Cell Res.* 83: 297, 1974.
5. GOLDSTEIN, S., J. W. LITTLEFIELD AND A. S. SOELDNER. Diabetes mellitus and aging: diminished plating efficiency of cultured human fibroblasts. *Proc. Natl. Acad. Sci. U.S.* 64: 155, 1969.
6. HARRIS, H., AND J. F. WATKINS. Hybrid cells derived from mouse and man: artificial heterokaryons of mammalian cells from different species. *Nature* 205: 640, 1965.
7. HAY, R. J., AND B. L. STREHLER. The limited growth span of cell strains isolated from the chick embryo. *Exptl. Gerontol.* 2: 123, 1967.
8. HAYFLICK, L. The limited in vitro lifetime of human diploid cell strains. *Exptl. Cell Res.* 37: 614, 1965.
9. HAYFLICK, L. The longevity of cultured human cells. *J. Am. Geriat. Soc.* 22: 1, 1974.
10. HAYFLICK, L., Cytogerontology. In: *Theoretical Aspects of Aging*, edited by M. Rockstein. New York: Academic 1974, p. 83.
11. HAYFLICK, L., AND P. S. MOORHEAD. The serial cultivation of human diploid cell strains. *Exptl. Cell Res.* 25: 585, 1961.
12. HOLLIDAY, R. Errors in protein synthesis and clonal senescence in fungi. *Nature* 221: 1224, 1969.
13. JINKS, J. L. Lethal suppressive cytoplasms in aged clones of *Aspergillus glaucus*. *J. Gen. Microbiol.* 21: 397, 1959.
14. KROHN, P. L. Review lectures on senescence: II. Heterochronic transplantation in the study of ageing. *Proc. Roy. Soc. London, Ser. B.* 157: 128, 1962.
15. LITTLEFIELD, J. W. Attempted hybridizations with senescent human fibroblasts. *J. Cellular Physiol.* 82: 129, 1973.
16. MARTIN, G. M., C. A. SPRAGUE AND C. J. EPSTEIN. Replicative life-span of cultivated human cells: effects of donor's age, tissue and genotype. *Lab. Invest.* 23: 86, 1970.
17. MUGGLETON, A., AND J. F. DANIELLI. Inheritance of the 'life-spanning' phenomenon in *Amoeba proteus*. *Exptl. Cell Res.* 49: 116, 1968.
18. ORGEL, L. E. The maintenance of the accuracy of protein synthesis and its relevance to aging. *Proc. Natl. Acad. Sci. U.S.* 49: 517, 1963.
19. ORGEL, L. E. Ageing of clones of mammalian cells. *Nature* 243: 441, 1973.
20. PONTEN, J. The growth capacity of normal and Rous-virus-transformed chicken fibroblasts in vitro. *Intern. J. Cancer* 6: 323, 1970.
21. SIMINOVITCH, L., J. E. TILL AND E. A. MCCULLOCH. Decline in colony forming ability of marrow cells subjected to serial transplantation into irradiated mice. *J. Cellular Comp. Physiol.* 64: 23, 1964.
22. SIMONS, J. W. I. M. A theoretical and experimental approach to the relationship between cell variability and aging in vitro. In: *Aging in Cell and Tissue Culture*, edited by E. Holeckova and V. J. Cristofalo. New York: Plenum, 1970, p. 25.
23. SMITH, J. R., AND I. RUBENSTEIN. Cytoplasmic inheritance of the timing of 'senescence' in *Podospora anserina*. *J. Gen. Microbiol.* 76: 297, 1973.
24. SONNEBORN, T. M., AND M. SCHNELLER. Age-induced mutations in paramecium. In: *The Biology of Aging*, edited by B. L. Strehler. Baltimore: Waverly, 1960, p. 286.
25. SONNEBORN, T. M., AND M. SCHNELLER. Measures of the rate and amount of aging on the cellular level. In: *Biology of Aging*, edited by B. L. Strehler. Baltimore: Waverly, 1960, p. 290.
26. STUDZINSKI, G. P., AND L. S. COHEN. Mitomycin-C induced increases in the activities of the deoxyribonucleases of HeLa cells. *Biochem. Biophys. Res. Commun.* 23: 506, 1966.

27. TODARO, G. J., AND H. GREEN. Quantitative studies of the growth of mouse embryo cells in culture and their development into established lines. *J. Cell Biol.* 17: 299, 1963.

28. WRIGHT, W. E. The production of mass populations of anucleate cytoplasms. In: *Methods in Cell Biology,* edited by D. Prescott. New York:

Academic Press, 1973, vol. VII, p. 203.

29. WRIGHT, W. E., AND L. HAYFLICK. Formation of anucleate and multinucleate cells in normal and S.V.$_{40}$ transformed WI-38 by cytochalasin B. *Exptl. Cell Res.* 74: 187, 1972.

30. WRIGHT, W. E., AND L. HAYFLICK. Enucleation of cultured human cells. *Proc. Soc. Exptl. Biol. Med.* 144: 587, 1973.

Aging of homeostatic control systems

Introductory remarks

PAOLA S. TIMIRAS

Department of Physiology–Anatomy
University of California, Berkeley, California 94720

One of the prevailing views of aging, and one that has been given ample exposure at this conference, is that aging results from cellular and molecular changes intrinsic to each cell in the body. However attractive this hypothesis might be, it does not appear to be substantiated in all cases, especially in higher organisms. Indeed, evidence is available to show that in these organisms, most cells of the body do *not* age because of intrinsic "pacemakers" of aging but, rather, because of changes in their environment. An indication that deterioration of control systems regulating interactions between the organism and its environment may be responsible for the aging process is provided by the findings of several investigators. For example, age-related alterations in cellular function can be eliminated by the administration of hormones and by appropriate neural stimulation. Changes in endocrine and autonomic nervous function associated with aging (and amply documented) may represent the cause for the many and diverse alterations that occur with age in cell function. Moreover, an alteration in neuroendocrine regulation might derive from imbalances in feedback mechanisms associated with the various "biological clocks" involved in homeostasis. (For a review on the subject of homeostasis and aging, see (1).)

The significance of undernutrition at critical periods during development is reviewed by Dr. Miller in terms of its repercussions on the resistance of the organism to different environmental conditions (e.g., infection) throughout the lifespan. Corollary to this research, Mr. Segall and Dr. Sandstead discuss the effects of specific dietary deficiencies, such as the lack of an essential amino acid (tryptophan) and an important dietary constituent (zinc) on growth, morbidity, and mortality.

Based on the knowledge that the nervous and endocrine systems play a major role in the adaptive responses of the organism to its environment, Dr. Vernadakis reaffirms the concept that the integration of the nervous system, as an expression of *cerebral* homeostasis, is essential for the internal ability of the organism to adapt, throughout life, to its changing environment. In discussing the integrative capacity of the brain, attention is centered on the significant neuronal-glial interactions occuring during development and aging, and their involvement in transmission.

Focusing more specifically on how endocrine factors regulate adaptive responses in the aging organism, Dr. Denckla reports recent experiments suggesting that a recently-described pituitary factor could be partially responsible for programming growth as well as aging, possibly by affecting thyroid-dependent systems necessary for sustaining life.

Moving from the more general timetable of the life-span, we are becoming increasingly cognizant that the concept of a biological clock that regulates development and aging is, in turn, comprised of a constellation of rhythmic processes occurring in the body and in the brain. Dr. Berger illustrates the way in which rhythmic clocks govern sleep and wakefulness patterns phylogenetically and ontogenetically, indicating with recent data that repeated inversions of the 12-hour light/dark cycles may dampen such rhythms and result in shortening the life-span.

Any study of the changes that occur with age in the central nervous system must take into consideration the possible deterioration of synaptic function in which neurotransmitter mechanisms play key roles. Several investigations in laboratory animals and humans seem to indicate that, indeed, the levels and metabolism of such neurotransmitters as the catecholamines, acetylcholine, and others may undergo alteration with advancing age, either in the brain as a whole or in specific regions of the brain. The presentation of Dr. Robinson is concerned with comparative studies of monoamine metabolism in different animal species and in humans, at selected ages. Dr. MacFarlane discusses the effects of pharmacological agents such as procaine HCl on the metabolism of catecholamines as a possible mechanism for their action on aging processes.

Each of the foregoing presentations —some full-length articles and others, short communications— selects to examine a different aspect of homeostatic function. The basic assumption of all, however, is that efficient and effective bodily responses are vital to homeostasis at all ages, and particularly in later life, when general functional competence declines and imbalances in control systems threaten survival. When discussing environmental challenges throughout the life-span, we generally think of those that endanger health and survival; it is also important to recognize that both physiological and psychologic stress have a strengthening effect; that is, noxious stimuli, as well as frustration and misfortune, test the resiliency of the organism and, within limits, are essential to the formation of adequate patterns of adaptive responses. The capacity of the individual to adapt to fluctuations in the environment, however, is not inexhaustible. In this respect, it is important that we intensify our experimental and clinical research efforts on the physiological mechanisms involved in adaptive reactions, their changes with age, and the consequences of such changes on the adaptability of the elderly.

REFERENCES

1. TIMIRAS, P. S. Decline in homeostatic regulation. In: *Developmental Physiology and Aging*. New York: Macmillan, 1972, p. 542–563.

Age-related changes in thermoregulatory capacity of tryptophan-deficient rats[1]

PAUL E. SEGALL[2] AND PAOLA S. TIMIRAS

Department of Physiology –Anatomy

University of California, Berkeley, California 94720

ABSTRACT

From a larger study seeking to develop indexes of physiological aging, the present experiment was designed *1*) to test thermoregulatory capacity in the aging and old rat subjected to 3 minutes of whole-body ice water immersion, and *2*) using this index of physiological age, to determine whether tryptophan deficiency from time of weaning can retard the onset of senescence. Results indicate a progressive prolongation of temperature recovery time from young to middle age to old, and tryptophan-deficient animals restored to commercial diet at middle age show the thermoregulatory capacity of young adults. The implications of tryptophan deficiency with respect to brain development, serotonin metabolism, and temperature regulation are also discussed in terms of the possibility of intervening with the aging process.—SEGALL, P. E. AND P. S. TIMIRAS. Age-related changes in thermoregulatory capacity of tryptophan-deficient rats. *Federation Proc.* 34: 83–85, 1975.

The present investigation is part of a larger study seeking to explore the involvement of neurotransmitter substances in the aging of the central nervous system (CNS) and, in turn, of the homeostatic functions of the whole organism. Our first effort was directed to measuring the time required for body temperature to be restored to 37 C following 3-min whole-body ice water immersion and, using this test as an index, to measure the degree of senescence in rats maintained from weaning on a long-term tryptophan-deficient diet, followed by refeeding on Purina Rat Chow.

Evidence indicates that serotonin levels and metabolism in the CNS

[1] From Session IV, *Aging of homeostatic control systems,* of the FASEB Conference on *Biology of Development and Aging,* presented at the 58th Annual Meeting of the Federation of American Societies for Experimental Biology, Atlantic City, N. J., April 10, 1974.

[2] Supported by Public Health Service traineeship HD 101.

play an important role in mechanisms of thermoregulation (11). It is also well-known that dietary tryptophan is the sole source of this putative neurotransmitter, and recent studies have shown that brain serotonin levels decrease in rats maintained on a tryptophan-deficient diet (3). In addition, it has been hypothesized and we concur, that the alterations observed in monoaminergic neurons with age may be ontogenetically programmed and responsible for numerous aging phenomena (4, 5). Given these relationships, it is reasonable to assume that one manifestation of such alterations in monoaminergic neurons over time may be the progressive loss of thermoregulatory competence. More significantly, by testing

TABLE 1. Age-related differences in recovery time following 3-min whole-body ice water immersion

Age groups	No. of animals	Recovery time, min ± SE
Adult (7–8 mo)	6	65.0 ± 2.2
Middle-aged (13–15 mo)	11	90.9 ± 5.7
Old (24–26 mo)	12	110.0 ± 6.9

P values: A/MA < 0.001; A/O < 0.001; and MA/O < 0.05

this hypothesis in tryptophan-deprived rats, we hope also to identify possible methods of interfering with the aging process.

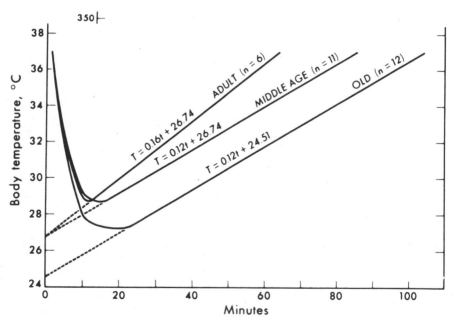

Figure 1. Age-related differences in body temperature changes following 3-min whole-body ice water immersion. Average body temperature plotted against time for three age groups. T represents body temperature and t represents time. Rats were immersed in ice water at 0 time, and removed 3 minutes later. Temperature loss and recovery profile for the three age groups were calculated by the method of the least squares (n = number of animals).

TABLE 2. Tryptophan-deficient diet (General Biochemicals, Incorporated TD-73319)

Ingredients	g/kg
Corn, ground yellow	500
Casein hydrolysate	200
Cornstarch	54
Sucrose	50
Gelatin	50
Jones-Foster salt mix	50
Vitamin mix (GBI)	30
Corn oil	25
Cod liver oil	25
Torula yeast	8
Desiccated liver	8

MATERIALS AND METHODS

Thermoregulatory competence was tested in control animals at three life stages—adult (7–8 mo), middle-aged (13–15 mo) and old (24–26 mo)—by comparing their speed of recovery to 37 C following 3-minute whole-body immersion in ice water. The life-span of this strain under our experimental conditions is approximately 30 mo. Speed of recovery is represented by the time required for restoration of normal body temperature following immersion.

Each animal was placed in a cylindrical restraining cage which was then immersed for 3 minutes in ice water such that only the eyes, nose and mouth could rise above the water level. On removal, the rats were placed in a sawdust-filled cage, a telethermometer probe was inserted rectally, and temperature readings were recorded at 5-min intervals.

RESULTS AND DISCUSSION

Average recovery times for restoration of normal body temperature for the three groups studied are presented in Table 1 and show pro-longed recovery with advancing age. The involvement of body weight as a factor in recovery time, both in the comparison of control animals of different ages and in comparison of control and experimental animals was tested and found not to be significant. Details of these calculations are beyond the scope of this communication and will be presented in a subsequent expanded publication.

When average body temperature is plotted against time for each of the three groups, using the method of least squares, each group shows a characteristic recovery curve. As indicated in Fig. 1, the drop in body temperature after ice water immersion is greater in old animals than in either middle-aged or adult rats. Furthermore, the slope of the curve indicates that young animals recover significantly faster than middle-aged or old, and that while the recovery rate is similar between the latter groups, body temperature of old animals remains lower than that of the other two groups throughout the test period.

The data from this first series of experiments suggest that homeostatic recovery is impaired by aging.

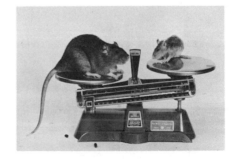

Figure 2. Effects of tryptophan deficiency on growth. Right: rat maintained on tryptophan-deficient diet for 405 days from weaning. Left: control of corresponding age.

In a second series of experiments, the same test was utilized in rats in which growth had been retarded by long-term tryptophan deficiency and subsequently restored by commercial diet. In this connection, a number of attempts to alter or delay the course of physiological senescence by the technique of caloric restriction have been reported (1, 2, 7–9, 12). McCay, in particular, was able to maintain weanling rats in a state of retarded development for over 1,000 days by restricting caloric intake. When re-

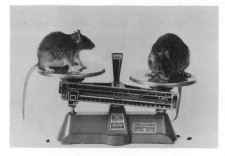

Figure 3. Effect of restoration of commercial diet (72 days) on growth (same notes as in Fig. 2: right, control, left, experimental).

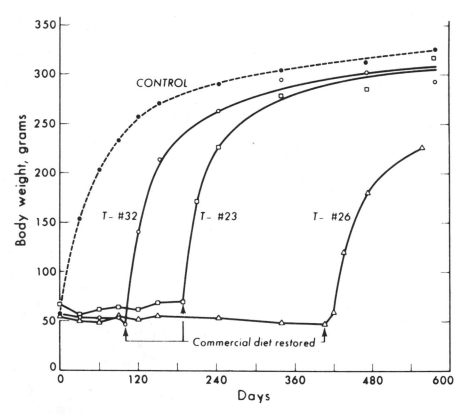

Figure 4. Body growth curves: in tryptophan deficiency (T −) and after restoration of commercial diet. Growth patterns of individual animals re-fed on commercial diet following varying periods of tryptophan deficiency. The curve on the farthest right describes the growth of the same experimental rat shown in Figs 2 and 3. This animal continued to grow after restoration of commercial diet and its body weight is now comparable to that of controls. In fact, this animal was mated, and, at 608 days of age, produced a litter of nine pups.

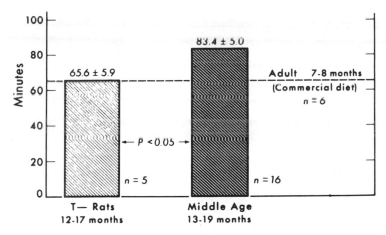

Figure 5. Comparison of recovery time between tryptophan-deficient rats restored to commercial diet and middle-age control animals. The animals exposed to long-term tryptophan deficiency and then placed on a commercial diet appear to recover at the same rate as the younger adult.

placed on a normal diet, some of these animals continued to live past 1,400 days of age, almost twice the average life-span of the strain of rat employed. He stated that the onset of tumor incidence and other forms of pathology were delayed as well (7–9). Some investigators have reported a similar growth arrest using a tryptophan-deficient diet (6, 10). Our intent was to explore whether the growth reduction association with tryptophan deficiency is reflected in a slowing of the aging process.

Our first effort was directed to establishing a tryptophan-deficient diet that would allow survival but retard growth. The final composition used is presented in Table 2 and its effects are illustrated in Figs. 2 and 3.

As shown graphically in Fig. 4, body weight gain resumes when the animal is returned to a commercial diet. At the time of reporting (April 1974), the weight of these animals corresponded to that of control rats comparable in *physiological* age. In subsequent months, their weight continued to increase and is approaching now (September 1974) that of control rats comparable in *chronological* age.

Comparing thermoregulatory competence of middle-aged tryptophan-deficient rats restored to commercial diets with that of control rats of corresponding age, Fig. 5 shows that their speed of recovery from ice water immersion was significantly faster—comparable, in fact, to values reported for adult controls.

These tentative findings support the hypothesis that suspension of growth consequent to long-term maintenance on a tryptophan-deficient diet retards physiological aging, at least with respect to temperature homeostatic capacity.

Inasmuch as tryptophan is equally important in protein synthesis as in neurotransmission, it remains to determine whether its effects are direct on neural regulatory processes or mediated through general effects on growth, or both. In addition, because of involvement of serotonin and other monoamines in various cyclical activities, it is interesting to speculate that tryptophan deficiency may stop the action of a "biological clock" governing both growth and aging.

REFERENCES

1. BERG, B. N. Nutrition and longevity in the rat. I. Food intake in relation to size, health and fertility. *J. Nutr.* 71: 242, 1960.

2. BERG, B. N., AND H. S. SIMMS. Nutrition and longevity in the rat. II. Longevity and onset of disease with different levels of food intake. *J. Nutr.* 71: 255, 1960.

3. FERNSTROM, J. D., AND R. J. WURTMAN. Effect of chronic corn consumption on serotonin content of rat brain. *Nature New Biol.* 234: 62, 1971.

4. FINCH, C. E. Enzyme activities, gene function and ageing in mammals (review). *Exptl. Gerontol.* 7: 53, 1972.

5. FINCH, C. E. Catecholamine metabolism in the brains of ageing male mice. *Brain Res.* 52: 261, 1973.

6. GORDON, R. S. Growth arrest through tryptophan deficiency in the very young chicken. *Sixth International Congress of Nutrition,* Edinburgh, Scotland, Abstract 471, 1963.

7. McCAY, C. M. Chemical aspects of ageing and the effect of diet upon ageing. In: *Cowdry's Problems of Ageing,* 3rd edition, edited by A. I. Lansing. Baltimore: Williams & Wilkins, 1952, p. 139.

8. McCAY, C. M., L. A. MAYNARD, G. SPERLING AND L. L. BARNES. Retarded growth, life span, ultimate body size and age changes in the albino rat after feeding diets restricted in calories. *J. Nutr.* 18: 1, 1939.

9. McCAY, C. M., G. SPERLING AND L. L. BARNES. Growth, ageing, chronic diseases and life span in rats. *Arch. Biochem.* 2: 469, 1943.

10. McROBERTS, M. R. Growth retardation of day old chickens and physiological effects at maturity. *J. Nutr.* 87: 31, 1965.

11. MYERS, R. D., AND T. L. YAKSH. The role of hypothalamic monoamines in hibernation and hypothermia. In: *Hibernation and Hypothermia, Perspectives and Challenges,* edited by F. E. South, et al. New York: American Elsevier, 1972, p. 551.

12. ROSS, M. H. Length of life and nutrition in the rat. *J. Nutr.* 75: 197, 1961.

Zinc deficiency and brain development in the rat[1,2]

HAROLD H. SANDSTEAD, GARY J. FOSMIRE,
JOAN M. McKENZIE[3] AND EDWARD S. HALAS

Human Nutrition Laboratory, Agricultural Research Service
United States Department of Agriculture, and
Departments of Biochemistry and Psychology
University of North Dakota, Grand Forks, North Dakota 58201

ABSTRACT

Effects of prenatal and postnatal zinc deficiency on the composition of the brain and on subsequent adult behavior were studied. Deficiency throughout the latter third of pregnancy resulted in decreased body and brain size without affecting total brain DNA, RNA, or protein. Adult males that had been subjected to intrauterine zinc deficiency displayed impaired shock avoidance. Zinc deficiency from birth until 21 days of age resulted in impaired growth, decreased brain size, diminished brain DNA, RNA and protein. Cerebellar lipid concentration was also diminished. Such male animals displayed impaired maze acquisition as adults.—SANDSTEAD, H. H., G. J. FOSMIRE, J. M. McKENZIE AND E. S. HALAS. Zinc deficiency and brain development in the rat. *Federation Proc.* 34: 86–88, 1975.

Current evidence suggests that biochemical events early in life can have a profound influence on the subsequent metabolic, physiological and behavioral characteristics of man and animals. To study these interactions we have chosen zinc deficiency in the rat as a model. Zinc deficiency seems particularly well suited for such studies because zinc is essential for the synthesis of nucleic acids (5, 16, 18, 19, 21, 22, 25) and protein (8, 12, 23, 24). In addition, the study of zinc deficiency in early life has practical implications, as there is evidence that some women do not consume optimal amounts of zinc during pregnancy (7).

[1] From Session IV, *Aging of homeostatic control systems*, of the FASEB Conference on *Biology of Development and Aging*, presented at the 58th Annual Meeting of the Federation of American Societies for Experimental Biology, Atlantic City, N. J., April 10, 1974.

[2] Supported in part by the USDA Cooperative Agreement 12-14-100-11, 178 (61), Amend. 1.

[3] Public Health Service, International Research Fellow.

167

In this paper we will summarize our observations on the abnormalities that occur when rats are exposed to zinc deficiency either during the latter third of gestation (6, 7, 13) or throughout the suckling period (1–3, 10, 18).

METHODS

Zinc deficiency was produced by feeding a biotin-enriched, 20% sprayed egg white diet containing <1.0 ppm zinc (2, 11) to dams from the 15th through the 21st day of gestation or from delivery through the 21st postnatal day. Zinc-adequate, pair-fed and ad libitum-fed dams were included in all experiments. The pair-fed and ad libitum-fed control animals were fed the same diet as the zinc-deficient animals. They were given supplemental zinc in their drinking water at a concentration of 50 or 100 ppm. The pair-fed animals were fed an amount of diet equivalent to the amount eaten by the zinc-deficient animals on the previous day. Thus they experienced semistarvation because, with the onset of zinc deficiency in the deficient group, the

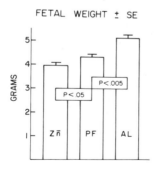

Figure 1. Effect of zinc deficiency (Zn) and of pair-feeding (PF) during the latter third of pregnancy on fetal weight (13). AL, ad lib-fed controls.

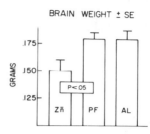

Figure 2. Effect of zinc deficiency and of pair-feeding during the latter third of pregnancy on fetal brain weight (13). Symbols as in Fig. 1.

typical anorexia and restriction of dietary intake occurred. Brains of pups were analyzed biochemically at intervals, and behavioral studies were done on rehabilitated young adult male offspring.

RESULTS

Zinc deprivation during the latter third of gestation (13) resulted in retarded fetal growth (Fig. 1) (zinc deficient versus pair fed, $P < 0.05$) which was greater than that which occurred as a consequence of pair feeding (pair fed versus ad libitum fed, $P < 0.005$). Brain weight of the zinc-deprived fetuses was less than that of either control group (Fig. 2) ($P < 0.05$). The total DNA, RNA and protein levels in the brains were not affected. On the other hand the concentrations of DNA, RNA and protein were increased in the zinc-deficient and pair-fed fetuses compared to normal fetuses. This finding may indirectly reflect an impaired synthesis of brain lipid in these two groups, as has been reported previously for the cerebellum of zinc-deficient and pair-fed suckling rats (18).

Postnatal zinc deficiency from birth through the 21st day of gestation (1, 3) resulted in growth depres-

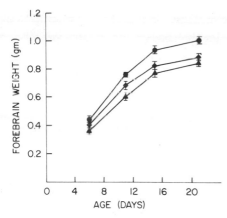

Figure 3. Effect of postnatal zinc deficiency and of semistarvation in the dam on weight of pups forebrain, ±SEM. Weights were derived from 12 brains in each group at 6 days, 8 in each group at 11 and 16 days, and 14 in each group at 21 days. Pups drawn from at least two litters for each test group are represented by each time point. The experimental groups are indicated by: ● — ● ad libitum controls; ◆ — ◆ pair-fed controls; ▲ — ▲ zinc deficient (1, 2).

polymerase was decreased by zinc deficiency (1), a finding consistent with earlier observations on liver (25). Preliminary work has also shown that the RNase activity of the forebrain (active, total and acid) was not increased by zinc deficiency (1). These latter findings are in conflict with observations reported on other tissues (15, 23), but are consonant with findings on the liver (4).

On the 12th postnatal day thymidine incorporation into DNA and sulfur incorporation into the trichloroacetic acid-precipitable fraction of the brain were reduced in brains of the zinc-deficient pups (18). Measurement of cerebellar lipids revealed that total lipids were decreased in the zinc-deficient animals (18).

Behavioral studies on the rehabilitated young adult males suggested that persistent adverse effects had been produced by the dietary manipulations. Shock avoidance condi-

sion (Figs. 3, 4). Pups of pair-fed dams were similarly affected. Zinc deficiency appeared to have a more adverse effect on forebrain growth and DNA content than did pair-feeding ($P < 0.05$), but pair-feeding also resulted in a decrease in these two parameters ($P < 0.05$). RNA content of the forebrain was also adversely affected by zinc deficiency as was protein content. Brains of the zinc-deficient pups contained less protein per milligram of DNA than did the brains of the pups nursed by the pair-fed control dams ($P < 0.05$) (2).

Sucrose density gradient profiles of brain polysomes showed that the ratio of monosomes to polysomes was increased in the zinc-deficient sucklings after 5 days of deficiency (1, 2). Preliminary studies have shown that the activity of brain RNA

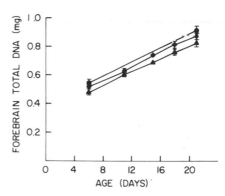

Figure 4. Effect of postnatal zinc deficiency and of starvation in the dam on the total DNA content of pup forebrain, ±SEM. The values are the means of 8 individual determinations at 6 days of age and 4 individual determinations at subsequent ages. The brains were obtained from two or more litters at each time point. The experimental groups are indicated as in Fig. 3 (1, 2).

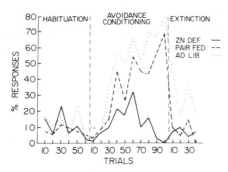

Figure 5. Effect of zinc deficiency and of pair-feeding during the latter third of pregnancy on avoidance conditioning of adult male offspring. Ten animals were used in each group. The animals were exposed to a 1 mA shock (6, 7).

tioning (6,7) was impaired ($P < 0.01$) by intrauterine zinc deficiency during the latter third of gestation (Fig. 5). A marginal effect on maze learning ($P = 0.06$) was observed in the zinc-deficient group (9). Avoidance was also decreased in the animals that had experienced intrauterine

starvation as a consequence of the dams being pair fed ($P < 0.05$). The animals that had been zinc deficient were also less tolerant of the 1 mA shock. Both the zinc-deficient and pair-fed groups extinguished avoidance better than did the normal controls ($P < 0.01$). They also were less active during the habituation period ($P < 0.01$).

Postnatal zinc deficiency was found to impair the acquisition (Fig. 6) of an elevated Tolman-Honzig maze ($P < 0.01$) (9, 10). The effect did not appear related to motivation as running times were similar in all three groups of animals.

DISCUSSION

These adverse effects of zinc deficiency on the brain support the hypothesis that the performance of an adult may be profoundly affected by nutritional and biochemical events that take place during the early development. Though we do not as yet understand the relation-

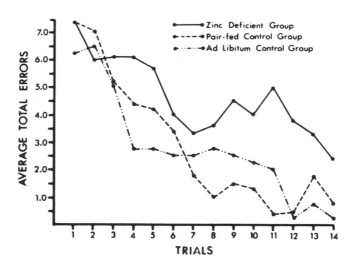

Figure 6. Effect of postnatal zinc deficiency and of semistarvation in the dam on acquisi-

tion of an elevated Tolman-Honzig maze by adult male offspring (10).

ship between the biochemical abnormalities and the behavioral findings, an association seems clear. We suspect that zinc deficiency during the critical period for brain growth not only decreases the total cellularity of the brain, but may also interfere with myelination and the formation of interconnections between neurons. Conceivably the "metabolic programming" which seems to occur during intrauterine and neonatal life may also be impaired.

In our introduction we suggest that our studies may have relevance to man. At present little is known about the zinc requirements of the human fetus. It has been estimated that approximately 750 µg of zinc must be retained daily by the pregnant woman during the latter half of pregnancy (17). To satisfy these needs the National Research Council has recommended that pregnant women consume 20 mg of zinc daily (14). This level substantially exceeds the amounts consumed by some women in the United States (17). It is unknown whether any of these women or their offspring experience undesirable effects from their presumed suboptimal intake of zinc.

A second condition for which these findings in experimental animals may be relevant is protein–calorie malnutrition in infants. Zinc deficiency has been reported in such infants (20). On the basis of our understanding of the importance of zinc for protein utilization (24) it seems possible that zinc deficiency may compound the effects of protein deprivation, and may in fact be partly responsible for the behavioral abnormalities that appear to be sequelae of severe protein–calorie malnutrition.

REFERENCES

1. FOSMIRE, G. J., Y. Y. AL-UBAIDI, E. S. HALAS AND H. H. SANDSTEAD. Proceedings of the ACS symposium on protein-metal interactions. *Adv. Exptl. Med. Biol.* 48: 329–345, 1974.
2. FOSMIRE, G. J., Y. Y. AL-UBAIDI AND H. H. SANDSTEAD. Some effects of postnatal zinc deficiency on developing rat brain. *Pediat. Res.* In press.
3. FOSMIRE, G. J., AND H. H. SANDSTEAD. Some effects of zinc deficiency on postnatal cerebellar development in the rat. *Federation Proc.* 33: 662, 1974.
4. FOSMIRE, M. A., G. J. FOSMIRE AND H. H. SANDSTEAD. Effects of zinc deficiency on polysomes. *Federation Proc.* 33: 699, 1974.
5. GREY, P. C., AND I. E. DREOSTI. Deoxyribonucleic acid and protein metabolism in zinc-deficient rats. *J. Comp. Pathol.* 82: 223–228, 1972.
6. HALAS, E. S., M. C. ROWE, O. R. JOHNSON, J. M. MCKENZIE AND H. H. SANDSTEAD. Effects of intra-uterine zinc-deficiency on subsequent behavior. In: *International Symposium on Trace Elements in Human Health and Disease,* edited by A. S. Prasad. New York: The Nutrition Foundation. In press.
7. HALAS, E. S., AND H. H. SANDSTEAD. Some effects of prenatal zinc deficiency on behavior of the adult rat. *Pediat. Res.* In press.
8. HSU, J. M., W. L. ANTHONY AND P. J. BUCHANAN. Zinc deficiency and incorporation of ^{14}C-labeled methionine into tissue proteins in rats. *J. Nutr.* 99: 425–432, 1969.
9. LOKKEN, P. M. Maze acquisition in the zinc deficient rat. M.S. Thesis. Grand Forks: Univ. of North Dakota, 1979.
10. LOKKEN, P. M., E. S. HALAS AND H. H. SANDSTEAD. Influence of zinc deficiency on behavior. *Proc. Soc. Exptl. Biol. Med.* 144: 680–682, 1973.
11. LUECKE, R. W., M. E. OLMAN AND B. V. BALTZER. Zinc deficiency in the rat: Effect on serum and intestinal alkaline phosphatase activities. *J. Nutr.* 94: 344–350, 1968.
12. MACAPINLAC, M. P., W. N. PEARSON, G. H. BARNEY AND W. J. DARBY. Protein and nucleic acid metabolism in the testes of zinc-deficient rats. *J. Nutr.* 95: 569–577, 1968.
13. MCKENZIE, J. M., G. J. FOSMIRE AND H. H. SANDSTEAD. Zinc deficiency in the prenatal rat. *Proc. N. Dakota Acad. Sci.* In press.
14. NRC/NAS Recommended Dietary Allowances, 1973.
15. PRASAD, A. S., AND D. OBERLEAS. Ribonuclease and deoxyribonuclease activities in zinc-deficient tissues. *J. Lab. Clin. Med.* 82: 461–466, 1973.

16. RUBIN, H. Inhibition of DNA synthesis in animal cells by ethylene diamine tetraacetate and its reversal by zinc. *Proc. Natl. Acad. Sci. U.S.* 69: 712–716, 1972.

17. SANDSTEAD, H. H. Zinc nutrition in the United States. *Am. J. Clin. Nutr.* 26: 1251–1260, 1973.

18. SANDSTEAD, H. H., D. D. GILLESPIE AND R. N. BRADY. Zinc deficiency: Effect on brain of the suckling rat. *Pediat. Res.* 6: 119–125, 1972.

19. SANDSTEAD, H. H., AND R. A. RINALDI. Impairment of deoxyribonucleic acid synthesis by dietary zinc deficiency in the rat. *J. Cellular Phys.* 73: 81–84, 1969.

20. SANDSTEAD, H. H., A. S. SHUKRY, A. S. PRASAD, M. K. GABR, A. EL HIFNEY, N. MOKHTAR AND W. J. DARBY. Kwashiorkor in Egypt. I. Clinical and biochemical studies, with special reference to plasma zinc and serum lactic dehydrogenase. *Am. J. Clin. Nutr.* 17: 15–26, 1965.

21. SCRUTTON, M. C., C. W. WU AND D. A. GOLDTHWAIT. The presence and possible role of zinc in RNA polymerase obtained from *Escherichia coli*. *Proc. Natl. Acad. Sci. U.S.* 68: 2497–2501, 1971.

22. SLATER, J. P., A. S. MILDVAN AND A. LOEB. Zinc in DNA polymerase. *Biochem. Biophys. Res. Comm.* 44: 37–43, 1971.

23. SOMERS, M., AND E. J. UNDERWOOD. Ribonuclease activity and nucleic acid and protein metabolism in the testes of zinc-deficient rats. *Australian J. Biol. Sci.* 22: 1277–1281, 1969.

24. SOMERS, M., AND E. J. UNDERWOOD. Studies of zinc nutrition in sheep. II. The influence of zinc deficiency in ram lambs upon the digestibility of the dry matter and the utilization of the nitrogen and sulphur of the diet. *Australian J. Agr. Res.* 20: 899, 1969.

25. TERHUNE, M. W., AND H. H. SANDSTEAD. Decreased RNA polymerase activity in mammalian zinc deficiency. *Science* 177: 68–69, 1972.

Neuronal–glial interactions during development and aging[1]

ANTONIA VERNADAKIS[2]

Departments of Psychiatry and Pharmacology

University of Colorado School of Medicine, Denver, Colorado 80220

ABSTRACT

Integration of the central nervous system is an expression of cerebral homeostasis that is essential for the internal ability of the organism to adapt to its changing environment throughout life. It is generally accepted that neurons undergo no further division after differentiation, whereas glial cells continue to proliferate throughout life. The increase in glial cells with advanced age may reflect a compensatory process of the brain to overcome neuronal loss or neuronal functional changes that may occur with age. Therefore, these neuronal–glial interactions during development and aging may play a key role in the integrative capacity of the brain. One of the mechanisms contributing to brain stability is the blood–brain barrier, which regulates the neuronal-glial microenvironment in the mature organism. Neuronal intercommunication is mediated via neurotransmitter substances and a shift may occur from excitation to inhibition and vice versa in some CNS areas with aging. Studies of some aspects of cholinergic, monoaminergic and amino acid neurotransmission show that their maturational patterns are CNS-area specific and that some neurotransmitter processes decline with advanced age. Glial cells, besides participating in the regulation of extraneuronal environment, are also proposed to be involved in neurotransmission mechanisms in the adult and aging CNS and since they are the major CNS cellular compartment that changes with age they may thus contribute significantly to the maintenance of CNS integrative ability and adaptation with age.—VERNADAKIS, A. Neuronal–glial interactions during development and aging. *Federation Proc.* 34: 89–95, 1975.

Neurons and glial cells are the structural units of the central nervous system, and their combined activity controls not only the complex functions of the higher organism, but also may underlie the integrative capacity of the organism. Central nervous system integration is an expression of cerebral homeostasis, and contributes to the internal

[1] From Session IV, *Aging of homeostatic control systems,* of the FASEB Conference on *Biology of Development and Aging,* presented at the 58th Annual Meeting of the Federation of American Societies for Experimental Biology, Atlantic City, N. J., April 10, 1974.

[2] Recipient of a Research Scientist Development Award KO2 MH-42479 from the National Institute of Mental Health.

Abbreviations: BuChe, butyrylcholinesterase; AChe, acetylcholinesterase; ChA, choline acetyltransferase.

ability of the organism to adapt to its changing environment. From a functional point of view, a similarity exists in the maturing and aging nervous system in that at both extremes of the life span CNS integration may not be adequate. This paper discusses the hypothesis that CNS integration, an expression of cerebral homeostasis, is determined by the neuronal–glial microenvironmental interrelationships. Evidence is presented that the balance of these brain cellular compartments changes with aging and thus may modify brain function and, in turn, total homeostasis.

NEURON–GLIA DISTRIBUTION WITH AGE

Despite the occurrence of mitotic activity after birth in some regions of the CNS (1, 2), it can be stated generally that neurons undergo no

further division after differentiation, whereas glial cells continue to proliferate throughout life (3). It is almost universally accepted that when neurons are lost they are not replaced by division of the remaining cells. In the cerebellum, approximately 20% loss of Purkinje cells in the aged rat has been reported (16). In contrast to this decrease in Purkinje cells in the aged rat, Brizzee and associates (3) have found no significant decreases in neuron density in the cerebral cortex. These authors, however, do not preclude the possibility that loss of neurons may occur at older age levels or in other CNS regions. Studies from our laboratory show that in both the cerebral hemisphere and cerebellum of chicks, DNA content decreases after 20 mo posthatching (Fig. 1, 2) (35). Based on the premise that DNA is located almost exclusively within the nucleus and is constant in amount within the diploid nucleus of

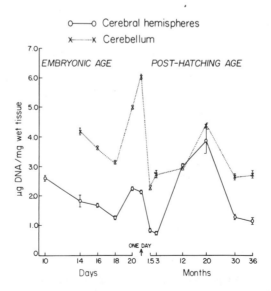

Figure 1. Changes in DNA content (μg/mg wet tissue) in the cerebral hemispheres and cerebellum of chicks during embryonic age (days) and post-hatching age (months). Points with bracketed vertical lines represent means ± standard errors. (From Vernadakis (32).)

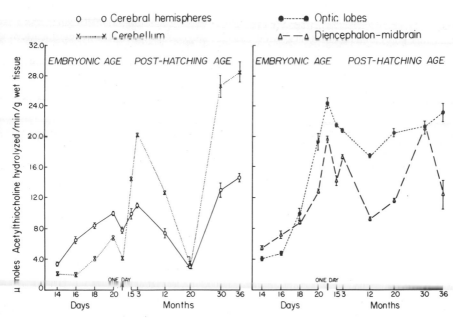

Figure 2. Changes in acetylcholinesterase activity expressed as μmoles of acetylthiocholine hydrolyzed per minute per gram wet tissue in the cerebral hemispheres and cerebellum of chicks during embryonic age (days) and post-hatching (months). Points as in Fig. 1. (From Vernadakis (33).)

a resting cell of any species (23), DNA content has been interpreted to reflect cell density. Thus, during early embryonic development, the decrease in DNA content observed in both the cerebral hemispheres and cerebellum (Fig. 1) reflects a decrease in cell density due to the growth in cell size, i.e., cell body and dendritic branching known to occur with maturation (4, 38). Correspondingly, the high rise in DNA content of the cerebellum between 20 days of embryonic age and 1 day after hatching is interpreted to reflect the marked increase in cell density, predominantly of granular cells and glial cells, during this period (11). Glial cell proliferation during this period is also evident from the marked increase· in the activity of butyrylcholinesterase (BuChe), an

enzyme predominantly found in glial cells (10), between 18 days of embryonic age and 1 day after hatching (32). The activity of BuChe also increases markedly in both the cerebral hemispheres and cerebellum of chicks from 20 mo up to 36 mo posthatching.

The increase in glial cells with aging is postulated to represent a compensatory process of the brain to overcome morphologic and functional neuronal loss or neuronal changes occurring with age. Such inverse relationships in neuronal–glial elements have been reported during various physiological states of CNS function (15). A time sequence and pattern of neuron–glial changes have also been shown in parkinsonism. Not only is parkinsonism manifested in older individuals, but some of its symptoms, such as the characteristic tremor-like phenomena, frequently occur in senile persons. Consequently, changes in neuronal–glial relationships in the specific extrapyramidal structures involved in the disease may be extrapolated to explain some of the alterations in motor function associated with old age. In biopsy material from the globus pallidus of patients suffering from parkinsonism, the large nerve cells and the surrounding glia were analyzed for RNA (15). At a very early stage of the disease, a highly aberrant RNA is found in the glia, whereas neuronal RNA at this time is less changed. The adenine value is greatly increased and that of guanine and uracil is decreased, and these changes persist for years. During the development of the disease, from the time the overt clinical symptoms emerge and progress, similar but less marked changes occur in neuronal RNA. Thus, to judge from the time sequence, the biochemical error first develops in the glia, which then seem to influence neurons both biochemically and functionally.

BLOOD–BRAIN BARRIER WITH AGE

It has long been suggested that the composition of the microenvironment of brain cells is maintained within closer limits than that of other tissue. This stability is supposed to be important for normal functioning of the nervous system, and to involve not only maintenance of a rather constant composition, but also the exclusion of harmful agents. The controlling mechanism of this microcellular stability is the blood–brain barrier. Functionally, the blood–brain barrier should be regarded as a system limiting the free exchange between blood and brain; it further

exerts its function on transport processes essential for the nutrition of the brain and on those involving the opposite direction from the brain into the blood. The blood–brain barrier is also effective as an intermediate system in humoral regulations of peripheral vegetative functions.

Early studies by Vernadakis and Woodbury (39) have shown that the development of the blood–brain barrier is a function of the neuronal–glial and interstitial compartments. During brain maturation the volume of the glial compartment increases at the expense of the interstitial and neuronal compartments. Also the permeabilities of the capillary–interstitial and the interstitial–glial interfaces decrease with development, whereas the permeability of the interstitial–neuronal interface does not change. The authors concluded that the development of the blood–brain barrier is due to age-dependent changes, both in the volume of cellular and extracellular compartments and in the permeabilities of these compartments. Recent work by Woodbury and associates (42) has shown that the relation between the cerebrospinal fluid (CSF) and the extracellular fluid of the brain is important in the development and function of the blood–brain barrier. The studies they report demonstrate that there is an intimate relationship between the CSF and the extracellular fluid of the brain.

That the blood–brain barrier regulates the stability of the brain is demonstrated in its implication in the development of kernicterus, resulting in mental retardation. It was recognized early that bilirubin staining of certain portions of the brain, particularly that of the basal ganglia, can frequently be seen in icteric newborn. On the other hand, adults, even with severe and long-lasting jaundice, do not show any bilirubin deposits in the CNS, except for that of the choroid plexuses and CSF. One of the explanations for this age difference with respect to the deposition of bile pigments is that the newborn brain is physiologically underdeveloped and its blood–brain barrier is more permeable, in contrast to the fully developed and "leakproof" blood–brain barrier of the mature brain.

Systematic studies of the blood–brain barrier mechanisms in the aging brain have not been reported. However, one can assume that such alterations may occur since glial cells proliferate and water decreases with advanced age (29), thus possibly re-

sulting in a decrease in extracellular space. Additionally, changes in the permeability of the cerebral capillaries with aging (29) can contribute to alterations of the blood–brain barrier at this time.

NEUROTRANSMITTER CHANGES WITH AGE

One of the biochemical substrates underlying integrative capacity in the maturating and aging CNS is that responsible for neurotransmission. Regardless of the speed with which information is transmitted from neuron-to-neuron or neuron-to-glia-to-neuron, it is assumed to involve neurotransmitter substances.

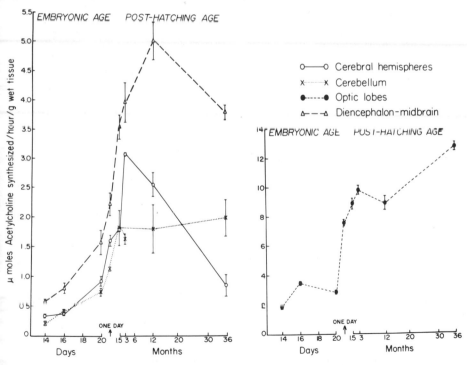

Figure 3. Changes in choline acetyltransferase activity expressed as μmoles of acetylcholine synthesized per hour per gram wet tissue in the four CNS structures of chicks during embryonic age (days) and post-hatching (months). Points as in Fig. 1. (From Vernadakis (33).)

Some aspects of cholinergic, mono-aminergic, and amino acid neuro-transmission and the changes oc-curring during development and aging will be discussed.

Cholinergic system

The activities of acetylcholinesterase (AChe) and choline acetyltransferase (ChA), the hydrolyzing and synthe-sizing enzymes of acetylcholine (ACh), respectively, have been used as indexes of cholinergic neuro-transmission. In the chick, the activity of AChe increases markedly in both the cerebral hemispheres and cere-bellum from embryonic age up to 3 mo after hatching, and from 20 mo up to 36 mo posthatching (Fig. 2) (33). The activity of ChA increases in the cerebral hemispheres up to 3 mo after hatching (Fig. 3), and then decreases reaching embryonic levels by 3 yr; in the cerebellum ChA increases up to 6 wk posthatching, and then levels off. Studies by

TABLE 1. Changes in choline acetyltrans-ferase activity in CNS areas of the rat with age[a]

Age, months	μMoles of [¹⁴C]acetylcholine synthesized/hour per g wet tissue		
	Cerebellum	Cerebral cortex	Spinal cord
2	0.56 ± 0.05[b] (16)	3.57 ± 0.23 (11)	6.39 ± 0.24 (13)
12	0.62 ± 0.04 (16)	3.65 ± 0.06 (16)	5.85 ± 0.30 (16) $P < 0.01$[c]
20	0.59 ± 0.03 (11)	3.29 ± 0.13 (11)	5.00 ± 0.26 (11) $P < 0.001$[c] $P < 0.05$[d]

[a] From Timiras (29). [b] Values are means ± SE (number of determinations shown in parentheses; one determination per animal.) [c] Significance of difference from 2-months-old. [d] Significance of difference from 12- to 14-months-old.

Timiras and associates (29) in the rat have also shown that ChA does not markedly change in the cerebellum and cerebral hemispheres from 2 mo up to 20 mo, whereas it markedly decreases with age in the spinal cord (Table 1). It is now generally ac-cepted that the presence of ChA is a more conclusive index for the pres-ence of ACh. On this basis the low levels of ChA activity in the aging cerebral hemispheres and spinal cord would suggest that cholinergic neurons are at a very low level of activity or have decreased in number.

Acetylcholinesterase has been proposed to have a dual function during maturation. Filogamo and Marchisio (9) speculate that the early ACh system, namely ACh itself, ChA and AChe, may be one of the path-ways involved in some way in the complex process of nervous system development through mechanisms that are not yet adapted to synaptic transmission. We further propose from our findings that the sharp rise in AChe activity with aging, particu-larly in cerebral hemispheres (Fig. 2), may present a function of AChe other that its role in neurotransmis-sion processes. For example, one can visualize the ACh system having a humoral function during aging and thus explain the high levels of AChe. The low levels of ChA in the cere-bral hemispheres during aging reflect a decrease in cholinergic neurons, a finding which supports the idea of a humoral role for AChe at this life stage.

Since glial cells markedly prolifer-ate during aging, another possibility that could explain the high levels of AChe is that glial cells may also contain AChe. Although Giacobini (10) has reported that glial cells do not contain specific ChE (AChe), the possibility that some AChe may be present in glial cells has not been

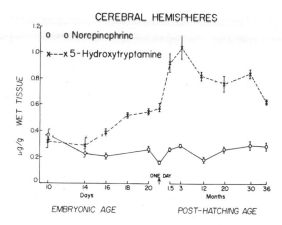

Figure 4. Changes in endogenous norepinephrine and 5-hydroxytryptamine expressed as μgrams per gram wet tissue in the cerebral hemispheres of chicks during embryonic age (days) and post-hatching (months). Points as in Fig. 1. (From Vernadakis (33).)

entirely excluded (12). Studies in our laboratory (37) using neurons and glial cells obtained through cell fractionation of chick cerebral hemispheres indicate that glial cells contain some AChe and that BuChe is higher in the glia than in the neurons as also reported by Giacobini (10). Moreover, glial cells in the aging CNS may display entirely different biochemical properties, including AChe, than those in the young or adult CNS. Such a shift in the role of glial cells during aging was discussed earlier.

Monoaminergic system

Total level of norepinephrine and 5-hydroxytryptamine with age

Three important putative neurotransmitter substances in the brain are ethylamine derivatives; two are catechol compounds, norepinephrine and dopamine and the third is an indole amine, 5-hydroxytryptamine. The maturational and aging changes in the levels of norepinephrine and 5-hydroxytryptamine in the cerebral hemispheres and cerebellum of the chick are presented in Fig. 4 and 5 (33). Beginning with high levels at 10 days of embryonic age, norepinephrine does not significantly change with age. In contrast, 5-hydroxytryptamine reaches peak activity at 3 mo posthatching and slightly decreases thereafter. In the cerebellum norepinephrine reaches peak activity at 3 mo posthatching whereas 5-hydroxytryptamine remains generally at a high level throughout embryonic age and posthatching. The high levels of 5-hydroxytryptamine in the early embryonic cerebellum and of norepinephrine in the cerebral hemispheres suggest that these two amines may have other functions than their proposed role in neurotransmission. Moreover, these findings suggest that the neurohumor involved in early cellular growth may differ from one CNS area to another, i.e., 5-hydroxytryptamine in the cerebellum, norepinephrine in the cerebral hemispheres. Monoamines have been proposed to have important functions during embryogenesis and may be involved in biochemical cellular differentiation (38).

If it is assumed that the levels of norepinephrine and 5-hydroxytryptamine represent noradrenergic and serotonergic neurons, respectively, then the finding that neither neurotransmitter level decreases with aging supports the view that nerve cell loss may be restricted to a few very specific cell types such as Purkinje cells of the cerebellum, the pyramidal cells of the cerebral cortex, and the motoneurons of the spinal cord, and that there are not significant overall losses of neurons (5).

Uptake and storage of norepinephrine with age

To further understand the maturation and aging of the monoaminergic system we have studied two processes that are involved in the storage of norepinephrine in the cerebral hemispheres and cerebellum of chickens during embryonic development and aging (34). In order to be stored within noradrenergic nerves, exogenous norepinephrine is first taken up across the neuronal

membrane and subsequently is taken up across the membrane of the storage granule in which it is stored. Slices from mammalian cerebral cortex have provided useful model systems for the study of the uptake, storage and metabolism of norepinephrine (21, 27, 28).

Uptake of ^{3}H-norepinephrine was measured in slices taken from the cerebral hemispheres or cerebellum of chicks ranging from 10 days of embryonic age up to 3 yr after hatching (Fig. 6 and 7). Uptake was studied in the presence and absence of cocaine, an agent known to inhibit neuronal uptake, and storage was studied in the presence and absence of reserpine, an agent that inhibits uptake of biogenic amines into storage granules. Accumulation of ^{3}H-norepinephrine increases during brain maturation and is attributed to maturation of the uptake and storage processes which appear to develop earlier in the cerebellum than in the cerebral hemispheres (Fig. 6 and 7). Although the endogenous level of norepinephrine is high in the cerebral hemispheres at 10 days of embryonic age (Fig. 4), these data

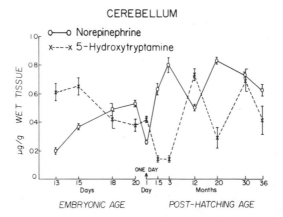

Figure 5. As in Fig. 4, except that the CNS structure is cerebellum.

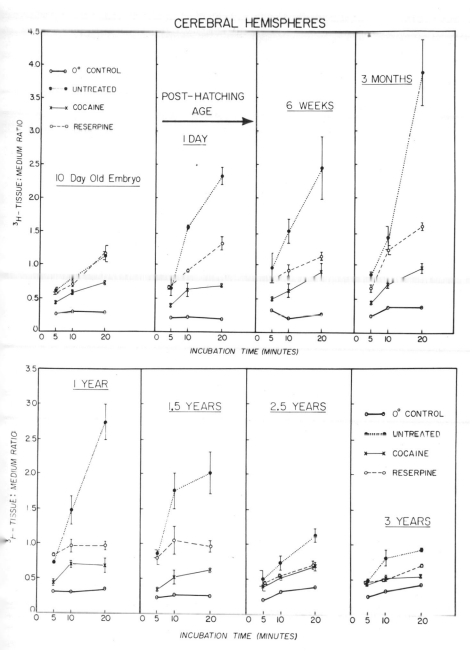

Figure 6. Uptake of ^{3}H-norepinephrine into slices of cerebral hemispheres taken from chick embryos at 10 days of age and from chicks at 1 day, 6 weeks, 3 months, and 1, 1.5, 2.5 and 3 years of age. The effects of cocaine (10 μg/ml) and reserpine (10^{-6}M) are illustrated. Results represent means ± SEM for five or six determinations. (From Vernadakis (34).)

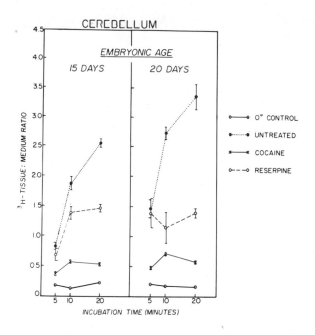

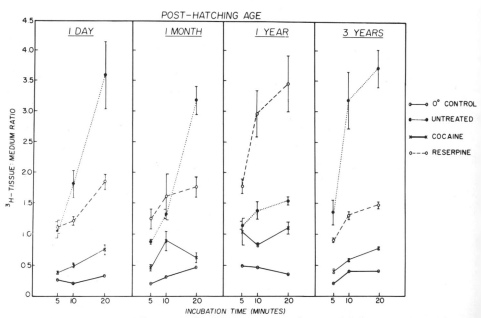

Figure 7. As in Fig. 6, except that uptake of ^{3}H-norepinephrine was into slices of cerebellum taken from chick embryos at 15 and 20 days, and from chicks at 1 day, 1 month and 1 and 3 years of age.

show that accumulation of ³H-norepinephrine is barely detectable in 10-day chick embryos (Fig. 6).

The decline in ³H-norepinephrine accumulation in the cerebral hemispheres of chicks with aging (Fig. 6) may represent neuronal loss as well as changes in uptake and storage processes with age. In contrast, the continued high ⁰H-norepinephrine accumulation in the cerebellum with aging (Fig. 7) reflects active uptake and storage processes and also maintenance of adrenergic neurons with age. It is of importance to recall here that the activity of ChA, the synthesizing enzyme of ACh, markedly declines with age in the cerebral hemispheres, but not in the cerebellum of chicks (Fig. 3). Thus, both adrenergic and cholinergic function, presumably excitatory, appears intact in the aging cerebellum of chicks and also of rats, as reported by Timiras and associates (29).

Extraneuronal uptake of norepinephrine

The continuous increase in ³H-norepinephrine accumulation during brain maturation is interpreted to reflect both maturation of the neuronal uptake and storage processes and possible accumulation of ³H-norepinephrine in glial cells. Evidence that norepinephrine accumulates in glial cells has been reported by Henn and Hamberger (14), who found that glial cell-enriched brain fractions accumulate norepinephrine in vitro. Iversen (17) has reported extraneuronal uptake (Uptake₂) of norepinephrine in the peripheral nervous system with different affinity properties from those of neuronal uptake (Uptake₁).

The role of glial cells in neurotransmission mechanisms is speculative at present. The fate of norepinephrine in the CNS and the proposed role of glial cells in norepinephrine metabolism is illustrated in Fig. 8 (35). When norepinephrine is released upon stimulation (Step 1 in Fig. 8), it acts on the postsynaptic factor (Step 2); norepinephrine may be inactivated by the reuptake process (Step 3); it may be degraded by catechol-*O*-methyltransferase (Step 4); the proposal is put forward here that norepinephrine also may be taken up by the glial cells (Step 5).

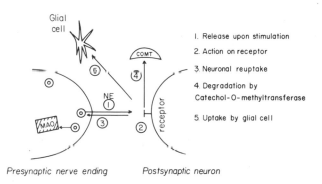

Glial cell

1. Release upon stimulation
2. Action on receptor
3. Neuronal reuptake
4. Degradation by Catechol-O-methyltransferase
5. Uptake by glial cell

COMT NE MAO

Presynaptic nerve ending   Postsynaptic neuron

Figure 8. A diagrammatic representation of the fate of norepinephrine in the central nervous system. (See text for details.) (From Vernadakis (35).)

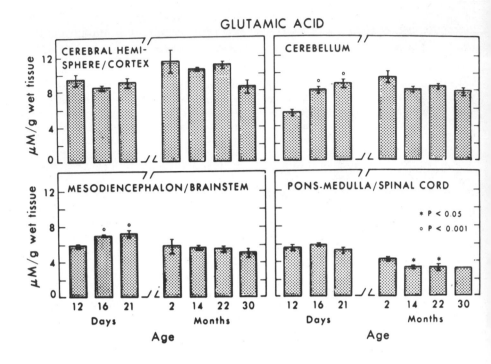

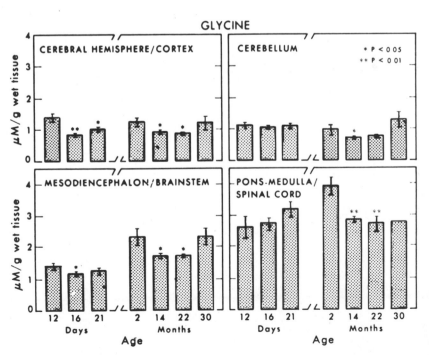

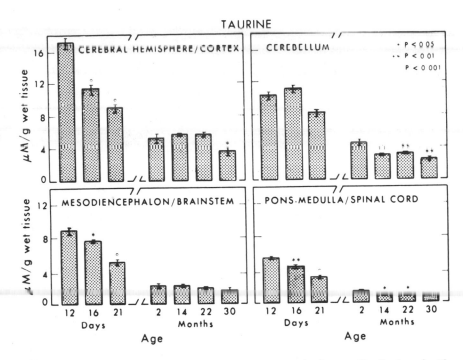

Figure 9. Glutamic acid (upper), glycine (middle), and taurine (lower) levels in μM/g wet tissue in selected CNS regions in rats at seven ages ranging from 12 days to 30 months of age. Bars with bracketed lines represent the mean ± standard errors. For P values the 16- and 21-day-old groups were compared with the 12-day-old group; all of the older groups were compared with the 2-month-old group. (From Timiras (30).)

Finally, it is proposed that glial cells modulate the level of brain excitability by their participation on neurotransmission mechanisms. For example, it is known that cortisol increases brain excitability (40, 41). The effect may be mediated via the action of cortisol on accumulation of norepinephrine in glial cells. Preliminary studies from this laboratory (36) have shown that cortisol inhibits the uptake of norepinephrine in neural explants removed from 16-day-old chick embryos and maintained in culture. We speculate that cortisol may affect extraneuronal uptake (glial cells) of norepinephrine since it occurs only with high concentrations of norepinephrine in the incubation medium. As shown by Iversen (17), extraneuronal uptake in the peripheral nervous system occurs with high concentrations of norepinephrine, and Iversen and Salt (18) have reported that cortisol inhibits extraneuronal uptake in the rat heart. Inhibition of norepinephrine uptake by cortisol in glial cells would result in high concentration of norepinephrine in the synaptic cleft to act on the postsynaptic receptor with subsequent enhanced effect. These findings further demonstrate that neuronal-glial interaction influences brain stability.

Amino acid neurotransmitters with age

A considerable volume of evidence suggests that some amino acids may be neurotransmitters in various CNS areas: glycine, γ-aminobutyric acid (GABA), and taurine as inhibitory transmitter substances and glutamic and aspartic acids as excitatory transmitters (6, 7, 13, 20, 22, 27). Changes therefore in these amino acids with age may be reflected on the integrative capacity of the brain with age.

Timiras and associates (30) have recently reported developmental and aging changes in CNS free amino acids in four CNS areas in the rat. Amino acid levels attain adult values according to different timetables specific to each CNS area. Glutamic acid, a proposed excitatory neurotransmitter (13, 20), appears to remain high in both the cerebral hemispheres and cerebellum from early postnatal life up to 30 months of age, whereas it decreases in the spinal cord with aging (Fig. 9). Glycine, proposed as a neurotransmitter in the spinal cord (6), progressively increases during early postnatal life, reaching a high level at 2 mo, decreases at 14 months of age, and remains at this level up to 30 months of age (Fig. 9). In the cerebral hemispheres, glycine is at the same level in rats at 12 days of age and 30 months of age. In contrast, in the cerebellum, glycine content appears to be the highest at 30 months of age (Fig. 9). Thus, it appears that inhibitory function represented in the cerebellum by glycine remains intact with age. However, in view of the known loss of Purkinje cells in the aging cerebellum, one would expect that the cell loss is a decrease in GABA, another inhibitory neurotransmitter (20) known to be in Purkinje cells (24, 25). The authors do not report GABA content in aging rats in this study. Taurine, another proposed inhibitory transmitter (19), is high during early postnatal development

and markedly decreases with aging, especially in the spinal cord (Fig. 9). Timiras and associates (30) suggest that perhaps during early postnatal development taurine may act in a nonspecific way to modulate or suppress the excitability of neuronal membranes, decreasing thereafter when functional inhibitory systems become established. Independently of whether cellular loss accompanies aging, definitive and widespread alterations do occur within the aged cell and may be related to changes in amino acid levels. In the spinal cord, for example, which matures earlier and ages earlier, amino acid levels show the most marked changes, and it is in this structure that others have noted significant morphological and functional deficits with aging (8).

CONCLUSIONS

Cerebral homeostasis is controlled by neuronal–glial cell interrelations and their microenvironment. The development of the blood–brain barrier is an expression of cerebral homeostasis in that it is through this mechanism that the brain can maintain its stability and plasticity throughout life of the organism. Alterations in the blood–brain barrier, such as in disease and in aging because of glial cell proliferation and capillary permeability, disrupt brain stability and may lead to dysfunction.

The biochemical substrates underlying aging of CNS integrative capacity are probably numerous. A primary factor, however, may be changes in neurotransmission mechanisms. Intercommunication of neurons involves neurotransmitter substances, which are synthesized and stored at the presynaptic neuron, are released by the arrival of the impulse and then act on the postsynaptic receptor. The molecular events occuring presynaptically, at the synaptic cleft, or on the postsynaptic membrane are not yet well understood and constitute one of the most intensively studied areas of research. The available evidence suggests that neuronal neurotransmitter uptake processes may not be functioning at optimal levels in the aging organism, i.e., neuronal permeability. Whether a decline in memory phenomena associated with aging can be implicated with maladaptation of neuronal chemical intercommunication remains to be studied.

The proliferation of glial cells with aging is the main cellular change observed, and may be regarded as a compensatory mechanism of the brain to maintain cellular equilibrium. That glial cells can undertake some of the neuronal functions during aging remains to be investigated. However, the available evidence suggests that glial cells may participate in neurotransmission mechanism and thus may modulate brain excitability.

REFERENCES

1. ALTMAN, J. In: *The Neurosciences*, edited by G. C. Quarton, T. Melnechuk and F. O. Schmidt. New York: Rockefeller Univ. Press, 1967, p. 723–743.
2. ALTMAN, J. In: *Handbook of Neurochemistry*, Vol. 2, edited by A. Lajtha. New York: Plenum, 1969, p. 137–182.
3. BRIZZEE, K. R., N. SHERWOOD AND P. S. TIMIRAS. *J. Gerontol.* 23: 289, 1968.
4. BRIZZEE, K. R., J. VOGT AND X. KHARETCHKO. *Progr. Brain Res.* 4: 136, 1964.
5. CRITCHLEY, M. In: *Problems of Aging*, edited by E. V. Cowdry. Baltimore: Williams & Wilkins, 1942.
6. CURTIS, D. R., J. HÖSLI, G. A. R. JOHNSTON AND I. H. JONSTON. *Brain Res.* 5: 112, 1967.
7. CURTIS, D. R., AND G. A. R. JOHNSTON. In: *Handbook of Neurochemistry*, Vol. 4, edited by A. Lajtha. New York: Plenum, 1970, p. 115–134.
8. DUNCAN, D. J. *J. Comp. Neurol.* 59: 47, 1934.
9. FILOGAMO, G., AND P. C. MARCHISIO. *Neurosci. Res.* 4: 29, 1971.
10. GIACOBINI, E. In: *Morphological and Biochemical Correlates of Neural Activity*, edited by M. M. Cohen and R. S. Snider. New York: Harper, 1964, p. 15–38.
11. HANAWAY, J. *J. Comp. Neurol.* 131: 1, 1967.
12. HEBB, C. *Nature* 192: 527, 1961.
13. HEDD, C. *Ann. Rev. Physiol.* 32: 165, 1970.
14. HENN, F. A., AND HAMBERGER, A. *Proc. Natl. Acad. Sci. U.S.* 68: 2686, 1971.
15. HYDÉN, H. In: *The Neurosciences*, edited by G. C. Quarton, T. Melnechuk and F. O. Schmidt. New York: Rockefeller Univ. Press, 1967, p. 765–771.
16. INAKAI, T. *J. Comp. Neurol.* 45: 1, 1928.
17. IVERSEN, L. L. *Brit. J. Pharmacol.* 41: 571, 1971.
18. IVERSEN, L. L., AND P. J. SALT. *Brit. J. Pharmacol.* 40: 528, 1970.
19. JACOBSEN, J. G. AND L. H. SMITH JR. *Physiol. Rev.* 48: 424, 1968.
20. JOHNSON, J. L. *Brain Res.* 37: 1, 1972.
21. KELLOGG, C., A. VERNADAKIS AND C. O. RUTLEDGE. *J. Neurochem.* 18: 1931, 1971.
22. KRNJEVIC, K. *Nature* 228: 119, 1970.
23. MIRSKY, A. E., AND H. RIS. *Nature* 163: 666, 1949.
24. OBATA, K., AND K. TAKEDA. *J. Neurochem.* 16: 1043, 1969.
25. OTSUKA, K., K. OBATA, Y. MIGATA AND Y. TANAKA. *J. Neurochem.* 18: 297, 1971.
26. ROBERTS, E., AND K. KURIYAMA. *Brain Res.* 8: 1, 1968.
27. RUTLEDGE, C. O. *J. Pharmacol. Exptl. Ther.* 171: 188, 1970.
28. RUTLEDGE, C. O., AND J. JONASON. *J. Pharmacol. Exptl. Ther.* 157: 493, 1967.
29. TIMIRAS, P. S. *Developmental Physiology and Aging*. New York: Macmillan, 1972, chapt. 26, p. 502–526.
30. TIMIRAS, P.S., D. B. HUDSON AND S. OKLUND. *Progr. Brain. Res.* 40: 267, 1973.
31. TIMIRAS, P. S., A. VERNADAKIS AND A. SHERWOOD. In: *Biology of Gestation*, edited by N. Assali. New York: Academic, 1968, p. 261–319.
32. VERNADAKIS, A. *J. Gerontology* 28: 281, 1973.
33. VERNADAKIS, A. *Progr. Brain Res.* 40: 1973, p. 231.
34. VERNADAKIS, A. *Mech. Ageing Develop.* 2: 371, 1973.
35. VERNADAKIS, A. In: *Drugs and the Developing Brain*, edited by A. Vernadakis

and N. Weiner. New York: Plenum, 1974, p. 133–148.

36. VERNADAKIS, A. In: *Proceedings of the Mie Conference of the International Society for Psychoneuroendocrinology*, edited by N. Hatotani. New York: Karger. 1974, p. 251–258.

37. VERNADAKIS, A., AND D. A. GIBSON. Abstracts, 4th Int. Mtg. Intern. Soc. Neurochem., Aug. 26–31, 1973, Tokyo, Japan.

38. VERNADAKIS, A., AND D. A. GIBSON. In: *Conferences on the Problems and Priorities in Perinatal Pharmacology*, edited by J. Dancis and J. C. Hwang. New York:

Raven. 1974, p. 65–76.

39. VERNADAKIS, A., AND D. M. WOODBURY. *Arch. Neurol.* 12: 284, 1965.

40. VERNADAKIS, A., AND D. M. WOODBURY. In: *Steroid Hormones and Brain Function*, edited by C. H. Sawyer and R. A. Gorski, UCLA Forum in Medical Sciences: Univ. of California Press, 1971, p. 35–42.

41. VERNADAKIS, A., AND D. M. WOODBURY. In: *Influence of Hormones on the Nervous System*, edited by D. H. Ford. Basel: Karger, 1971, p. 85–97.

42. WOODBURY, D. M. *Progr. Brain Res.* 29: 297, 1968.

Pituitary inhibitor of thyroxine

W. DONNER DENCKLA

Roche Institute of Molecular Biology
Nutley, New Jersey 07110

ABSTRACT

A description is given of a new pituitary function. It is suggested that the new function acts to decrease gradually the responsiveness of the peripheral tissues to thyroid hormones throughout life. It is suggested that the postulated relative hypothyroidism of older animals might contribute to their loss of viability. — Denckla, W. D. Pituitary inhibitor of thyroxine. *Federation Proc.* 34: 96, 1975.

The hypothesis that hypothyroidism might contribute to the pathogenesis of old age has been considered earlier in this century and more recently has been discredited (1). Originally the hypothesis was formulated because of the striking similarity between some of the symptoms of hypothyroidism in young persons and the symptoms of "normal" old age. In addition a supposedly specific assay for the thyroid state of the peripheral tissues, the basal metabolic rate (BMR), was found to decline with age. The hypothesis was discredited because: *a)* treatment of older persons with thyroid hormones failed to restore youthful vigor, *b)* the BMR was found to be a nonspecific test, and *c)* plasma levels of free thyroid hormones were found to be relatively constant throughout life.

The discovery of a new function of the pituitary and a new physiological parameter, minimal O_2 consumption (MOC), tends to weaken the arguments against the original hypothesis.

MINIMAL O_2 CONSUMPTION

In extensive experiments with most of the major known endocrine hormones and their secretory glands, the MOC, unlike the BMR, was found to be a relatively specific assay for the thyroid state of peripheral tissues (2). However, the MOC, like the BMR, also declined with age (1).

---

[1] From Session IV, *Aging of homeostatic control systems*, of the FASEB Conference on *Biology of Development and Aging*, presented at the 58th Annual Meeting of the Federation of American Societies for Experimental Biology, Atlantic City, N.J., April 10, 1974.

PITUITARY FACTOR

In a series of endocrine ablation and replacement experiments it was concluded that most of the age-associated decline in the MOC could be attributed to a new function of the pituitary (1). Partial isolation of the active material from bovine pituitaries has been accomplished (1).

Experiments with the pituitary factor suggested the following model. At the onset of puberty the pituitary appears to secrete in significant amounts a material which gradually throughout life depresses the response of peripheral tissues to endogenous thyroid hormones. This conclusion was drawn from experiments with rats in which it was shown that the response to either thyroxine (T_4) or triiodothyronine (T_3) was decreased approximately threefold with advancing age as determined by the effects on MOC. Removal of the pituitary in adult rats restored the response to the hormones and injection of a pituitary fraction into prepuberally hypophysectomized rats depressed the response.

It is suggested that in the presence of a postulated antagonist to the peripheral effects of thyroid hormones it is not surprising that thyroid hormone administration failed to rejuvenate the elderly. In addition, if such an antagonist exists, constant plasma levels of the thyroid hormones cannot be used as a criterion for euthyroidism. It is apparent that much more data must be obtained to indicate whether the pituitary factor depresses other thyroid-dependent functions necessary for life as it depresses the MOC.

REFERENCES

1. DENCKLA, W. D. *J. Clin. Invest.* 53: 572, 1974.
2. DENCKLA, W. D. *Endocrinology* 93: 61, 1973.

Bioenergetic functions of sleep and activity rhythms and their possible relevance to aging[1,2]

RALPH J. BERGER

Thimann Laboratories
University of California, Santa Cruz 95060

ABSTRACT

The hypothesis is proposed that sleep constitutes a period of dormancy in which energy is conserved to partially offset the increased energy demands of homeothermy. Phylogenetic data indicate that the complete physiological and behavioral manifestations of sleep are unique to homeotherms; furthermore "ontogeny recapitulates phylogeny" in the parallel development of slow wave sleep and thermoregulation as exemplified in the opossum. Thus, sleep constitutes a state of reduced metabolism that may represent a variation on the theme of dormancy, functionally lying on a continuum of energy conservation processes, ranging from inactivity and estivation to torpor and hibernation. The high amounts of sleep in infancy may involve conservation of energy and its consequent availability for growth. Decreased amounts of *stage 4* and total sleep with aging in humans may represent reduced energy demands reflected by parallel declines in basal metabolic rate and physical activity. Disruptions of circadian rhythms of sleep and wakefulness in humans produce impairments in mood and performance independent of total amounts of sleep obtained, and reduce the amplitude of physiological rhythms. It is suggested that aging processes might also be affected by such disruptions in activity rhythms. BERGER, R. J. Bioenergetic functions of sleep and activity rhythms and their possible relevance to aging. *Federation Proc.* 34: 97–102, 1975.

A schoff (5) has already drawn attention to the survival value of diurnal rhythms in allowing animals to do the right thing at the right time, thereby making use of most favorable and avoiding unfavorable conditions for survival. My intention, however, is to focus on the bioenergetic properties of activity rhythms, and to discuss how these have survival value to the organ-

[1] From Session IV, *Aging of homeostatic control systems*, of the FASEB Conference on *Biology of Development and Aging*, presented at the 58th Annual Meeting of the Federation of American Societies for Experimental Biology, Atlantic City, N.J., April 10, 1974.

[2] Research described herein was supported by National Institute of Mental Health Grant MH 18928.

Abbreviations: SWS, slow wave sleep; PS, paradoxical sleep; EMG, electromyogram; EOG, electrooculogram.

191

ism. In particular, I shall concentrate on sleep as an alteration in physiological and behavioral activity that might best be considered adaptive in terms of energy conservation, rather than in having a restorative role for waking functions.

In poikilothermic animals activity patterns are largely determined by the ambient temperature. The selective advantage of homeothermy in mammals and birds lies in providing a constant internal body temperature independent of exogenous temperature fluctuations, so that these animals can become active at any point of the 24-hour cycle, within limits. Naturally, homeothermy has to be paid for in terms of food calories, and the advantages gained by temperature independence have to be realized in terms of an increased food intake beyond that required to produce endogenous body heat. In times of food shortage or low temperature it is well known that some warm-blooded animals are capable of reverting to the poikilothermic condition, whereby their body temperature follows the ambient temperature down to a certain point, but no further. This occurs during states of torpor and hibernation. In this way energy is conserved at times when activity of the animal would be ineffective.

I now wish to present some data concerning the characteristics of sleep which indicate that sleep represents one of a continuum of energy conservation processes ranging from inactivity to hibernation, and may be unique to homeotherms.

PHYLOGENY OF SLEEP

All mammals and birds studied thus far have exhibited unequivocal slow wave sleep (SWS); SWS is defined as a period of behavioral inactivity accompanied by a high voltage slow wave EEG pattern (23), reduced reactivity, but rapid reversibility to wakefulness in response to sufficiently strong sensory stimulation. Amphibians studied to date, the bullfrog (23) and salamander (39), did not exhibit these signs of SWS. The status of SWS or even REM sleep (7) in reptiles remains unclear and a controversial issue. Tauber et al. (66) described sleep in the lizard as mainly characterized by a reduction in EEG amplitude and decreased behavioral activity. Behavioral immobility, high voltage spiking occurring over a background of low voltage EEG activity, and decreased EMG activity have been described in the chameleon (65). Others claimed to have seen SWS (22) or both SWS and paradoxical sleep (PS) in the tortoise (72). Pyrethon and Dusan-Pyrethon (49) studied a representative from each of three reptilian orders (python, caiman, and turtle) and described the presence of SWS in each of them. Finally, Karmanova and Churnosov (34) reported diminished slow wave activity during sleep in the swamp turtle.

All of these studies failed to measure adequately arousal thresholds during periods of slow wave EEG activity and/or behavioral quiescence. Furthermore, none of them demonstrated unambiguous electrophysiological characteristics of sleep similar to those observed in mammals and birds.

Because of these contradictory and inconclusive results, we pursued the question of sleep in reptiles by studying the tortoise, for which claims for the presence of sleep based on earlier results appeared the least equivocal (74).

Several 24-hour recordings of electromyogram (EMG), EKG, electrooculogram (EOG), and electroencephalogram (EEG) as well as behavioral observations were made on seven adult tortoises (*Testudo denticulata*). Two distinct electrophysiological states were observed (Fig. 1): *1*) high tonic and phasic EMG associated with low voltage–fast frequency (predominately 6–10 cps, <40 µV) EEG activity and a heart rate of 20–30 beats/min; *2*) reduced tonic EMG, and EEG of high voltage (00–150 µV) spikes superimposed on low voltage–fast frequency activity and a decreased heart rate (10–20 beats/min). Electroencephalogram spiking was present during behaviorally inactive periods and disappeared on arousal. Thresholds of arousal did not differ between these two electrophysiological states and neither did oxygen consumption when EMG activity was constant. Rate of EEG spiking and to some extent heart rate and EMG activity were directly related to the ambient temperature. All spiking disappeared when the temperature was lowered to 16 C. Behavioral postures of heliothermic reptiles such as the tortoise

are known to be contingent on thermal conditions. Therefore it appears that, to a large extent, both electrophysiological and behavioral activity are passive reflections of changes in ambient temperature.

Other recent studies on the American alligator (76) and the sea turtle (59) failed to confirm the presence of electrophysiological signs of sleep in reptiles and are consistent with the hypothesis that the complete physiological and behavioral manifestations of sleep are unique to homeotherms and possibly evolved in parallel with homeothermy and the consequent need for energy conservation. In this respect, sleep may be viewed as a variation on the theme of dormancy analogous to hibernation, daily torpor, and estivation, all of which presumably evolved as energy conservation processes.

ONTOGENY OF SLEEP

It is of theoretical interest that those mammals in which slow wave sleep

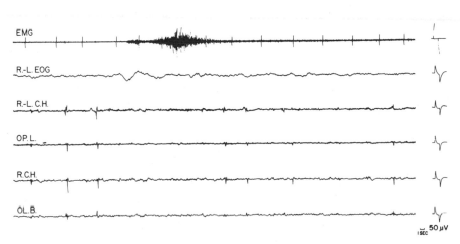

Figure 1. Two electrophysiological states of EEG spiking and non-spiking accompanying behavioral inactivity and arousal, respectively, in the tortoise. Note the disappearance of EEG spiking activity with increased EMG activity and arousal, and that the low voltage–fast frequency EEG activity remains unchanged during arousal (R = right, L = left, C.H. = cerebral hemisphere, OP.L. = optic lobe, OL.B. = olfactory bulb.

is not evident at birth but develops within the first few weeks of life also lack complete thermoregulation at birth. In the rat, SWS first appears at approximately 12 days of age, developing into adult-like EEG patterns of sleep with only minor variations at approximately 18 days (29, 46). Concurrently, the ability of newborn rats to maintain a relatively constant body temperature in the cold develops at approximately 2 weeks of age (19) and is fairly well established by the age of 3 weeks (67). The dog, which is essentially poikilothermic at birth, exhibits SWS beginning at 13 days of age (20), developing coincidentally with the animal's ability to maintain a constant temperature in a cold environment (26). The rabbit, which has poor thermal stability at birth, develops SWS in conjunction with thermoregulation during the first week of life (1, 57). Those animals exhibiting thermoregulation shortly following birth, such as the guinea pig (16), lamb (3) and rhesus monkey (15), all exhibit SWS soon after birth (26, 39, 46). There are incomplete data on the ontogenesis of sleep in birds but that which exists indicates that the same relationship as observed in mammals between the development of SWS and thermoregulation holds for this species as well. The chicken manifests thermoregulation on hatching, and heat production probably begins during late embryonic development (52). Slow wave EEG activity is also evident during late stages of incubation (68) and SWS has been described during the first day following hatching (13, 14). The pigeon, which is poikilothermic on hatching, is able to maintain effective temperature control at approximately 11 days of age (21). The EEG in the pigeon is isoelectric until 5 days of age and not until between 10 and 14 days of

age does slow wave activity similar to sleep appear (68).

Although it is difficult to draw comparisons between studies designed to investigate different issues in ontogenesis, these results do indicate a close correlation between the development of SWS and homeothermy.

For this reason we recently investigated the development of SWS and homeothermy in an American marsupial, the opossum (*Didelphis virginiana*). The EEG, EOG, EMG, and respiration were recorded from young opossums in their mothers' pouches. Concurrently, electrophysiological recordings were also taken together with rectal temperature from a littermate placed in a small chamber at ambient temperatures of 25 ± 1 C and 30 ± 1 C. Recordings lasted from 4 to 6 hours and were obtained from animals between 55 and 80 days of age, four animals being sampled at each age (two in the mother's pouch and two in the chamber). The records obtained from the infants in the mothers' pouches were coded, and visually scored without knowledge of each animal's age for the presence of distinct electrophysiological patterns of wakefulness, SWS, and REM sleep. Heat production at the two different ambient temperatures in the chamber was also measured. Heat production developed simultaneously with 1–3 cps high voltage slow waves and spindles in the EEG. Incipient slow wave activity first appeared at approximately 65 days, with transient episodes of SWS appearing at approximately 70 days. Well-developed SWS consisting of high voltage slow wave activity and 10–15 cps spindles was firmly established by 75 days of age (Fig. 2). In older animals (95–115 days), in which there were prolonged episodes of both REM sleep and SWS, we measured relative oxygen consumption and observed large decreases during both SWS and REM sleep as compared to the waking state (Fig. 3). Oxygen consumption was closely related to muscle tension and was lowest during REM sleep. Reynolds (50) described increases in oxygen consumption of approximately 1,300% between the ages of 75 and 85 days. However, during this same period the body weight of opossums only increases by approximately 80%. This tremendous increase in oxygen consumption represents the energetic cost of homeothermy. Thus, SWS appears at that point in the opossum's development when, because of the large energy expenditures involved in the production of metabolic heat, it would appear profitable to conserve

energy. These data indicate that SWS and heat production develop simultaneously in the opossum, and that SWS is uniquely associated with homeothermy.

METABOLISM AND PERIODIC DORMANCY

Muscular activity and heart rate diminish during sleep (36). Both body temperature and oxygen consumption also decrease during the course of the night in humans (37) with the magnitude of oxygen consumption reduced 10–22% below waking levels (42, 51). Furthermore, depth of sleep (excluding REM sleep) as indicated by the incidence of EEG slow waves is inversely related to the

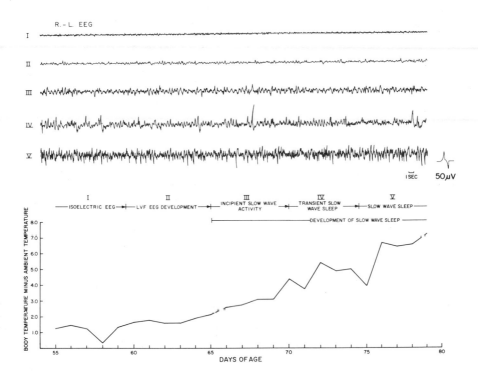

Figure 2. Heat production of infant opossums and associated characteristics of the EEG with increasing age. Note the marked rise in body temperature at about 65 days of age when slow wave activity first begins to appear in the EEG (LVF = low voltage–fast frequency).

rate of oxygen consumption (8). Zepelin and Rechtschaffen (76) reviewed previous phylogenetic studies and found a strong positive correlation between basal metabolic rate and length of time spent asleep, perhaps indicating that in animals with high metabolic rates there is a greater need for energy conservation. Decreases in body temperature accompany both sleep and hibernation although the magnitude of change is much greater in hibernation. Furthermore, there is an inverse relationship between core temperature and the duration of hibernation (48, 69). Significantly, this relationship can be extended to include sleep so that the length of dormancy as represented by hibernation, partial hibernation and sleep is inversely proportional to the body temperature of the animal (69). These data support the notion of a continuum from sleep to hibernation and the question has been raised that hibernation might be a deeper stage of sleep possibly regulated by the same regions of the brain that control normal sleep (55). Sleep, however, provides the advantage of rapid reversibility of state to wakefulness, allowing critical reactivity to such dangers as predators. There is some evidence, although not conclusive, indicating that animals enter hibernation from a

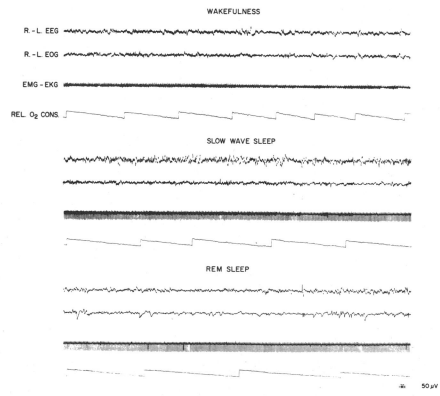

Figure 3. Relative rates of oxygen consumption during wakefulness, SWS and REM sleep in a 85-day-old opossum.

state of sleep (57); and vice versa, the EEG in the birchmouse (4) and hamster (12) changes from an iso-electric pattern to slow wave activity during the early phases of arousal from hibernation.

If, indeed, sleep evolved by virtue of its energy-conserving functions, then we see that sleep is merely one of several different ways of solving the same central problem that confronts warm-blooded animals. Thus some mammals can survive cold winters during food shortage without lowering their body temperature appreciably, by entering "Winterruhe" (10, 25) (also called "partial hibernation" and "seasonal lethargy"), which may merely be an extended period of sleep. Other homeotherms hibernate and some remain active throughout the winter period because they still manage to either find or draw upon stores of food. Most homeotherms sleep at night but there are a few exceptions. Animals of very small body weight with high rates of heat loss, such as the hummingbird, cannot maintain an energy balance by sleeping at night if it is extremely cold or if they have failed to take in adequate food during the prior day (11). Such animals enter torpor at night, when their body temperatures fall with the ambient temperature within certain limits. At times, when the energy demands are not so critical, they sleep at night; presumably because sleep provides sufficient energy conservation without the disadvantages of lack of reactivity to external stimuli that results from torpor. Still another homeotherm, the shrew, of extremely small body size and having a very high metabolic rate, may solve the energy problem by remaining awake and taking in food throughout the 24-hour period, since in preliminary investigations no clear signs of sleep were observed in this animal (71). The generaliza-

tion can probably be made that homeotherms with high rates of metabolism must maintain an energy balance either by constant food intake or by reduction of metabolism during inactive periods by entering the states of sleep, torpor or hibernation.

It is conceivable that the main reason that the function of sleep has remained a biological puzzle is that sleep is most often considered as being subservient to the waking state, revitalizing processes that have deteriorated during prior wakefulness. The impetus for this line of thought is based on findings that sleep deprivation produces psychological and performance deficits as well as subsequent "rebounds" of sleep. Although loss of sleep produces unmistakable effects on waking psychophysiology and behavior (27), the results of recent studies in our laboratory indicate that disturbance of an established circadian rhythm of sleep and wakefulness in itself produces similar impairments in waking mood and performance independent of the total amount of sleep obtained. Therefore, the integrity of waking functions may depend not so much on an absolute amount of sleep as on the maintenance of a regular sleep–wakefulness rhythm. We previously found that performance on vigilance and psychomotor tasks was severely affected by allowing regular 8-hour sleepers to extend their sleep beyond their habitual amounts (61, 64), as is typically observed following partial or total sleep deprivation (75). If the function of sleep is to restore the integrity of waking functions, it is difficult to understand why sleep is not self-limiting, so that it automatically terminates itself when maximum waking potential has been restored. Furthermore, it was found that shifting the time in the circadian rhythm when habitual 8-hour periods of sleep are taken also impairs subsequent waking performance (Fig. 4) and mood (62). Results from a similar study on habitual 9–10 hour sleepers indicate similar effects (63). Therefore, it appears that the detrimental effects of deprivation and extension of habitual sleep can be largely attributed to the disturbance of an established circadian rhythm, and the length of sleep itself may be relatively less important.

SLEEP, ACTIVITY, ONTOGENESIS, AND AGING

What might be the possible significance of this foregoing analysis for questions of ontogenesis and aging? Growth is, of course, one of the most important aspects of infancy, and since the rate of metabolism is directly related to the temperature, which in turn, therefore, influences the rate of growth, the importance of warm temperatures for optimal growth is apparent. In toads, for example, it has been shown that a body temperature of 27 C produces

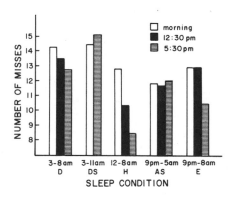

Figure 4. Number of misses on an auditory vigilance task after extended (E), advanced-shift (AS), habitual (H), deprivation (D) and delayed-shift (DS) sleep conditions. (From Taub and Berger (62).)

maximal rates of growth, and immature toads when placed in a temperature gradient select a temperature of 27 C (39). However, if they are starved, they select a much lower temperature and thereby conserve energy, but at the expense of decreased growth. Analogously, it seems that sleep offers an alternate method for homeotherms to conserve energy without a retardation of growth. It is a universal characteristic for sleep to be maximal in infancy, and to decrease with age; and in mammals there tends to be a sharp drop in the amount of sleep at the time of weaning (28). Increases in *stages 3* and *4* sleep in adult humans following 2 days starvation were recently described in two independent studies (32, 37). Here again, sleep seems to serve an energy conserving function when food is limited. The increased secretion of growth hormones observed during sleep in adults (33, 47, 54, 60) is also consistent with the notion that sleep and growth are related. However, this relationship is not so markedly apparent in infants whose growth hormone levels tend to be high throughout the 24-hour period (18, 56, 73).

Finally what possible functional significance might activity rhythms have in relation to aging? This is a relatively unexplored area, but some definitive findings are beginning to emerge. It has been well established in humans that the rate of both brain and body metabolism declines with increasing age (17). Paralleling this decline is the decrease in total sleep time as well as the proportion of sleep spent in *stage 4* (2, 18, 30, 31) —considered the deepest stage of sleep and the one in which metabolism is at its lowest levels (8). If the overall rate of metabolism is a direct reflection of aging in the body then it follows that there might be an associated decreased "need" for sleep, especially *stage 4* sleep, if sleep serves an energy conserving function. Even in young adults it appears that sleep is somewhat labile relative to the energy expenditures during prior wakefulness. Baekeland and Lasky (6) reported increased amounts of *stages 3* and *4* sleep following prior exercise during the day, and Hobson (24) and Matsumoto et al. (43) described increased slow wave sleep in cats and rats, respectively, following enforced exercise.

I have focused my discussion on activity and sleep and wakefulness rhythms, but these constitute only a minute fraction of the total constellation of rhythmic processes occurring in the body and brain. These range in the length of their period from one millisecond for the nerve action potential to as long as 1 year for sexual, migratory and hibernation activities. Now aging may be considered as a rhythm in itself. It is also conceivable that artificial disruption of the body's rhythms may reflect back onto the basic aging process so as to change its period. As mentioned earlier, disruption of circadian rhythms has been observed to have detrimental effects on both behavior and psychological functions and appears to dampen the amplitude of physiological rhythms within the body (35). That such a dampening might also occur for processes underlying aging is suggested by results of a preliminary study in mice indicating that repeated inversions of 12-hour light–dark cycles reduced their life-span (41). The recognition of temporal factors in physiology and behavior has been a relatively recent event in psychobiology. We are increasingly coming to realize that not only does an animal evolve to fit into a spatial ecological niche but also into a temporal one that is reflected in the ordered interrelations between its various internal biological rhythms. An increased recognition of the significance of these temporal rhythms for the viability of the organism may also help us to understand the process of aging.

The author wishes to thank James M. Walker for his valuable contributions to this paper.

REFERENCES

1. ADAMSON, K. Breathing and the thermal environment in young rabbits. *J. Physiol., London* 149: 144, 1959.
2. AGNEW, H. W., JR., W. B. WEBB AND R. L. WILLIAMS. Sleep patterns in late middle age males: An EEG study. *Electroencephalog. Clin. Neurophysiol.* 23: 168, 1967.
3. ALEXANDER, G. Temperature regulation in the new-born lamb. III. Effect of environmental temperature on metabolic rate, body temperature, and respiratory quotient. *Australian J. Agr. Res.* 12: 1152, 1961.
4. ANDERSEN, P., K. JOHANSEN AND J. KROG. Electroencephalogram during arousal from hibernation in the birchmouse. *Am. J. Physiol.* 199: 535, 1960.
5. ASCHOFF, J. Survival value of diurnal rhythms. *Zool. Soc. Lond. Symp.* 13: 79, 1964.
6. BAEKELAND, F., AND R. LASKY. Exercise and sleep patterns in college athletes. *Percept. Motor Skills* 23: 1203, 1966.
7. BERGER, R. J. Oculomotor control: a possible function of REM sleep. *Psychol. Rev.* 76: 144, 1969.
8. BREBBIA, D. R., AND K. Z. ALTSHULER. Oxygen consumption rate and electroencephalographic stage of sleep. *Science* 150: 1621, 1965.
9. BRODY, E. B. Development of homeothermy in suckling rats. *Am. J. Physiol.* 139: 230, 1943.
10. CADE, C. J. Observations on torpidity in captive chipmunks of the genus *Eutamias*. *Ecology* 44: 255, 1963.
11. CALDER, W. C., AND J. BOOSER. Hypothermia of broad-tailed hummingbirds during incubation in nature with ecological correlations. *Science* 180: 751, 1973.
12. CHATFIELD, P. O., C. P. LYMAN AND D. P. PURPURA. The effects of temperature on the spontaneous and induced electrical activity in the cerebral cortex of the golden hamster. *Electroencephalog. Clin. Neurophysiol.* 3: 225, 1951.

13. CORNER, M. A., J. J. PETERS AND P. R. VAN DER LOEFF. Electrical activity patterns in the cerebral hemisphere of the chick during maturation, correlated with behavior in a test situation. *Brain Res.* 2: 274, 1966.

14. CORNER, M. A., J. P. SCHADÉ, J. SEDLACEK, R. STOECKART AND A. P. C. BOT. Developmental patterns in the central nervous system of birds. I. Electrical activity in the cerebral hemisphere, optic lobe, and cerebellum. *Progr. Brain Res.* 26: 145, 1967.

15. DAWES, G. S., H. N. JACOBSON, J. C. MOTT AND H. J. SHELLEY. Some observations on foetal and new-born rhesus monkeys. *J. Physiol., London* 152: 271, 1960.

16. FAZEKAS, J. F., F. A. D. ALEXANDER AND H. F. HIMWICH. Tolerance of the newborn to anoxia. *Am. J. Physiol.* 134: 281, 1941.

17. FEINBERG, I., AND V. R. CARLSON. Sleep variables as a function of age in man. *Arch. Gen. Psychiat.* 18: 239, 1968.

18. FEINBERG, I., R. L. KORESKO AND N. HELLER. EEG sleep patterns as a function of normal and pathological ageing in man. *J. Psychiat. Res.* 5: 107, 1967.

19. FINKELSTEIN, J. W., T. F. ANDERS, E. J. SACHAR, H. P. ROFFWARG AND L. D. HELLMAN. Behavioral state, sleep stage and growth hormone levels in human infants. *J. Clin. Endocrinol. Metab.* 32: 368, 1971.

20. FOX, M. F. *Integrative Development of Brain and Behavior in the Dog.* Chicago: Univ. of Chicago Press, 1971.

21. GINGLINGER, A., AND C. KAYSER. Etablissement de la thermorégulation chez les homéothermes au cours du development. *Ann. Physiol. Physicochim. Biol.* 5: 710, 1929.

22. HERMAN, H., M. JOUVET AND M. KLEIN. Etude polygraphique du sommeil chez la tortue. *Compt. Rend. Soc. Biol.* 158: 2175, 1964.

23. HOBSON, J. A. Electrographic correlates of behavior in the frog with special reference to sleep. *Electroencephalog. Clin. Neurophysiol.* 22: 113, 1967.

24. HOBSON, J. A. Sleep after exercise. *Science* 162: 1503, 1968.

25. HUDSON, J. W., AND G. A. BARTHOLOMEW. Terrestrial animals in dry heat: estivators. In: *Handbook of Physiology: Adaptation to the Environment*, edited by D. B. Dill, E. F. Adolph and C. G. Wilber. Washington, D.C.: Am. Physiol. Soc., 1964, sect. 4, chapt. 34, p. 541–550.

26. JENSEN, C., AND H. E. EDERSTROM. Development of temperature regulation in the dog. *Am. J. Physiol.* 183: 340, 1955.

27. JOHNSON, L. C. Physiological and psychological changes following total sleep deprivation. In: *Sleep: Physiology and Pathology*, edited by A. Kales. Philadelphia: Lippincott, 1969, p. 206.

28. JOUVET-MOUNIER, D. Ontogenèse des états de vigilance chez quelques mammifères. (Thèse de Médecine.) Lyon: Beaux-Arts. 1968.

29. JOUVET-MOUNIER, D., L. ASTIC AND D. LACOTE. Ontogenesis of the states of sleep in rat, cat, and guinea pig during the first postnatal month. *Develop. Psychobiol.* 2: 216, 1970.

30. KAHN, E., AND C. FISHER. The sleep characteristics of the normal aged male. *J. Nervous Mental Disease* 148: 477, 1969.

31. KALES, A., T. WILSON, J. D. KALES, A. JACOBSON, M. J. PAULSON, E. KOLLAR AND R. D. WALTER. Measurements of all-night sleep in normal elderly persons: effects of aging. *J. Am. Geriat. Soc.* 15: 405, 1967.

32. KARACAN, I., A. L. ROSENBLOOM, J. H. LONDONO, P. J. SALIS, J. I. THORNBY AND R. L. WILLIAMS. Sleep and the sleep-growth hormone (GH) response during acute fasting. *Sleep Res.* 2: 197, 1973.

33. KARACAN, I., A. L. ROSENBLOOM, R. L. WILLIAMS, W. W. FINLEY AND C. J. HURSCH. Slow wave sleep deprivation in relation to plasma growth hormone concentration. *Behav. Neuropsychiat.* 2: 11, 1971.

34. KARMANOVA, I. G., AND E. V. CHURNOSOV. Electrophysiological investigation of natural sleep and wakefulness of turtles and chickens. *Zh. Evol. Biokhim. Fiziol* 8: 59, 1972.

35. KLEIN, K. E., H. M. WEGMANN AND B. I. HUNT. Desynchronization of body temperature and performance circadian rhythm as a result of outgoing and homegoing transmeridian flights. *Aerospace Med.* 43: 119, 1972.

36. KLEITMAN, N. *Sleep and Wakefulness.* Chicago: Univ. of Chicago Press, 1963.

37. KREIDER, M. B., E. R. BUSKIRK AND D. E. BASS. Oxygen consumption and body temperatures during the night. *J. Appl. Physiol.* 12: 361, 1958.

38. LEWIS, S. A., U. M. MACFADYEN AND I. OSWALD. Starvation and human slow wave sleep. *J. Appl. Physiol.* 35: 391, 1973.

39. LILLYWHITE, H. B., P. LICHT AND P. CHELGREN. The role of behavioral thermoregulation in the grown ener-

getics of the toad, *Bufo boreas*. *Ecology* 54: 375, 1973.

40. LUCAS, E., M. B. STERMAN AND D. J. MCGINTY. The salamander EEG: A model of primitive sleep and wakefulness. *Psychophysiology* 6: 230, 1969.

41. LUCE, G. G. *Body time: Physiological rhythms and social stress*. New York: Pantheon, 1971, p. 37.

42. MAGNUSSEN, G. *Studies on the respiration during sleep. A contribution to the physiology of the sleep function*. London: H. K. Lewis, 1944.

43. MATSUMOTO, J., T. NIHISHO, T. SUTO, T. SADAHIRO AND M. MIYOSHI. Influence of fatigue on sleep. *Nature* 218: 177, 1968.

44. MEIER, G. W., AND R. J. BERGER. Development of sleep and wakefulness patterns in the infant rhesus monkey. *Exptl. Neurol.* 12: 257, 1965.

45. NELSON, R. A., M. W. WAHNER, J. D. JONES, R. D. ELLEFSON AND P. E. ZOLLMAN. Metabolism of bears before, during, and after winter sleep. *Am. J. Physiol.* 224: 491, 1973.

46. OISHI, H., AND S. IWAHARA. A development study of brain waves and spontaneous motor activity in white rats. *Japan. Psychol. Res.* 13: 82, 1971.

47. PARKER, D. C., J. F. SASSIN, J. W. MACE, R. W. GOTLIN AND L. G. ROSSMAN. Human growth hormone release during sleep: Electroencephalographic correlation. *J. Clin. Endocrinol Metab.* 29: 871, 1969.

48. PENGELLEY, E. T., AND K. C. FISHER. Rhythmical arousal from hibernation in the golden-mantled ground squirrel *Citellus lateralis tescorum*. *Can. J. Zool.* 39: 105, 1961.

49. PYRETHON, J., AND D. DUSAN-PYRETHON. Etude polygraphique du cycle veille-sommeil chez trois genres de reptiles. *Compt. Rend. Soc. Biol.* 162: 181, 1968.

50. REYNOLDS, H. C. Studies on reproduction in the opossum (*Didelphis virginiana*). *Univ. Calif. Berkeley Publ. Zool.* 52: 232, 1952.

51. ROBIN, E. D., R. D. WHALEY, C. H. CRUMP AND D. M. TRAVIS. Alveolar gas tensions, pulmonary ventilation and blood pH during physiological sleep in normal subjects. *J. Clin. Invest.* 37: 981, 1958.

52. ROMANOFF, A. L. Development of homeothermy in birds. *Science* 94: 218, 1941.

53. RUCKEBUSCH, Y. Development of sleep and wakefulness in the foetal lamb. *Electroencephalog. Clin. Neurophysiol.* 32: 119, 1972.

54. SASSIN, J. F., D. C. PARKER, J. W. MACE, R. W. GOTLIN, L. C. JOHNSON AND L. G. ROSSMAN. Human growth hormone release: relation to slow-wave sleep and sleep-waking cycles. *Science* 165: 513, 1969.

55. SATINOFF, E. Hibernation and the central nervous system. In: *Progress in Physiological Psychology*, edited by E. Stellar and J. M. Sprague. New York: Academic, 1970, vol. 3, p. 201.

56. SHAYWITZ, B. A., J. FINKELSTEIN, L. HELLMAN AND E. D. WEITZMAN. Growth hormone in newborn infants during sleep-wake periods. *Pediatrics* 48: 103, 1971.

57. SHIMIZU, A., AND H. E. HIMWICH. The ontogeny of sleep in kittens and young rabbits. *Electroencephalog. Clin. Neurophysiol.* 24: 307, 1968.

58. SOUTH, F. E., J. E. BREAZILE, H. D. DELLMANN AND A. D. EPPERLY. Sleep, hibernation and hypothermia in the yellow-bellied marmot (*M. flaviventris*). In: *Depressed Metabolism*, edited by X. J. Mosacchia and J. F. Saunders. New York: American Elsevier, 1969, p 277.

59. SUSIC, V. Electrographic and behavioral correlations of the rest-activity cycle in the sea turtle, *Caretta caretta* L. (Chelonia). *J. Exptl. Marine Biol. Ecol.* 10: 81, 1972.

60. TAKAHASHI, Y., D. M. KIPNIS AND W. H. DAUGHADAY. Growth hormone secretion during sleep. *J. Clin. Invest.* 47: 2079, 1968.

61. TAUB, J. M., AND R. J. BERGER. Extended sleep and performance: The Rip Van Winkle effect. *Psychonomic Sci.* 18: 82, 1969.

62. TAUB, J. M., AND R. J. BERGER. Performance and mood following variations in the length and timing of sleep. *Psychophysiology* 10: 559, 1973.

63. TAUB, J. M., AND R. J. BERGER. Behavioral effects of extended sleep, sleep deprivation, and shifted sleep in habitual long sleepers. *Sleep Res.* 2: 192, 1973.

64. TAUB, J. M., G. G. GLOBUS, E. PHOEBUS AND R. DRURY. Extended sleep and performance. *Nature* 233: 142, 1971.

65. TAUBER, E. S., H. P. ROFFWARG AND E. D. WEITZMAN. Eye movements and electroencephalogram activity during sleep in diurnal lizards. *Nature* 212: 1612, 1966.

66. TAUBER, E. S., J. ROJAS-RAMIREZ AND R. HERNANDEZ-PEON. Electrophysiological and behavioral correlates of wakefulness and sleep in the lizard, *Ctenosaura pectinata*. *Electroencephalog. Clin. Neurophysiol.* 24: 424, 1968.

67. TAYLOR, P. M. Oxygen consumption in new-born rats. *J. Physiol., London* 154: 153, 1960.

68. TUGE, H., Y. KANAYAMA AND C. H. YUEH. Comparative studies on the development of EEG. *Japan. J. Physiol.* 10: 211, 1960.

69. TWENTE, J. W., AND J. A. TWENTE. Regulation of hibernating periods by temperature. *Proc. Natl. Acad. Sci. U.S.* 54: 1058, 1965.

70. VAN TWYVER, H. Polygraphic studies of the American alligator. *Sleep Res.* 2: 87, 1973.

71. VAN TWYVER, H., AND T. ALLISON. EEG study of the shrew (*Blarina brevicauda*): A preliminary report. *Psychophysiology* 6: 231, 1969.

72. VASILESCU, E. Sleep and wakefulness in the tortoise (*Emys orbicularis*). *Rev. Roumaine Biol. Ser. Zool.* 15: 177, 1970.

73. VIGNERI, R., AND R. D'AGATA. Growth hormone release during the first year of life in relation to sleep-wake periods. *J. Clin. Endocrinol. Metab.* 33: 561, 1971.

74. WALKER, J. M., AND R. J. BERGER. A polygraphic study of the tortoise (*Testudo denticulata*): Absence of electrophysiological signs of sleep. *Brain Behav. Evol.* 8: 453, 1973.

75. WILKINSON, R. T. Sleep deprivation: Performance tests for partial and selective sleep deprivation. *Progr. Clin. Psychol.* 8: 28, 1968.

76. ZEPELIN, H., AND A. RECHTSCHAFFEN. Relationships between mammalian sleep parameters and other constitutional variables. *Sleep Res.* 2: 89, 1973.

Changes in monoamine oxidase and monoamines with human development and aging[1,2,3]

D. S. ROBINSON[4]

Clinical Pharmacology Unit
Departments of Pharmacology and Medicine
University of Vermont College of Medicine
Burlington, Vermont 05401

ABSTRACT

A series of studies of monoamines and their metabolism in a variety of human tissues indicate that there are aging effects that may alter neurotransmitter substances. Monoamine oxidase (MAO) activity has a significant positive correlation with age in plasma and blood platelets of normal subjects and patients suffering from depressive disorders. Monoamine oxidase and age correlate positively in hindbrain and in eight separate areas of human brains from patients who died from a variety of causes. Hindbrain norepinephrine concentration progressively decreases with advancing age ($r = -0.44$, $P < 0.01$) while no changes were noted for serotonin (5-HT) and 5-hydroxyindoleacetic acid (5-HIAA). Hindbrain norepinephrine concentration has a significant negative correlation with MAO ($r = -0.41$, $P < 0.025$) and hindbrain 5-HIAA has a significant positive correlation with MAO ($r = +0.66$, $P = <0.05$). These studies suggest that aging processes may significantly affect monoamine mechanisms and be a predisposing factor to the development of clinical diseases in man such as depression, parkinsonism and other disorders of central nervous system homeostasis.—ROBINSON, D. S. Changes in monoamine oxidase and monoamines with human development and aging. *Federation Proc.* 34: 103–107, 1975.

[1] From Session IV, *Aging of homeostatic control systems*, of the FASEB Conference on *Biology of Development and Aging*, presented at the 58th Annual Meeting of the Federation of American Societies for Experimental Biology, Atlantic City, N.J., April 10, 1974.

[2] Some of the data presented have been previously published (25, 29, 30) and the studies referred to were done in collaboration with Drs. A. Nies, J. M. Davis, and C. L. Ravaris.

[3] The support of Public Health Service grants 1 R01 MH15533, 5 S01 RR-05429, and T02 05935 and awards from the Burroughs Wellcome Fund, Research Triangle Park, N.C., The Pharmaceutical Manufacturers Association Foundation, Washington, D.C. and The Warner-Lambert Charitable Foundation, Morris Plains, N.J., are acknowledged.

[4] Burroughs Wellcome Scholar in Clinical Pharmacology.

203

There has been extensive interest in two sectors of central nervous system (CNS) investigation, biogenic amine metabolism and age-related biochemical changes in brain tissues. In light of recent evidence relating amine metabolism in human brain to aging (25, 29, 30), these two areas of research interest now overlap and are interrelated. Other recent discoveries of similar significance that tie biochemical changes in the CNS to advancing age include reduced neuronal uptake of ^{3}H-norepinephrine by the cerebral cortex (37); increased butyrylcholinesterase activity in the CNS suggesting increased proliferation of glial cells with aging (38); and altered levels of amino acids with possible neurotransmitter functions in the brain (35).

The importance of the physiological roles played by the biologically active amines in the CNS has received wide recognition and review (2, 8, 14). Recent work to be summarized in this paper strongly suggests that the biogenic amines are influenced by the aging process in man. Studies in our laboratory have centered around the biogenic amines and their metabolism in the CNS and in peripheral tissues. Some of the work described was done in collaboration with others, including Drs. A. Nies, J. M. Davis, L. S. Harris, I. Kay, C. L. Ravaris, S. Spector and K. L. Lamborn. These studies were an outgrowth of our interest in biologic phenomena relating to CNS functions and in the biogenic amine hypothesis which puts forth a role for certain monoamines (norepinephrine, serotonin, dopamine) in the etiology of depression, mania, and parkinsonism (11, 33). The evidence for this hypothesis has been largely indirect; for example, agents that deplete neuronal amines, such as reserpine and methyldopa, can precipitate depressive illness, particularly in patients with a past history or family history of depression. In addition, pharmacologic agents that are useful in the treatment of depression, such as the tricyclic antidepressants and monoamine oxidase inhibitors, significantly alter the metabolism and function of biogenic amines in the CNS. Parkinsonism, a disorder caused by a defect in dopamine metabolism, has been successfully treated by the administration of pharmacologic doses of the amino acid precursor of dopamine (10).

Both parkinsonism and the depressive disorders show a definite relation to aging with increased incidence and prevalence associated with advancing age (7, 28). It is generally accepted that major depressive illnesses are more common in women than in men (28, 34). The possibility that there might be a biochemical determinant related to age and sex predisposing to the development of a depressive illness is intriguing.

The enzyme, monoamine oxidase (MAO), which catalyzes one of the major pathways for degrading the biogenic amines serotonin and the catecholamines, could be one of the mediating factors in these disorders of aging. Previous reports of the relationship of MAO to development and to aging in animal studies generally failed to detect any changes in brain MAO levels except for initial increases either in embryonic stages or during early maturation and development (3, 24). While an age-related change was not detected in rat brain MAO activity in several studies, heart MAO was found to increase with aging (15, 19, 20, 27) and in one report with the development of cardiac hypertrophy (12). Because animal models for many disorders of man are imperfect and in some cases nonexistent, animal studies often have serious limitations, especially in biologic psychiatry. Consequently alterations in amine metabolism relating to clinical disease might only be expected in higher animals susceptible to the illness. This led us to carry out a series of studies of monoamines and their metabolism in human tissues.

Until the recent development of a sensitive radioassay for MAO activity (31) it had been difficult or impractical to carry out direct tissue studies in man so that it was usually necessary to assess monoamine metabolism by indirect means such as measuring metabolites in blood and urine. This approach had the obvious drawbacks that such data might reflect largely dietary factors or only local metabolism of amines by the kidney or the gastrointestinal tract rather than the more relevant but less accessible areas such as nervous tissue. With the recent capability of direct assay of MAO levels in man we have investigated this enzyme in three human tissues — blood platelets, plasma, and brain.

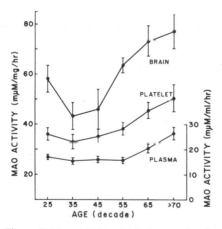

Figure 1. Mean MAO activities by age decade in three human tissues. Vertical bars = SEM. The upper curve shows the mean enzyme activities for hindbrains from 26 patients. The lower curves represent the means of platelet and plasma MAO activities of 162 normal subjects.

HUMAN PLASMA AND PLATELET MAO ACTIVITIES

Monoamine oxidase levels were determined in platelets and plasma of 71 normal men and 91 normal women, 21 to 84 years of age. Individuals who volunteered from local industries and civic organizations were selected on the basis of absence of a personal or family history of psychiatric illness, no concurrent medication, and never having received a major psychotropic drug. Specimens were processed and MAO assayed using benzylamine as substrate as previously described (29, 31). When mean enzyme activities of these normal subjects are determined according to age decade, there is a consistent trend of higher activity with increasing age (lower two curves, Fig. 1). The Pearson correlation coefficient of MAO activity and age for these individuals is 0.39 for platelets ($P < 0.001$) and 0.47 for plasma ($P < 0.001$). In a separate study reported elsewhere (25) a similar age–activity relationship for both platelets and plasma has been observed in patients with depressive disorders, supporting the view that this MAO–age pattern is a general one in man.

There is further evidence for a sex as well as for an age difference such that for a given age women have a higher mean platelet and plasma MAO than men. This sex difference in enzyme activity, if it proved to be a general biologic phenomenon in man, would have important implications which are consistent with the clinical observations that women have a greater predisposition to depressive illness (25, 29). Thus, in contrast to animal studies, which have been largely negative with respect to age–MAO changes except for heart tissue, a high correlation of MAO activity with aging has been observed in two human tissues, platelets and plasma.

Long-term chronological studies in man will be required to establish whether individuals do develop higher blood MAO levels as they age. The fact that the age–activity relationship holds both for the plasma and platelet enzymes is also interesting because of the diverse nature of these two enzymes including dissimilarities of solubility, cofactor requirements and inhibitor characteristics (31), suggesting separate origins and functions.

HUMAN BRAIN MAO

Brain specimens were obtained at autopsy from 55 patients who died from a variety of medical illnesses. Hindbrains (rhombencephalon) were prepared by removing the cerebellum and cutting the cerebral peduncles flush with the base of the brain. The hindbrain was stripped of vessels and membranes, placed in a carbon dioxide atmosphere, rapidly frozen, and stored for varying periods of time until thawed and prepared for assay. Studies in our laboratory have shown that under these conditions length of storage time does not influence MAO activity. At the time of assay the hindbrain was hemisectioned in the sagittal plane, and one hemisection from each brain specimen was selected at random for homogenization in 0.15 M phosphate buffer pH 7.4 and quickly refrozen. Subsequently specimens were assayed for MAO activity as previously described (31) with ^{14}C-benzylamine as substrate.

Twenty-six of the hindbrain hemisections were assayed for MAO activity, and the resulting means of enzyme activities grouped according to age decade are shown in Fig. 1 (top curve). The plot of brain MAO activity and age rather closely parallels those for platelet and plasma

MAO except for a more exaggerated secondary peak in the 20–29 year bracket. The correlation of hindbrain MAO activity with age is 0.57 (P < 0.005). When the results were analyzed according to sex, it is interesting that women had slightly higher mean values than men, but this difference did not achieve statistical significance.

Since this age–activity pattern appeared to be clearly established for plasma, blood platelets and whole hindbrain, it seemed important to determine whether a similar relationship of enzyme activity to age held for the brain cortex and for specific subcortical regions with high monoamine concentrations. It was also deemed important to measure enzyme activities using more than one substrate since brain MAO isoenzymes have been described which differ in substrate characteristics (9, 39). Brain specimens were obtained at autopsy from 13 patients dying from a variety of causes including accidental death and various medical illnesses. After opening the dura, the brain was rapidly dissected and uniform specimens were obtained from each of the following regions: globus pallidus, thalamus, hypothalamus, hippocampus, substantia nigra, reticular activating system (floor of the fourth ventricle), orbital cortex, and caudate nucleus. Specimens were immediately placed in a nitrogen atmosphere, rapidly frozen, and stored at −10 C. The tissue was subsequently thawed, homogenized in sufficient 0.2 M phosphate buffer pH 7.4 to yield a final protein concentration of approximately 5 mg/ml. The crude homogenates were refrozen, stored at −10 C, and thawed just prior to MAO assay using ^{14}C-benzylamine and ^{14}C-tryptamine as substrates as previously described (31).

Of the 13 brain specimens assayed, 6 of the patients were younger than 45 years of age and 7 were over 45 years of age. The mean MAO activities of each brain area comparing the two age groups are shown with benzylamine (Fig. 2) and tryptamine (Fig. 3) as substrates. For each area and for both substrates the mean MAO activity was greater for the older patient group than for the younger one. Correlations of age and MAO activity for the eight brain areas were all positive, ranging from 0.25 to 0.63 for benzylamine and from 0.23 to 0.40 for tryptamine. Similar results were obtained whether enzyme activities were calculated on the basis of activity per milligram of protein or per gram wet weight of brain tissue. Thus the MAO–age relationship observed for whole hindbrain tissue seems to hold for a variety of discrete brain areas and differing substrates as well.

These findings suggest that this age–activity relationship for this

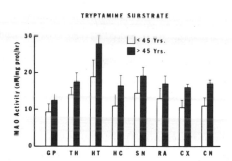

Figure 3. Mean MAO activities with tryptamine as substrate of eight brain areas from 6 patients under 45 years of age compared to 7 patients over 45 years old. Vertical bars = SEM. Symbols defined in Fig. 2 legend.

enzyme is common to many tissues in man presumably secondary to aging processes. Work is in progress to examine the extent and significance of these aging mechanisms on monoamine oxidase and monoamine metabolism in discrete brain areas especially those where monoaminergic neurons have been localized. Preliminary results in our laboratory indicate that while aging may alter MAO activity, other brain enzymes important in amine synthesis and degradation, such as tyrosine hydroxylase and catechol-O-methyltransferase, are unaffected by age.

BRAIN MONOAMINES AND AGING

The possibility that MAO activity and monoamines may be interrelated in the brain was examined in two ways. Hindbrain hemisections from the 55 patients were assayed for serotonin (5-HT) by the method of Bogdanski et al. (5), norepinephrine by a modification of the method of Anton and Sayre (1), and 5-hydroxyindoleacetic acid (5-HIAA) by the method of Udenfriend et al. (36). Mean concentrations of each of these substances were calculated by age decade. The

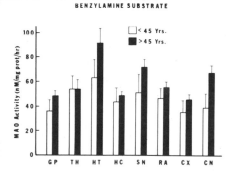

Figure 2. Mean MAO activities with benzylamine as substrate of eight brain areas from 6 patients under 45 years of age compared to 7 patients over 45 years old. Vertical bars = SEM. GP = globus pallidus; TH = thalamus; HT = hypothalamus; HC = hippocampus; SN = substantia nigra; RA = reticular activating system (floor of IVth ventricle); CS = cortex (orbital); CN = caudate nucleus.

relationship of human hindbrain norepinephrine concentration and age is shown in Fig. 4. Hindbrain norepinephrine concentration progressively decreased with age, correlating negatively ($r = -0.44$, $P < 0.01$). Hindbrain 5-HT and 5-HIAA content, on the other hand, did not vary in relation to age (Fig. 5), the correlations with age not differing from zero for either substance. Thus, hindbrain norepinephrine as well as MAO appears to be related to the aging process in a manner consistent with the hypothesis of biogenic amine depletion and the clinical epidemiology of depressive disorders. Studies of amines and their metabolites are currently in progress to determine whether the age–norepinephrine relationship extends to discrete areas with high monoamine concentrations within the CNS.

To further evaluate the possible role of MAO in regulating monoamine metabolism in brain, it seemed important also to examine the relationship of hindbrain amine content to MAO activity. In the 26 patients

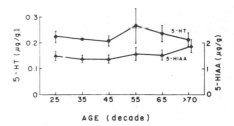

Figure 5. Mean serotonin (5-HT) and 5-hydroxyindoleacetic acid (5-HIAA) concentrations by age decade in hindbrains from 55 patients. Vertical bars = SEM. There is no correlation between age and either 5-HT or 5-HIAA.

for whom both MAO activities and amine concentrations were determined in corresponding hindbrain hemisections, correlations of enzyme activity to monoamine content were carried out. Significant correlations were found between MAO activity and both hindbrain norepinephrine and 5-HIAA content (Fig. 6). Norepinephrine correlated negatively with MAO ($r = -0.41$, $P < 0.025$) while 5-HIAA correlated positively with MAO activity ($r = 0.66$, $P < 0.05$). Hindbrain 5-HT content did not correlate with MAO. The fact that norepinephrine concentrations correlated negatively and 5-HIAA concentrations positively with hindbrain MAO activity suggests that this enzyme may play a major role in regulating intracellular concentrations of biogenic amines in the CNS.

DISCUSSION

On the subject of the biological concomitants of aging, the effects of age on enzyme activity in a variety of tissues and species has been dealt with in several recent reviews (4, 13, 40). A confounding problem in many studies has been confusion in distinguishing between maturational and aging changes.

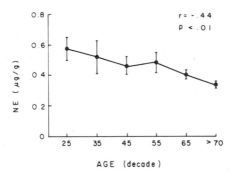

Figure 4. Mean norepinephrine (NE) concentrations by age decade in hindbrains from 55 patients. Vertical bars = SEM. Norepinephrine and age have a significantly negative correlation ($r = -0.44$, $P < 0.01$). (From Nies, Robinson, Davis and Ravaris (25) with permission of Plenum Publishing Corporation.)

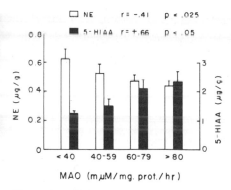

Figure 6. Relationship of MAO activity to norepinephrine (NE) and 5-hydroxyindoleacetic acid (5-HIAA) concentrations in corresponding hindbrain hemisections from 26 patients. Grouped data by quartiles of MAO activity are shown with vertical bars indicating SEM. Norepinephrine concentration has a significant negative correlation with MAO ($r = -0.41$, $P < 0.025$) and 5-HIAA concentration has a significant positive correlation with MAO ($r = +0.66$, $P < 0.05$).

There is a general tendency in both animals and primates for enzymatic activities to be enhanced during development and maturation of the fetus and in early infancy. It would appear that the majority of enzymes studied maintain relatively constant levels throughout the life-span of the adult organism although many have a tendency to decrease gradually in association with the aging process.

Monoamine oxidase changes associated with maturation have been described in the developing rat brain (3, 21, 23, 24) but not during aging in the adult animal (15, 19, 20, 27). In the rat brain monoamines also increase during the prenatal period and early infancy (3, 21, 24). The consistent finding in our studies of a significantly positive age–MAO correlation in several human tissues may be a reflection of either the longer life-span or a true species difference. It is interesting that in another primate, the rhesus monkey, MAO activity was found to increase progressively over the age span from 3 to 18 yr, in two brain areas, cortex and caudate (32). These authors also detected a corresponding and progressive decrease in norepinephrine content in hypothalamus and brainstem of the monkey over the same age range. Thus, present evidence suggests these age-related changes in brain MAO and monoamines are phenomena of primates but not of lower animals.

We have failed to observe any differences in brain MAO activities from adult values in children as young as 4 years of age. However, there is a tendency for a modest peak in enzyme activity during late adolescence, which we have observed in platelet, plasma and brain MAO. This transient effect of early adulthood presumably reflects a maturational process. Changes in plasma MAO associated with pregnancy and the menstrual cycle also have been previously described (16, 22) suggesting hormonal influences on this enzyme.

Psychobiologic studies of amine metabolites in cerebrospinal fluid also have revealed age-related changes (6, 18) such that monoamine metabolites are present in higher concentrations in older patients, consistent with our findings of increasing MAO activity in brain with aging. It is important to take into account and to control for the biologic consequences of aging in future investigations of CNS amine metabolism.

The regional MAO studies of human brain also would indicate that the age changes may be a general biologic phenomenon that is not limited to specific areas or tissues with high amine concentrations or specialized functions. The similar age–MAO patterns observed in tissues other than brain, human plasma and blood platelets (26, 29, 30) support the view that the increasing enzyme activity is a general aging process. The activity of another plasma enzyme, dopamine beta hydroxylase, involved in catecholeamine synthesis and thought to be an index of sympathetic nervous system activity, has been reported recently to have a positive correlation with age (17). Thus, selected enzymes involved in the synthesis and in the degradation of monoamines appear to undergo age changes in at least one or more human tissues. It is quite possible that dopamine beta hydroxylase and MAO in neural tissues are interrelated, with primary changes in one enzyme inducing activity changes in the other as a compensatory mechanism secondary to increased amine turnover rates.

Another explanation for these changes in enzyme activity would be decreasing levels of an inhibitor with advancing age, but there is little evidence to support this. Additional work will be required to extend these investigations to other neural tissues and to more specific brain regions so as to characterize their effects on monoaminergic neurotransmission and on vital physiological functions such as control of blood pressure, emotions, behavior, and so on.

Our findings to date are compatible with the other body of evidence that CNS amine depletion is a contributing factor to the development of depressive disorders. Hindbrain norepinephrine content is negatively correlated with both MAO activity and age in a large sample of patients who died from a variety of causes including accidental death and nonpsychiatric medical problems. The importance of developing a better understanding of affective disorders is emphasized by the fact that they represent one of the most common medical problems in clinical practice, equal to if not exceeding in incidence most other medical problems including hypertension and coronary artery disease.

REFERENCES

1. ANTON, A. H., AND D. F. SAYRE. A study of the factors affecting the aluminum oxide-trihydroxyindole procedure for the analysis of catecholamines. *J. Pharmacol. Exptl. Therap.* 138: 360, 1962.
2. AXELROD, J. Metabolism of epinephrine and other sympathomimetic amines. *Physiol. Rev.* 39: 751, 1959.
3. BENNETT, D. S., AND N. J. GIARMAN. Schedule of appearance of 5-hydroxytryptamine (serotonin) and associated enzymes in the developing rat brain. *J. Neurochem.* 12: 911, 1965.
4. BJORKSTEN, J. Enzymes and cellular metabolism. In: *Enzymes and Mental Health*, edited by G. J. Martin and B. Fisch. Philadelphia: Lippincott, 1966.
5. BOGDANSKI, D. F., A. PLETSCHER, B. B. BRODIE AND S. UDENFRIEND. Identification and assay of serotonin in brain. *J. Pharmacol. Exptl. Therap.* 117: 82, 1956.
6. BOWERS, M. B., AND F. A. GERBODE. Relationship of monoamine metabolites in human cerebrospinal fluid to age. *Nature* 219: 1256, 1968.
7. BRAIN, W. R., AND J. N. WALTON. Brain's *Diseases of the Nervous System*. London: Oxford Univ. Press, 1969, p. 522–534.
8. BRODIE, B. B., D. F. BOGDANSKI AND L. BONOMI. In: *Comparative Neurochemistry*, edited by D. Richter. Oxford: Pergamon, 1964, p. 367.
9. COLLINS, G. G. S., M. SANDLER, E. D. WILLIAMS AND M. B. H. YOUDIM. Multiple forms of human brain mitochondrial monoamine oxidase. *Nature* 225: 817, 1970.
10. COTZIAS, C. G., M. H. VAN WOERT AND L. M. SCHIFFER. Aromatic amino acids and the modification of parkinsonism. *New Engl. J. Med.* 276: 374, 1967.
11. DAVIS, J. M. Theories of biological etiology of affective disorders. *Intern. Rev. Neurobiol.* 12: 145, 1970.
12. DE CHAMPLAIN, J., L. R. KRAKOFF AND J. AXELROD. Increased monoamine oxidase activity during the development of cardiac hypertrophy in the rat. *Circ. Res.* 23: 361, 1968.

13. FORD, D. H. Neurobiological Aspects of Maturation and Aging. In: Prog. Brain Res. Vol. 40: 1973.

14. FUXE, K. Evidence for the existence of monoamine neurons in the central nervous system. Acta Physiol. Scand. 64: suppl. 37, 247, 1965.

15. GEY, K. F., W. P. BURKARD AND A. PLETSCHER. Variation of the norepinephrine metabolism of the rat heart with age. Gerontologia 11: 1, 1965.

16. GILMORE, N. J., D. S. ROBINSON, A. NIES, D. SYLWESTER AND C. L. RAVARIS. Blood monoamine oxidase levels in pregnancy and during the menstrual cycle. J. Psychosomatic Res. 15: 215, 1971.

17. GOLDSTEIN, M., R. EPSTEIN AND L. S. FREEDMAN. Dopamine-B-hydroxylase as an index of sympathetic activity. Presented at the 12th annual meeting of the Am. Col. Neuropsychopharmacol., Palm Springs, Cal., Dec. 7, 1973.

18. GOTTFRIES, C. G., I. GOTTFRIES, B. JOHANNSON, R. OLSSON, T. PERSSON, B. E. ROOS AND R. SJÖSTRAM. Acid monoamine metabolites in human cerebrospinal fluid and their relations to age and sex. Neuropharmacology 10: 655, 1971.

19. HORITA, A. The influence of age on the recovery of cardiac monoamine oxidase after irreversible inhibition. Biochem. Pharmacol. 17: 2091, 1968.

20. HO-VAN-HAP, A., L. M. BARBINEAU AND L. BERLINGUET. Hormonal action on monoamine oxidase activity in rats. Can. J. Biochem. 45: 355, 1967.

21. KARKI, N., R. KNUTMAN AND B. B. BRODIE. Storage, synthesis, and metabolism of monoamines in the developing brain. J. Neurochem. 9: 53, 1962.

22. KLAIBER, E. L., Y. KOBAYASHI, D. M. BROVERMAN AND F. HALL. Plasma monoamine oxidase activity in regularly menstruating women and in amenorrheic women receiving cyclic treatment with estrogens and a progestin. J. Clin. Endocrinol. 33: 630, 1971.

23. KUZUYA, H., AND T. NAGATSU. Flavins and monoamine oxidase activity in the brain, liver and kidney of the developing rat. J. Neurochem. 16: 123, 1969.

24. NACHMIAS, J. T. Amine oxidase and 5-hydroxytryptamine in developing rat brain. J. Neurochem. 6: 99, 1960.

25. NIES, A., D. S. ROBINSON, J. M. DAVIS AND C. L. RAVARIS. Changes in monoamine oxidase with aging. In: Psychopharmacology and Aging, edited by C.

Eisdorfer and W. F. Fann. New York: Plenum, 1974, p. 41.

26. NILSSON, S. E., N. TRYDING AND G. TUFVESSON. Serum monoamine oxidase (MAO) in diabetes mellitus and some other internal diseases. Acta Med. Scand. 184: 105, 1968.

27. PRANGE, A. J., J. E. WHITE, M. A. LIPTON AND A. M. KINKEAD. Influence of age on monoamine oxidase and catechol-O-methyltransferase in rat tissues. Life Sci. 6: 581, 1967.

28. RAWNSLEY, K. Epidemiology of affective disorders. In: Recent Development in Affective Disorders. British Journal of Psychiatry Special Publication No. 2, 1968, p. 227.

29. ROBINSON, D. S., J. M. DAVIS, A. NIES, et al. Relation of sex and aging to monoamine oxidase activity of human brain, plasma and platelets. Arch. Gen. Psychiat. 24: 536, 1971.

30. ROBINSON, D. S., J. M. DAVIS, A NIES, et al. Ageing, monoamines, and monoamine oxidase levels. Lancet 1: 290, 1972.

31. ROBINSON, D. S., W. LOVENBERG, H. KEISER AND A. SJOERDSMA. Effects of drugs on human blood platelet and plasma amine oxidase activity in vitro and in vivo. Biochem. Pharmacol. 17: 109, 1968.

32. SAMORAJSKI, T., AND C. ROLSTEN. Age and regional differences in the chemical composition of brains of mice, monkeys and humans. In: Neurobiological Aspects of Maturing and Aging, edited by D. H. Ford. New York: American Elsevier, 1973.

33. SCHILDKRAUT, J. J., AND S. S. KETY. Biogenic amines and emotion. Science 156: 21, 1967.

34. SILVERMAN, C. The Epidemiology of Depression. Baltimore: Johns Hopkins Press, 1968.

35. TIMIRAS, P. S., D. B. HUDSON AND S. OKLUND. Changes in central nervous system free amino acids with development and aging. In: Neurobiological Aspects of Maturing and Aging, edited by D. H. Ford. New York: American Elsevier, 1973.

36. UDENFRIEND, S., H. WEISSBACH AND B. B. BRODIE. Assay of serotonin and related metabolites, enzymes and drugs. In: Methods of Biochemical Analysis, edited by D. Glick. New York: Wiley-Interscience, 1958.

37. VERNADAKIS, A. Comparative studies of neurotransmitter substances in the maturing and aging central nervous

system of the chicken. In: *Neurobiological Aspects of Maturing and Aging*,
edited by D. H. Ford. New York:
American Elsevier, 1973.

38. VERNADAKIS, A. Changes in nucleic
acid content and butyrylcholinesterase
activity in CNS structures during the
life-span of the chicken. *J. Gerontol.*

28: 281, 1973.

39. YOUDIN, M. B. H. Multiple forms of
mitochondrial monoamine oxidase.
Brit. Med. Bull. 29: 120, 1973.

40. ZORZOLI, A. Enzymes and cellular metabolism. In: *Men, Molecules and Aging*,
edited by S. Bakerman. Springfield, Ill.:
Thomas, 1967.

Procaine HCl (Gerovital H3): A weak, reversible, fully competitive inhibitor of monoamine oxidase[1,2]

M. DAVID MacFARLANE[3]

School of Pharmacy
University of Southern California
Los Angeles, California 90007

ABSTRACT

A specially stabilized form of procaine hydrochloride (Gerovital H3) has been shown to be a more potent inhibitor of monoamine oxidase than procaine HCl itself and a weaker inhibitor of this enzyme than iproniazid. This preparation was studied to determine its mode of interaction with monoamine oxidase using purified rat brain mitochondrial monoamine oxidase as the enzyme source. Reaction velocities were determined spectrophotometrically by quantitating the rate of appearance of 4-hydroxyquinoline from kynuramine. Dilutional studies comparing the mechanism of inhibition of monoamine oxidase produced by Gerovital H3 and by iproniazid demonstrated that Gerovital H3 was a reversible inhibitor of monoamine oxidase. Analysis of studies using Lineweaver-Burk and Dixon plots revealed that Gerovital H3 was a fully competitive inhibitor of monoamine oxidase. That Gerovital H3 is a weak, reversible, competitive inhibitor of monoamine oxidase may explain the absence of adverse reactions associated with the clinical use of Gerovital H3 as compared to the severe adverse reactions that have been associated with the use of irreversible monoamine oxidase inhibitors.—MACFARLANE, M. D. Procaine HCl (Gerovital H3): A weak, reversible, fully competitive inhibitor of monoamine oxidase. *Federation Proc.* 34: 108–110, 1975.

[1] From Session IV, *Aging of homeostatic control systems*, of the FASEB Conference on *Biology of Development and Aging*, presented at the 58th Annual Meeting of the Federation of American Societies for Experimental Biology, Atlantic City, N.J., April 10, 1974.

[2] Supported in part by a grant from Rom- Amer Pharmaceuticals, Beverly Hills, California.

[3] Current address: Meyer Laboratories, 1900 West Commercial Blvd., Ft. Lauderdale, FL. 33309.

Abbreviations: GH3 = Gerovital H3; MAO = monoamine oxidase.

Previously reported studies (8, 12) were designed to elucidate a possible mechanism of action for the compound Gerovital H3 (GH3), a drug which has been shown to be useful for the treatment of some of the manifestations of old age (1, 4, 18). The results of these studies showed that GH3 was an inhibitor of the enzyme monoamine oxidase (MAO) (8, 12). When the ability of GH3 to inhibit MAO was compared with that of procaine hydrochloride (Novocain), it was found that GH3 produced a significantly greater inhibition of MAO than did procaine. The GH3 used in these pharmacological studies, in geriatric individuals, and in the studies reported herein was composed of a 2% solution of procaine hydrochloride that had been altered during the manufacturing process by the addition of various substances which have been said to increase the half life of the active ingredient, procaine hydrochloride (for exact composition of GH3, see ref 1).

In addition to comparing the activity of GH3 with that of procaine, the ability of GH3 to inhibit MAO was compared with iproniazid. Iproniazid was chosen as a standard of comparison in these studies since it is a classical inhibitor of MAO about which much is known concerning its mechanism of action.

Table 1 presents the results of experiments comparing the MAO inhibiting activity of GH3 and iproniazid. These data demonstrated that iproniazid was a more potent inhibitor of MAO than was GH3 with all the concentrations of the compounds studied. The data in the third row of Table 1 present the percent difference in inhibition of MAO produced by these two compounds. Statistical analysis of these differences showed that iproniazid produced a significantly greater inhibition of MAO than did GH3.

The difference in the ability of GH3 and iproniazid to inhibit MAO could be explained in a number of ways. For one, the weaker inhibition of MAO produced by GH3 may be due to a different mechanism of interaction between GH3 and MAO than has been reported for iproniazid and MAO. It has been demonstrated that iproniazid is an irreversible (23), mixed noncompetitive–competitive inhibitor of MAO (5, 14) that has been speculated to produce inhibition by combining with sulfhydryl and metal groups at the active site of the enzyme (9). In contrast, it might be possible to explain the weaker inhibition of MAO produced by GH3 by postulating that GH3 interacts in a reversible, competitive manner with the active site on MAO. In order to determine the validity of this hypothesis concerning the mode of enzyme inhibition produced by GH3, a series of studies were performed to determine the nature of the interaction between the drug GH3 and the enzyme MAO.

METHODS

These studies were conducted using rat brain mitochondrial MAO obtained by differential centrifugation techniques. The method of prepara-

TABLE 1. Percent inhibition of kynuramine hydrolysis by MAO produced by Gerovital H3 and iproniazid[a,b]

	Concentration of Inhibitor		
Inhibitor	1×10^{-2}	3.3×10^{-3}	1×10^{-4}
Gerovital H3	86.5 ± 2.6	50.6 ± 2.2	32.3 ± 2.0
Iproniazid	99.4 ± 0.1	85.6 ± 1.3	62.7 ± 1.5
Difference, %	12.9[c]	35.0[c]	30.4[c]

[a] Percent inhibition was calculated from the rate of hydrolysis of kynuramine with and without inhibitors present.   [b] Each value represents the average of 5 experiments ± SE.   [c] Significant difference: $P < 0.05$.   (After MacFarlane (12). Courtesy of *J. Am. Geriat. Soc.*)

tion of the mitochondrial MAO was that of Seiden and Westley (19) who showed that this enzyme preparation had high MAO activity with only 60% of the total protein. The isolation procedure resulted in approximately a 10-fold purification of the MAO.

The enzyme substrate used in these studies was kynuramine and the activity of the enzyme was determined using the spectrophotometric method of Weissbach et al. (22). In these studies the velocity of the enzymatic reaction was quantitated by measuring the appearance of 4-hydroxyquinoline, a metabolite of kynuramine, in micromoles/milligram protein/hour. Protein determinations were performed as described by Lowry and co-workers (11).

The protocol used in experiments to determine the reversibility of the interaction between GH3 and MAO included incubation of the enzyme with one of the two inhibitors for 15 min at 37 C after which the enzyme–inhibitor complex was diluted three times with buffer prior to adding the substrate kynuramine and determining the degree of inhibition. (For further details of the methodology used in these studies, see ref 13.) The percent inhibition of MAO produced in the diluted, preincubated solutions was compared with other appropriate solutions to determine if dilution of the enzyme–inhibitor complex resulted in decreased inhibition of the enzyme, thus indicating the type of drug–enzyme complex formed. According to the experimental protocol, it was established that if the percent inhibition produced in solution #1 was equal to that in solution #2 the interaction between the inhibitor and the enzyme was reversible. On the other hand, if the percent inhibition produced in solution #1 was the same as that observed in solution #3, the interaction between the enzyme and the inhibitor was irreversible.

TABLE 2. Inhibition of rat brain MAO by Gerovital H3 and iproniazid

Inhibitor	Solution #	Percent Inhibition $\pm$ SE[a]
Gerovital H3	1 GH3	49.5 $\pm$ 5.6
Gerovital H3	2 GH3	50.6 $\pm$ 5.2
Gerovital H3	3 GH3	86.5 $\pm$ 2.6[b]
Iproniazid	1 Ipr	99.4 $\pm$ 0.1
Iproniazid	2 Ipr	85.6 $\pm$ 1.3[c]
Iproniazid	3 Ipr	99.4 $\pm$ 0.1

Reversible inhibition: percent inhibition in #1 = #2. Irreversible inhibition: percent inhibition in #1 = #3.   [a] Each value represents the average of 5 experiments.   [b] Significantly different from solutions 1 GH3 and 2 GH3: $P < 0.01$.   [c] Significantly different from solutions 1 Ipr and 3 Ipr: $P < 0.05$.   (After MacFarlane and Besbris (13). Courtesy of *J. Am. Geriat. Soc.*)

RESULTS

Table 2 shows the results of experiments designed to determine whether GH3 was a reversible or irreversible inhibitor of MAO. In these experiments, GH3 was compared with iproniazid, a known irreversible inhibitor of MAO. The data presented in Table 2 show that the percent inhibition of MAO produced by GH3 in solutions #1 and 2 were for all intents and purposes equal and the inhibition produced in these solutions was significantly less than the inhibition produced by GH3 in solution #3. These data were interpreted to indicate that the inhibition of MAO produced by GH3 was reversible. In the experiments in which iproniazid was used, drug-induced inhibition of MAO was the same in solutions #1 and 3 and the percent inhibition produced in solution #2 was significantly less than that observed in solutions #1 and 3. These results demonstrated that iproniazid was an irreversible inhibitor of MAO.

Since the results of these experiments indicate that GH3 is a reversible inhibitor of MAO, it would be desirable to determine if GH3 is a competitive or noncompetitive inhibitor of the enzyme. It was felt that it was important to obtain this information since competitiveness would indicate that GH3 is reacting with the active site of the enzyme. On the other hand, if the inhibition is noncompetitive, then this would indicate that GH3 may be acting at a nonspecific site to prevent essential conformational changes of the active site of the enzyme.

Figure 1 shows the results of enzyme kinetic studies plotted according to the method described by Lineweaver and Burk (10). When the reciprocal of the substrate concentration was plotted against the reciprocal of the velocity, the intercept of the

control and inhibited enzyme plots on the ordinate coincided. Thus, GH3 had no effect on V_{max} but did cause an increase in the K_m. This is interpreted to indicate that GH3 interacts competitively with MAO. The concentrations of GH3 used in these studies were 1×10^{-4}, 5×10^{-5} and 2.5×10^{-5}M. The K_m for the uninhibited reaction was 5.0×10^{-4} and the K_i was 8.9×10^{-5}M.

In order to obtain additional information relating to the type of interaction occurring between GH3 and MAO, the inhibition kinetics were analyzed according to Dixon (6). The results of this assessment are presented in Fig. 2. Reciprocals of the rates of the inhibited reactions obtained using kynuramine concentrations of 1×10^{-4} and 2×10^{-4}M were

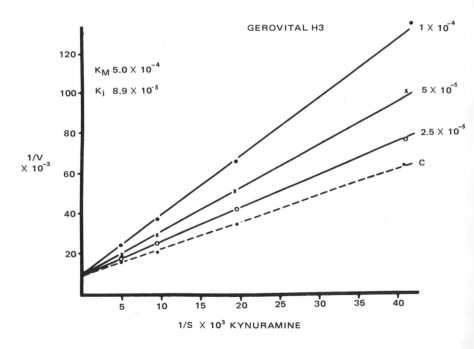

Figure 1. Kinetics of inhibition of purified rat brain mitochondrial MAO produced by GH3. The Lineweaver-Burk plot shows competitive inhibition. V is the rate of production of 4-hydroxyquinoline from kynuramine and is expressed as micromoles/milligram protein/hour. (After MacFarlane and Besbris (13). Courtesy of *J. Am. Geriat. Soc.*)

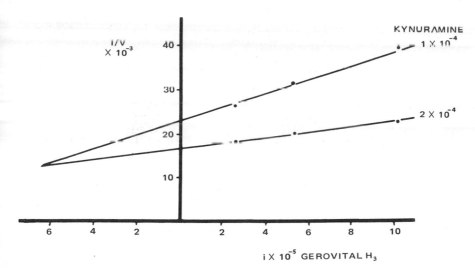

Figure 2. Kinetics of inhibition of purified rat brain mitochondrial MAO produced by GH3. The Dixon plot shows fully competitive inhibition. V is the rate of production of 4-hydroxyquinoline from kynuramine and is expressed as micromoles/milligram protein/hour. (After MacFarlane and Besbris (13). Courtesy of *J. Am. Geriat. Soc.*)

plotted against various inhibitor concentrations. The lines so obtained were straight and did not intersect on the abscissa. This indicates that GH3 and the substrate kynuramine combine with the same active site on the surface of MAO and not with another site sufficiently close to the active site to reduce the affinity of the enzyme for the substrate.

DISCUSSION

The data presented here indicate that GH3 is a weak, reversible, fully competitive inhibitor of MAO. This mode of action is in marked contrast to that exhibited by other known inhibitors of MAO that are used clinically for the treatment of depression and hypertension. For example, it has been demonstrated that compounds like pargyline (Eutonyl) (7, 21), phenelzine (Nardil) (21) and tranylcypromine (Parnate) (2) are irreversible inhibitors of MAO and

produce, for all intents and purposes, a noncompetitive inhibition, probably due to formation of covalent bonds between the drug and MAO (15).

It has been widely reported that patients who are given irreversible inhibitors of MAO may experience hypertensive reactions manifested by chest pain, headache, and, on occasion, fatal intracranial hemorrhage; particularly after eating certain tyramine-containing foods such as cheese and wine, after taking tricyclic antidepressants, and after ingesting certain commonly used sympathomimetic amines that are found in common cold remedies (3, 20). On the other hand, hypertensive reactions have not been reported to occur in patients being treated with GH3, and consequently, there are no restrictions as to the types of food that may be enjoyed while taking GH3.

The absence of hypertensive reactions with GH3 therapy may be related to the reversible, competitive inhibition of MAO produced by this agent. With the use of this type of inhibitor, the presence of additional and/or excessive quantities of substrate for MAO such as tyramine, norepinephrine, or serotonin could result in alleviation of the GH3-induced inhibition of MAO with displacement of the drug from its binding sites on the enzyme. This would allow the enzyme to metabolize and reduce the elevated levels of substrate and thereby prevent a hypertensive reaction that may be hazardous to the patient.

Robinson et al. (16, 17) have shown that there is an age-dependent increase in MAO activity of human brain, plasma and platelets and a corresponding decrease in central monoamines. These correlations could explain some of the manifestations of aging, especially as related to CNS function. The ability of GH3 to inhibit MAO may explain why this agent is effective in the alleviation of some of the signs and symptoms of aging.

The author gratefully acknowledges the technical expertise of Mr. Richard E. Brown and Ms. Priscilla Lucas.

REFERENCES

1. ASLAN, A. *Therapiewoche* 7: 14, 1956.
2. BARBATO, L. M., AND L. G. ABOOD. *Biochim. Biophys. Acta* 67: 531, 1963.
3. BLACKWELL, B., E. MARLEY, J. PRICE AND D. TAYLOR. *Brit. J. Psychiat.* 113: 349, 1967.
4. COHEN, S. 20th Annual meeting of the Academy of Psychosomatic Medicine, 1973.
5. DAVIDSON, A. N. *Biochem. J.* 67: 316, 1957.
6. DIXON, M. *Biochem. J.* 55: 170, 1953.
7. HELLERMAN, L., AND V. E. ERWIN. *J. Biol. Chem.* 243: 5234, 1968.
8. HRACHOVEC, J. P. *Federation Proc.* 31: 604, 1972.
9. KUROSAWA, A. *Chem. Pharm. Bull. Tokyo* 17: 43, 1969.
10. LINEWEAVER, H., AND D. BURK. *J. Am. Chem. Soc.* 56: 658, 1934.
11. LOWRY, O. H., N. J. ROSEBROUGH, A. I. FARR AND R. J. RANDALL. *J. Biol. Chem.* 193: 265, 1951.
12. MACFARLANE, M. D. *J. Am. Geriat. Soc.* 21: 414, 1973.
13. MACFARLANE, M. D., AND H. BESBRIS. *J. Am. Geriat. Soc.* 22: 365–371, 1974.
14. MCEWEN, C. M., G. SASAKI AND D. C. JONES. *Biochemistry* 8: 3963, 1969.
15. ORELAND, L., H. KINEMUCHI AND B. Y. YOO. *Life Sci.* 13: 1533, 1973.
16. ROBINSON, D. S., J. M. DAVIS, A. NIES, R. W. COLBORN, J. N. DAVIS, H. R. BOURNE, W. E. BONNEY, D. M. SHAW AND A. J. COPPEN. *Lancet* 1: 290, 1972.
17. ROBINSON, D. S., J. N. DAVIS, A. NIES, C. L. RAVARIS AND D. SYLVESTER. *Arch. Gen. Psychiat.* 24: 536, 1971.
18. SAKALIS, G., D. OH, S. GERSHON AND B. SHOPSIN. *Current Therap. Res.* 16: 59, 1974.
19. SEIDEN, L. S., AND J. WESTLEY. *Biochim. Biophys. Acta* 58: 363, 1972.
20. SJOQVIST, F. *Proc. Roy. Soc. Med.* 58: 967, 1965.
21. TAYLOR, J. D., A. A. WYKES, C. GLADISH AND W. B. MARTIN. *Nature* 187: 941, 1960.
22. WIESSBACH, H., T. E. SMITH, J. W. DALY, B. WITKOP AND S. ODENFRIEND. *J. Biol. Chem.* 235: 1160, 1960.
23. ZELLER, E. A., J. BARSKY AND E. R. BERMAN. *J. Biol. Chem.* 214: 267, 1955.

Discussion of papers on aging of homeostatic control systems

Questions presented to individual panel members brought out the following additional points:

PAUL E. SEGALL: Subsequent to the preparation of the findings reported, 2 out of 3 tryptophan-deficient rats, restored to commercial diet and mated at 18–20 months of age, gave birth to normal litters of 8 and 9 pups each. In 11 controls of corresponding age, no offspring were produced. Although limited, these findings indicate that in terms of reproductive capability, the physiological age of tryptophan-deprived rats corresponded to that of significantly younger animals.

Evidence of behavioral aberrations (severe trembling and even convulsions) supports the proposition that serotonin metabolism was affected in those tryptophan-deficient animals. Brain 5-HT levels will soon be measured in our experimental rats, and their significance in relation to sleep regulation is recognized as a useful parameter to investigate in aging studies.

The weight of the animal does not alter its rate of recovery from cold immersion within the range tested (280–370 g).

HAROLD H. SANDSTEAD: I am not aware of any correlation between zinc deficiency and increased convulsibility.

WILLIAM D. DENCKLA: Eighteen hormones were tested directly and indirectly, but whether the hormone postulated is another known pituitary hormone will depend on its subsequent purification and molecular identification. It is not likely, based on our findings, to be somatomedin.

If this pituitary factor, thought to inhibit peripheral effects of thyroid hormone, plays an important role in the aging process, one might wonder whether pituitary insufficiency in human beings might affect aging; however, since humans cannot be hypophysectomized,

this aspect remains unexplained. In rats, in which hypophysectomy can be effected surgically, the pituitary will often regenerate, and one of the hormones restored is the pituitary hormone in question. If regeneration is prevented by treatment of the sella turcica with 40% formaldehyde, one might expect some degree of rejuvenation. These experiments would be interesting to undertake.

DONALD S. ROBINSON: Although I have not studied cholinergic systems, others have done work which shows that these systems also can be altered in aging. In considering changes in neurotransmitter activity, we must remember that these changes can occur in different degrees, depending on the brain region. In addition, absolute changes in level and activity might be less meaningful in functional terms than relative changes in the balance of the several neurotransmitters characteristic of each brain region.

With respect to the ratio of Type a to Type b MAO isoenzyme activities with aging, although we did not calculate it, one can make deductions based on the activities of tryptamine, supposedly a substrate for MAO a, and of benzylamine as a substrate for MAO b.

It may, indeed, be useful to study MAO levels in animals of long life-span, such as parrots and tortoises.

M. DAVID MACFARLANE: When comparing Gerovital H3 with procaine HCl in terms of MAO inhibition, procaine produces greater inhibition, but only slightly.

As I published previously, both Gerovital and procaine HCl contain 2% procaine, but in Gerovital benzoic acid, para-amino acid as well as some other salts and buffers have been added, and the pH is slightly lower. I have had a physical chemist look into Gerovital and the possibility of its forming a complex with benzoic

219

acid, and such complexing evidently is possible. I have some preliminary evidence to indicate that benzoic acid and procaine form a complex at the ester linkage in procaine, and this may protect the procaine from hydrolysis by pseudocholinesterase, although we have not worked out experiments to determine this yet. Our assumption is that the active ingredient is procaine.

Ontogeny of mouse T-lymphocyte function

DONALD E. MOSIER AND PHILIP L. COHEN

Laboratory of Immunology
National Institute of Allergy and Infectious Diseases
National Institutes of Health
Bethesda, Maryland 20014

ABSTRACT

The development of lymphocytes within the fetal and neonatal BALB/c mouse thymus is reviewed with particular emphasis on the maturity of immunologic functions. Fetal thymocytes respond by vigorous proliferation to stimulation by allogeneic lymphoid cells or by phytohemagglutinin. Such reactivity is much diminished in neonatal thymus or thymic-derived (T) cells in neonatal spleen. Splenic T cells seem to mature more slowly than immunoglobulin-bearing B lymphocytes in the neonatal spleen, but the finding is confounded by the presence of large numbers of "suppressor" T cells in the neonatal spleen. For example, the in vitro antibody response to the T-independent antigen dinitrophenyl-lysine-Ficoll is optimal by 2 or 3 weeks of age, but the in vitro response to T-dependent sheep erythrocytes does not reach adult levels until 6 weeks of age, suggesting a deficiency in T "helper cells." The response of neonatal spleen cells to sheep erythrocytes cannot be reconstituted by adult T cells however, unless neonatal splenic T cells are first depleted by anti-Thy 1 serum and complement. The target of this T suppressor cell seems to be only B cells, and not other T cells. The overall sequence of T lymphocyte maturation in the mouse seems to start with large numbers of reactive T cells during intrauterine life, to proceed to an excess of suppressor T cells as well as some functionally active helper or effector T cells in early neonatal life, and finally to achieve a stable equilibrium between T cell subpopulations between 5 and 6 weeks of age.—MOSIER, D. E. AND P. L. COHEN. Ontogeny of mouse T-lymphocyte function. *Federation Proc.* 34: 137–140, 1975.

L ymphocytes that differentiate within the thymus or under thymic influence acquire unique functions and surface markers. This population of cells has been called "T lymphocytes" in recent years to distinguish it from other lymphocyte populations with different functions and characteristics. Within the population of cells called T lymphocytes there are undoubtedly several subpopulations of cells with different functional properties or in different stages of maturation. Many T lymphocytes seem to be involved in regulation of immune responses. At least some T lymphocytes must bear anti-gen-specific receptor molecules on their surfaces. These receptors may or may not be immunoglobulin in nature, but their specificity is shown by the "carrier effect" in antibody formation to hapten-protein conjugates, by the hapten specificity of delayed hypersensitivity and by recognition of cellular alloantigens in the mixed lymphocyte reaction, cell-mediated cytotoxicity, and graft-versus-host reaction. So, despite their common origin in the thymus, individual T cells show great heterogeneity in terms of specificity and function.

Studies carried out in our laboratory over the last 2 years have focused on the ontogeny of T lymphocyte function in the BALB/c mouse (6, 7). The original impetus for this work sprang from the obvious hetero-geneity of T-cell function in the adult, and the hope that during ontogeny different T-cell subpopulations, and hence different functions, might appear at different times. Before discussing our data, however, I will review briefly the work of others regarding the origin of thymic lymphocytes in the mouse (5, 9), which is summarized in Fig. 1.

Lymphocytes first develop in the mouse thymus at 12–14 days of gestation. The first lymphocytes are derived from yolk sac or primitive blood island stem cells that differentiate in the environment of the thymic epithelial rudiment (4). Several investigators have produced evidence to suggest that the interaction of epithelial and lymphoid stem cells is required for lymphopoiesis in the thymus (1, 8). Between 14 and 18 days of gestation, the number of thy-

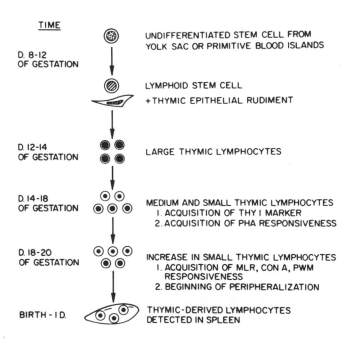

Figure 1. Ontogeny of thymus-derived lymphocytes in mice.

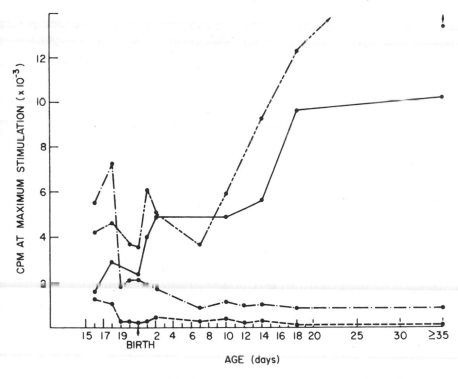

Figure 2. The reactivity of BALB/c fetal, neonatal, or adult thymocytes to phytohemagglutinin (● —·—·—·— ●), concanavalin A (● — — — — — — — ●), pokeweed mitogen (● ——— ●), or no phytomitogen (● – – – ●).

mus lymphocytes increases greatly, mainly by proliferation of groups of large cells in the thymic area destined to become cortex, and several differentiation antigens, e.g., Thy 1 (θ), Ly 1, Ly 2/Ly 3, Ly 5, appear on their surface (2). The ability to respond to the plant lectin phytohemagglutinin (PHA) is acquired at about 16 days of gestation in the BALB/c mouse. By 18 days of gestation, the thymus is rich in lymphocytes which have begun to express some of the functional activities of their adult counterparts, as will be discussed below. Emigration of T cells to peripheral lymphoid tissue begins about the time of birth in the mouse, with lymph nodes developing signifi-

cant numbers of Thy-1-positive cells before the spleen (10). Although these first peripheral T cells may come from the thymus, there is some evidence to suggest that fetal liver also may be a source of T lymphocytes during late embryonic life (11).

By about 16 days of gestation, it is possible to obtain enough cells from fetal BALB/c thymus to assay their reactivity to a variety of stimulants in microculture. We have stimulated such fetal cells with plant lectins,

---

Abbreviations: PHA, phytohemagglutinin; Con A, concanavalin A, DNP-Ficoll, dinitrophenyl-lysine substituted Ficoll.

bacterial lipopolysaccharide or allogeneic spleen cells, and assayed proliferation by incorporation of tritiated thymidine into acid-precipitable material.

Lipopolysaccharide failed to stimulate proliferation at any time. This is not surprising since lipopolysaccharide seems to stimulate primarily bone marrow-derived immunoglobulin-bearing lymphocytes, and only 4–5 such cells per 1,000 lymphoid cells were detected in 18-day fetal thymus.

The results of stimulating fetal or neonatal thymocytes with phytohemagglutinin (PHA), concanavalin A (Con A), or pokeweed mitogen (PWM) are shown in Fig. 2. The curves for mitogen reactivity were drawn by pooling data from a large number of experiments. In any individual experiment, mice of several ages were examined, and six replicate microcultures were performed per experimental group. Only pokeweed mitogen at 16 days

of gestation failed to show significant ($P < 0.05$) stimulation of proliferation. Fetal thymocytes were quite reactive to PHA, in fact more so than normal thymocytes at any other time in the life of the animal. Prior to birth, however, reactivity to PHA begins to decline and stabilizes at a low level at about one week of age.

Reactivity of thymocytes to Con A and pokeweed mitogen increases slowly during late fetal and early neonatal life and reaches adult levels between 2 and 3 weeks of age. The ability of BALB/c thymocytes to react to mitomycin-treated allogeneic C57BL/6 spleen cells is shown in Fig. 3. By the 19th or 20th day of gestation, fetal thymocytes give a mixed lymphocyte reaction equal in magnitude to that of adult thymocytes. The ability of neonatal thymocytes to give a mixed lymphocyte reaction diminishes during the first 2 weeks of life, then returns to adult levels. The reactivity against syn-

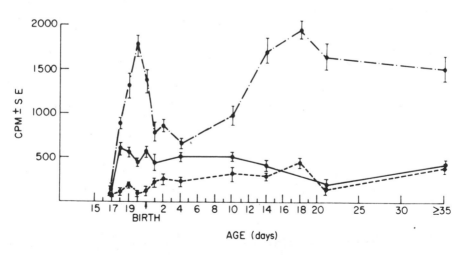

Figure 3. The reactivity of BALB/c thymocytes to mitomycin-treated allogeneic (C57BL/6) or syngeneic spleen cells. Legend: + allogeneic spleen cells (●—·—·—●); + syngeneic spleen cells (● —— ●); + syngeneic thymocytes (● – – – ●).

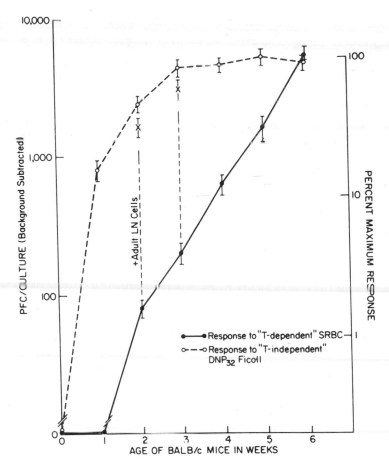

Figure 4. IgM plaque-forming cell response of BALB/c spleen cells cultured 4 days with sheep erythrocytes (SRBC) or dinitrophenyl-lysine Ficoll (DNP$_{32}$Ficoll).

genetic adult spleen is also shown, and, as previously reported by others, fetal or neonatal thymocytes mixed with adult spleen cells result in more proliferation than the mixture of adult thymus and spleen cells. Whether this so-called "isogeneic lymphocyte reaction" is a meaningful analogue of allogeneic recognition of H-2 and Ia-associated antigens is not clear.

As mentioned above, Thy 1-bearing lymphocytes of apparent thymic origin appear in the spleen shortly after birth. At the same time, numbers of immunoglobulin-bearing lymphocytes are increasing to the 30–40% of lymphoid cells characteristic of adult spleen. To examine the ontogeny of T lymphocyte function in the spleen, it was therefore necessary to take into account the reactivity of splenic B lymphocytes.

We have examined the reactivity of neonatal BALB/c spleen cells to mitogens as well as their ability to respond to "thymic-dependent" and "thymic-independent" antigens by producing antibody in vitro.

Reactivity of BALB/c spleen cells to the T-dependent mitogens PHA and Con A reaches adult levels between 3 and 4 weeks of age, whereas B-cell proliferation induced by lipopolysaccharide has achieved adult magnitude by 2 weeks of age.

Further evidence that splenic B cells are functionally mature before T cells is shown in Fig. 4. The ability of 1×10^7 spleen cells from BALB/c mice of different ages to respond to sheep erythrocytes or dinitrophenyl-lysine substituted Ficoll (DNP-Ficoll) in Mishell-Dutton cultures was determined. In adult BALB/c mice, sheep erythrocytes require T lymphocytes to generate a plaque-forming cell response, that is, are "T-dependent," and the response to DNP-Ficoll is unaffected by depletion of T cells, and is "T-independent" by current nomenclature. Cells releasing IgM antibody were detected by plaque-formation against sheep erythrocytes or trinitrophenyl-substituted sheep erythrocytes after 4 days in culture. Spleen cells from mice less than 24 hours old did not respond to either antigen. Thereafter, the ability of spleen cells to respond to the T-independent antigen DNP-Ficoll clearly preceded the ability to respond to T-dependent sheep erythrocytes. The magnitude of the plaque-forming cell response to DNP-Ficoll had attained adult levels by 3 weeks of age, whereas the maximum response to sheep erythrocytes was not attained until 6 weeks of age in this experiment. In other replicate experiments, mice 4 to 6 weeks old gave a maximal plaque-forming cell response to sheep erythrocytes, but at least a 2-week lag between optimal DNP-Ficoll and sheep erythrocyte responsiveness was always observed.

Our initial interpretation of these findings was that B cells are functionally mature earlier than T cells in the spleen, at least in terms of contributing to antibody formation. To test this hypothesis, peripheral lymph node cells from adult BALB/c mice were added to neonatal spleen cells to serve as a source of mature T lymphocytes. The response to sheep erythrocytes and DNP-Ficoll was determined. Although large numbers (5×10^6) of adult lymph node cells significantly improved the sheep erythrocyte plaque-forming cell response of 2-week-old spleen cells, smaller numbers (1×10^6) had little if any effect. This result was puzzling since 1×10^6 lymph node cells fully reconstituted the sheep erythrocyte response of anti-Thy 1-treated adult spleen cells. In order to test the possibility that neonatal T lymphocytes were interfering with the activity of the adult lymph node T cells, neonatal spleens were treated with anti-Thy-1 serum and complement prior to adding 1×10^6 adult peripheral lymph node cells. Using this experimental protocol, we were able to show full reconstitution of the sheep RBC response as shown by the vertical dashed lines in Fig. 4. Pretreatment of 2-week-old spleen with anti-Thy 1 and complement also slightly enhanced the response to DNP-Ficoll (data not shown). Our tentative interpretation of these results is that neonatal T lymphocytes are not only very poor in providing "helper function" for antibody formation but also possess a nonspecific suppressor activity, which is anti-Thy 1-sensitive, and which inhibits the expression of helper activity by adult T cells as well as whatever helper function the neonatal T cells may possess. This interpretation was strengthened by the data generated in the following set of experiments. Spleen cells from BALB/c mice 1 or 2 weeks old were mixed with adult

BALB/c spleen cells in varying ratios, but with the total number of cells in culture kept constant at 1×10^7/ml. To simplify interpretation, only the T-independent response to DNP-Ficoll was measured so that maturity or efficiency of T helper cells did not contribute to responsiveness. Figure 5 shows the result of one such mixing experiment. The expected line illustrates the magnitude of the response anticipated if neonatal and adult cells interact neither synergistically nor antagonistically. The addition of small numbers of neonatal cells reduced the DNP-specific plaque-forming cell response more than expected. That this antagonistic or suppressor activity was due to T cells in neonatal spleen was shown

in the same experiment. Neonatal BALB/c spleen cells were passed over a nylon wool column. The column-passed cells contained 3% immuno-globulin-positive cells (T cell enriched) and the cells eluted from the column were 80% immunoglobulin-positive (B cell enriched). The same mixing experiment was done with these T and B cell-enriched fractions, and the DNP-Ficoll response measured. Enriching for T cells increased the suppressive activity of neonatal spleen cells, while the B-cell fraction gave an enhanced response, suggesting elimination of suppressor activity. Small numbers of neonatal thymocytes also suppress both the sheep erythrocyte and DNP-Ficoll plaque-forming cell responses of

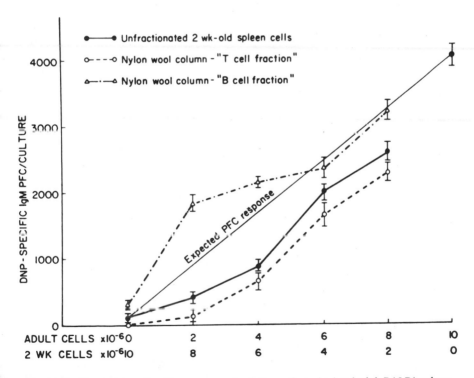

Figure 5. Plaque-forming cell response of mixtures of neonatal and adult BALB/c spleen cells to DNP-Ficoll.

adult spleen to a much greater extent than equal numbers of adult thymocytes, suggesting again that the cell in neonatal spleen capable of suppressing antibody formation in vitro is thymus-derived.

Several observations suggest that the neonatal T lymphocytes that suppress antibody formation are capable of regulating B cells but not other T cells. These observations are all negative experiments, but taken together they suggest that the putative regulatory T cell has a limited specificity allowing it to distinguish T and B lymphocytes. The experiments involved mixing 2-week-old and 8-week-old BALB/c spleen cells in varying ratios, just as was done when antibody synthesis in vitro was as-

sayed, and determining the ability of the cell mixture to respond to phyto mitogens, to respond to allogeneic cells in the mixed lymphocyte reaction or in the generation of cytotoxic lymphocytes, and to induce splenomegaly in neonatal (BALB/c × C57BL/6)F$_1$ hybrids (unpublished observations of D. E. Mosier, R. E. Tigelaar and H. C. Morse III). In none of these mixing experiments was there any suggestion that neonatal cells suppressed the reactivity of adult cells.

Figure 6 depicts a hypothetical scheme for T lymphocyte differentiation in the adult mouse. Many of the differentiation or emigration pathways are speculative, but an attempt was made to incorporate most

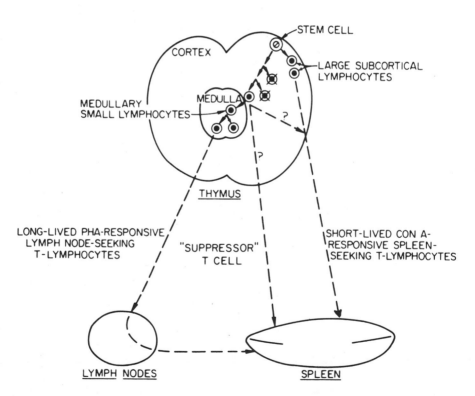

Figure 6. Hypothetical scheme for differentiation of T-cell subpopulations.

of the available data into the model. Blood-borne stem cells immigrate into the thymic cortex where, under the stimulatory and perhaps regulatory influence of thymic epithelial cells, cell division and differentiation begin. The subcapsular region thus contains large numbers of rapidly-dividing blast-like cells.

These cells have been assumed to be precursors of thymic lymphocytes only, but the possibility that short-lived spleen-seeking lymphocytes are derived from this supposedly immature pool is supported by some preliminary evidence (I. Weissman, personal communication, and P. L. Cohen and D. E. Mosier, unpublished observations). The thymic cortex is a mitotically active area, but at least some of the cells arising by division are eliminated by cell death. The purpose of the simultaneous high rate of division and cell death is unknown.

Cells reaching the corticomedullary junction may encounter a branch point in further differentiation pathways (3). Some cells may enter the medulla to undergo another cycle of division and join a small, highly-reactive, stable pool of lymphocytes. Cells also may emigrate from the region of the corticomedullary junction to the periphery, and these cells are good candidates for regulatory or suppressor T cells. Some long-lived lymph node-seeking lympho-cytes probably emigrate from the medulla, but at a much lower rate than cortical thymocytes. An anal-ogous cell population may be present in the fetal thymus, but cell types later represented in the cortex begin to dominate lymphopoiesis in the thymus of neonatal animals. Implicit in this scheme is the concept that several relatively independent lines of lymphocyte differentiation may be occurring simultaneously in the adult thymus.

In summary, we have shown signifi-cant T lymphocyte function in the fetal thymus in terms of PHA and mixed lymphocyte reaction activity. Between 2 and 3 weeks of age, reactivity to all the T cell mitogens and in the mixed lymphocyte reac-tion increases to adult levels in the thymus. Shortly thereafter, T-cell function seems to mature in the spleen for all functions measured ex-cept T-dependent antibody synthesis. The apparent lag in responsiveness to T-dependent antigens may be ex-plained, however, by the transitory appearance of T cells capable of regulating B-cell function. Although our initial hope of finding a time in ontogeny when pure T cell sub-populations exist has not been fully realized, it is clear that T–T- and T–B-cell interactions are important in regulating differentiation during ontogeny as well as differentiation during the course of an immune response. Indeed, the precedent for regulation may be set during estab-lishment of control over self-reactive cells. Finally, further study of the early events of T-lymphocyte func-tional differentiation would seem a promising route for understanding the final behavior of the differen-tiated product.

REFERENCES

1. AUERBACH, R. *Develop. Biol.* 2: 271, 1960.
2. BOYSE, E. A., M. MIYAZAWA, T. AOKI AND L. J. OLD. *Proc. Roy. Soc. London Ser. B* 170: 175, 1968.
3. JOEL, D. D., M. W. HESS AND H. COTTIER. *J. Exptl. Med.* 135: 907, 1972.
4. METCALF, D., AND M. A. S. MOORE. In: *Haemopoietic Cells.* Amsterdam: North-Holland, 1971, p. 278–284.
5. MOORE, M. A. S., AND J. J. T. OWEN. *J. Exptl. Med.* 126: 715, 1967.
6. MOSIER, D. E. *Nature New Biol.* 242: 184, 1973.
7. MOSIER, D. E. *J. Immunol.* 112: 305, 1974.
8. MOSIER, D. E., AND C. W. PIERCE. *J. Exptl. Med.* 136: 1484, 1972.
9. OWEN, J. J. T., AND M. C. RAFF. *J. Exptl. Med.* 132: 1216, 1970.

10. RAFF, M. C., AND J. J. T. OWEN. *European J. Immunol.* 1: 27, 1971.

11. YUNG, L. L. L., T. C. WYN-EVANS AND E. DIENER *European J. Immunol.* 3: 224, 1973.

Differentiation of thymus cells[1,2]

IRVING L. WEISSMAN,[3] MYRA SMALL,[4]
C. GARRISON FATHMAN[5] AND LEONARD A. HERZENBERG
*Laboratory of Experimental Oncology, Department of Pathology
and Department of Genetics, Stanford University
School of Medicine, Stanford, California 94305*

The process of cellular differen- tiation in the thymus presum ably leads to the development of im- munocompetent peripheral "T" lym- phocytes (1, 6). Although there are considerable data showing the exist- ence of a small pool of immunocom- petent cortisone-resistant, medullary thymocytes which, as a population, bear low concentration of Thy 1.2, lack TL antigens, and exhibit high concentrations of H-2, the identifica- tion of their immediate precursors is not yet known (1). Under conditions of parenteral hydrocortisone admin- istration it has been demonstrated that at least some of the cortisone-re- sistant medullary thymocytes are de- rived from an intrathymic pool of cortisone-sensitive cortical precur- sors (7). In this paper we demon- strate the in vivo maturation of at least three lines of "mature" thymus cells from a precursor subclass using selective labeling of these precursors in situ as a marker.

MATERIALS AND METHODS

We used two methods of cell sorting to define and analyze thymocyte sub- populations—sedimentation velocity

(5) and a fluorescence and light acti- vated cell sorter (FACS) (3, 4). The latter technique (FACS) allows sepa- ration of cell subpopulations on the basis of size (by monitoring the inten- sity of low angle light scattering) or concentration of cell-surface anti- gens (by monitoring intensity of fluorescence emitted by cells binding specific fluorescence antiserum). These techniques are described in full in a previous publication (2).

[1] From Session V, *Development and Aging in Organ Systems*, of the FASEB Conference on *Biology of Development and Aging*, presented at the 58th Annual Meeting of the Federation of American Societies for Experimental Biology, Atlantic City, N.J., April 11, 1974.

[2] Supported by Public Health Service Grants AI-09072 and GM-17367.

[3] Faculty Research Awardee, American Can- cer Society. Sabbatical address: Salk Institute, P.O. Box 1809, San Diego, CA 92112.

[4] Stanley McCormick Fellow; present address, Department of Cell Biology, Weiz- mann Institute for Science, Rehovoth, Israel.

[5] Present address, National Cancer Institute, Bethesda, Md.

RESULTS

Size distribution of normal thymocytes separated by velocity sedimentation and the FACS

The distribution of cells obtained by 1-*g* sedimentation is shown in Fig. 1. (Total cell recovery in that experiment was 87.7% of input cell numbers.) It is apparent that the modal cell number lies in the small lymphocyte region (labeled A in Fig. 1), containing ~80% of the total re-

covered cell population, whereas fractions 1 to 32 contain large to medium cells. Nonviable cells appear in increasing numbers after fraction 45; in this experiment they constitute 7.1% of recovered cells.

Sedimentation and scatter analysis of cortisone-resistant thymocytes

Since cortisone-resistant thymocytes appear to be derived (at least in part) from cortisone-sensitive precursors, experiments were performed to

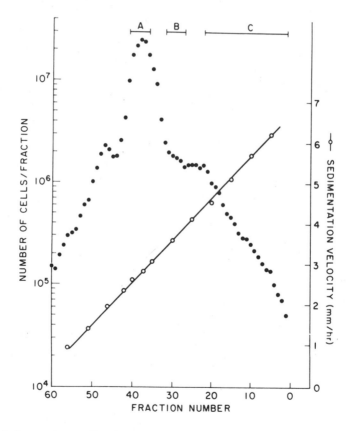

Figure 1. Sedimentation profile of a 5-week-old BALB/c donor's thymocyte suspension: 2×10^8 cells were layered over an FBS-CSM gradient as described in Materials and Methods, and allowed to sediment at 4 C for 12 hours. The ordinate is the logarithm of the number of cells per fraction, and the abscissa the fraction number. Pools A, B and C, as indicated, were removed for scatter analysis.

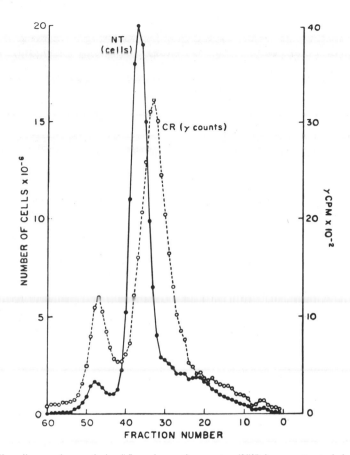

Figure 2. Cosedimentation analysis of 5-week-old BALB/c donor thymocytes: 2×10^7 ^{51}Cr-labeled cortisone-resistant (CR) thymocytes were cosedimented with 2×10^8 unlabeled thymocytes (NT) from untreated donors. On the ordinate, either ^{51}Cr or cell counts are recorded for each of the indicated fractions.

determine what size categories were enriched after administration of cortisone in vivo. Those thymus cells remaining 48 hours after intramuscular injection of 5 mg hydrocortisone acetate in adults or 2.5 mg in 5-day-old BALB/c mice were suspended, and cosedimented with "marker" normal thymocytes. A typical curve of cosedimented normal thymocytes and cortisone-resistant cells is shown in Fig. 2. It is apparent that the peak of cortisone-resistant cells is at a higher sedimentation velocity (fraction 34, ~3.1 mm/hr) than the modal peak of normal thymocytes (fraction 37, ~2.8 mm/hr), although there is considerable overlap.

Fluorescence analysis of αThy 1.2 stained BALB/c thymocytes

When unfractionated normal thymocytes are stained with fluoresceinated αThy 1.2 (Θ), and then analyzed for fluorescence intensity (excluding dead cells from analysis by electronic "gating" methods (4)) one obtains the distribution shown in Fig. 3. Three major peaks are seen, all with fluorescence above background (AKR/J thymocytes stained with fluoresceinated αThy 1.2 served as background controls for fluorescence). The dimmest peak corresponds with cortisone-resistant cells (which are shown superimposed in Fig. 3). Fluorescence analysis of cells in 1-*g* gradient fractions A, B and C (Fig. 1), after staining with fluoresceinated αThy 1.2, gives curves shown in Fig. 4. Pool A, which consists of small thymocytes, coincides with the middle fluorescence peak in Fig. 3, while pool B (cortisone-resistant cell enriched) contains mostly dim cells. The large and medium cells in pool C are mostly contained in the brightest

fluorescence peak. By calculation, the modal fluorescence per cell of pool C cells is approximately 1.3 × that of pool A, and 3.2 × that of the dim pool B cells.

Subclass maturation pathways

In the foregoing sections we have defined at least four distinct and separable subclasses of BALB/c thymocytes: *1*) dead or fragile cells; *2*) small thymic lymphocytes; *3*) large and medium thymic lymphocytes; and *4*) a class of thymocytes which share anti-Thy 1.2 fluorescence, scatter-intensity and sedimentation properties with cortisone-resistant thymocytes. It is the object of the following sections to analyze intersubclass maturation pathways, by selectively labeling in vivo a single subclass of cells.

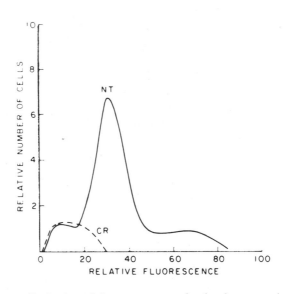

Figure 3. Frequency distribution of fluorescence intensity of normal thymocytes (NT) stained with anti-Thy 1.2 compared with a frequency distribution of the fluorescence intensity of cortisone-resistant (CR) thymocytes that has been superimposed. Note the correlation of CR-fluorescence intensity with the dullest subpopulation of the total thymocyte fluorescence distribution.

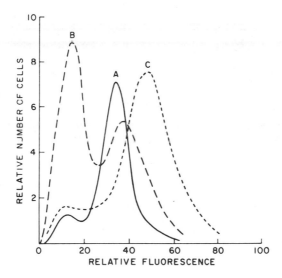

Figure 4. Frequency distribution of fluorescence intensity of the pooled 1-g cell populations (as displayed in Fig. 1). Note the relatively large fraction of dull cells seen in pool B. These cells correspond in fluorescence intensity and in size to cortisone-resistant thymocytes. Note the relative depletion of dull cells from Pools A and C. Again the ordinate portrays relative number of cells per fraction.

Sedimentation analysis of surface-labeled neonatal mouse thymus

A previous observation had indicated that ^{3}H-thymidine applied to the surface of the thymus could be detected initially in cells of the outer cortex and, under conditions of cold thymidine chase, subsequently in cells of the deeper cortex and the medulla (7).

In Fig. 5 it can be seen that 1 hour after application of ^{3}H-thymidine to the surfaces of neonatal thymus, label is concentrated in pool C (i.e., larger cells). It is thus apparent that dividing lymphocytes of the subcapsular zone of the thymic cortex vary in size from the largest to medium large. By 24 hours after administration of ^{3}H-thymidine, most of the label has shifted to the smaller cell fractions (pools A, B), with some residual counts in region C. After 48 or 72 hours, ^{3}H-thymidine is almost exclusively in the fractions of smaller thymocytes (pools A and B, Fig. 1), suggesting that the cells initially labeled had divided or differentiated to progeny of smaller size.

Fluorescence and scatter analysis of surface-labeled neonatal BALB/c thymus

The thymuses of 4- to 5-day-old BALB/c mice were labeled topically in situ as in the previous experimental section. At varying times thereafter, thymus cell suspensions were prepared, and sorted by scatter or fluorescence intensity. In the former, scatter peaks 1 (dead cells), 2 (small cells = Pool A), and 3 (large and medium cells = Pool C) were analyzed as to the relative percentage of labeled cells per subclass, as compared (as a ratio) to unfractionated cells (Fig. 6). The label is limited to cells in peak 3 30 min after application of ^{3}HTdR, and by 24 hours, the proportion of labeled cells is increasing in peaks 1 and 2, and decreasing in peak 3. High proportions of labeled cells are limited to peaks 1 and 2 by 48 and 72 hours after thymidine application. Since peak 1 represents dead cells, it is of interest that this peak contains rare (or no) labeled cells at 30 min, but increasing proportions of labeled cells at later times. It is evident that the dead cells do not become labeled until the appearance of label in the viable small cell population. This raises the interesting possibility that these cells

have died in vivo, although selective fragility of small cells has not been ruled out in this study.

In the final set of separation experiments, we compared the labeling index of the anti-Thy 1.2 brightest (large and medium) and dimmest (cortisone-resistant cell-like) fractions at varying intervals after topical administration of ^{3}HTdR. The results are shown in Fig. 7. Dull cells are not labeled immediately after topical administration of ^{3}HTdR, whereas the brightest fractions are. With increase in time, the labeling index of dull cells increases, while the labeling index of bright cells decreases. Thus, dull cells also represent progeny of

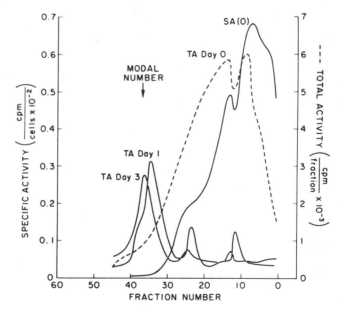

Figure 5. Sedimentation analysis of in situ labeled 5-day-old donor BALB/c thymus cells as a function of time after topical labeling with ^{3}HTdR. The data are graphed as either total activity (TA = cpm/fraction) or specific activity (SA = cpm/100 cells). Every fraction was tested, but the data points are removed for clarity of presentation. (The graphs represent connections of all data points.) In all three experiments, the modal cell peak was at fraction 37. Two modes of total activity were seen 1 hour after labeling (Day 0), at fractions 7 and 14. By day 1 the modal total activity was at fraction 35, and by day 3, fraction 37.

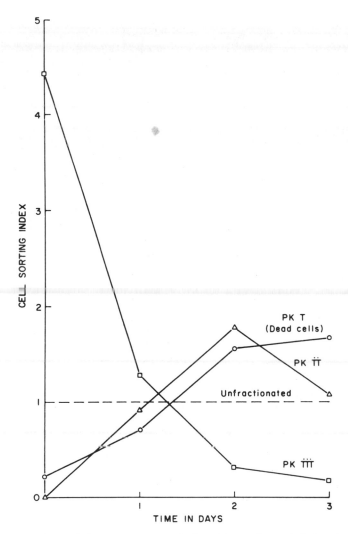

Figure 6. A comparison of the appearance of label within different scatter-defined subpopulations as a function of time after labeling. The ratio of the labeling index of test cells to unfractionated cells is plotted on the ordinate, and labeling to sacrifice interval on the abscissa. Note only peak 3 (large) cells are labeled at time zero. There then follows a disappearance of label in peak 3 coincident with the appearance of label in peaks 1 and 2. Peaks 1 and 2 label in parallel.

large, high Thy 1.2 (by fluorescence) cells.

SUMMARY AND CONCLUSIONS

Sedimentation, scatter, and fluorescence (with fluoresceinated anti-Thy 1.2) analysis of BALB/c thymocytes reveals several distinctive subclasses: *1*) dead (or fragile) cells; *2*) small cells with intermediate Thy 1.2

fluorescence; *3*) a broad peak of large cells which exhibit very bright Thy 1.2 fluorescence; and *4*) mid-size cells with low, but above background Thy 1.2 fluorescence. Labeling of thymus outer cortical DNA synthetic cells by topical application of ^{3}HTdR in situ initially labels only subclass 3 of these cells. These large bright cells serve as progenitors for all three of the other subclasses during the 1–3 days following initial labeling. It

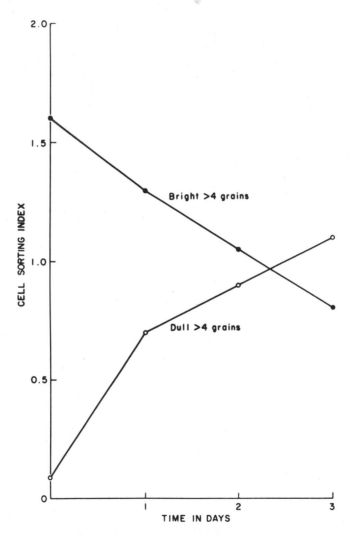

Figure 7. The comparison of appearance of label in cells fractionated in the fluorescence and light activated cell sorter by anti-Thy 1.2 fluorescence intensity over time. Only bright cells label at time zero and then the label appears in dull cells (cortisone-resistant) as it disappears from the bright fraction over 3 days.

should be noted that pathways of maturation which derive from cells other than subpopulation 3 are not susceptible to this method of analysis, and therefore we may be missing other important maturation sequences. It also should be noted that this analysis did not reveal a difference in maturation time from subclass 3 to the other three subclasses. This brings up the important point that there is no evidence here presented that sequential maturation from subclass 3 must proceed through any subclass to any other subclass. Therefore, it is possible that the three "mature" subclasses could be descendants of either common or independent "immature" progenitor cells in the outer cortex. Furthermore, we do not know if subclass 1 represents cells that are dead in situ, and therefore represent a late event in thymus cell maturation, are selectively radiosensitive to the doses of incorporated ^{3}H (calculated to be less than 10 rads per cell), or are merely more susceptible than other subpopulations to possible damage in the preparation of thymus cell suspensions.

Ms. Libuse Jerabek and Ms. Emi Kusaba provided excellent technical assistance, Ms. Lois Johnson provided excellent histological and autoradiographic preparations. We are indebted to George Gutman and David Korn for criticism of this manuscript.

REFERENCES

1. CANTOR, H., AND I. L. WEISSMAN. Development and function of subpopulations of thymocytes and T lymphocytes. *Progress in Allergy* In press.

2. FATHMAN, C. G., M. SMALL, L. A. HERZENBERG AND I. L. WEISSMAN. Thymus cell maturation, II. Differentiation of three "mature" subclasses in vivo. *Cellular Immunol.* In press.

3. HULETT, H. R., W. A. BONNER, R. G. SWEET AND L. A. HERZENBERG. Development and application of a rapid cell sorter. *Clin. Chem.* 19: 813, 1973.

4. JULIUS, M. H., R. G. SWEET, C. G. FATHMAN, AND L. A. HERZENBERG. Fluorescence activated cell sorting and its applications. Los Alamos, N.M. Oct. 17–19, 1973. AEC Symposium Series (C.O.N.S. 73–1007), 1974.

5. MILLER, R. G., AND R. A. PHILLIPS. Separation of cells by velocity sedimentation. *J. Cellular Physiol.* 73: 191, 1969.

6. WEISSMAN, I. L. Thymus cell migration. *J. Exptl. Med.* 126: 291, 1967.

7. WEISSMAN, I. L. Thymus cell maturation, studies on the origin of cortisone-resistant thymic lymphocytes. *J. Exptl. Med.* 137: 504, 1973.

Development of B lymphocytes[1,2]

R. G. MILLER AND R. A. PHILLIPS

*Department of Medical Biophysics, University of Toronto
and the Ontario Cancer Institute, Toronto, Ontario M4X 1K9 Canada*

ABSTRACT

A rough outline of the development pathway of stem cells to B lymphocytes in mammals is beginning to emerge. The stem cell is most probably either identical to or closely related to the spleen colony-forming unit or hemopoietic stem cell. The stem cell appears not to be specificity-restricted and to lack Ig surface receptors. Whether part of B-cell development in mammals takes place in a specialized lymphoid environment, analogous to the bursa of Fabricius in birds, is still unresolved. The bone marrow does not form such an environment. The bone marrow and spleen, but not the lymph nodes, of mice contain a nondividing B-cell precursor population at an intermediate stage of development between the stem cell and B cell. This population has Ig surface receptors and is specificity-restricted. It cannot be initiated into differentiating into antibody-producing cells. However, under appropriate conditions, it can give rise to functional B cells within 3 days. Newly-formed B cells (designated B_1) are physically different from mature B cells (designated B_2) and appear to be a dividing population of cells differentiating from the B-cell precursor to B_2 nondividing cell populations.—MILLER, R. G. AND R. A. PHILLIPS. Development of B lymphocytes. *Federation Proc.* 34: 145–150, 1975.

The cells involved in the humoral immune response can be conveniently divided into three functionally distinct compartments (35): the effector cell compartment, which contains mature antibody-producing cells; the "antigen-sensitive unit," which comprises B lymphocytes and any other cells required for their development into antibody-producing cells; and the stem cell compartment, which repopulates the antigen-sensitive unit as required. B lymphocytes are specificity-restricted prior to contact with antigen and express their specificity through antigen-specific immunoglobulin surface receptors. For many antigens, T lymphocytes

[1] From Session V, *Development and Aging in Organ Systems,* of the FASEB Conference on *Biology of Development and Aging,* presented at the 58th Annual Meeting of the Federation of American Societies for Experimental Biology, Atlantic City, N.J., April 11, 1974.

[2] Supported by the Medical Research Council of Canada (MT-3766) and the National Cancer Institute of Canada.

are also required. These are also specificity-restricted prior to contact with antigen.

Both B and T cells appear to have a life-span much shorter than that of their host and are being continuously replaced throughout adult life by proliferation and differentiation from more primitive precursors. These are thought not to be specificity-restricted. It is difficult to consider B-cell development without also considering T-cell development. In birds, they develop in anatomically discrete locations, B cells in the bursa of Fabricius and T cells in the thymus. Each site is seeded by stem cells from the marrow. In mammals, to which this review will largely be restricted, the situation is not so clear. Stem cells are found in the bone marrow. T-cell development appears to occur from stem cells that seed the thymus but there is no convincing evidence for the existence of a bursa-equivalent. Bone marrow itself and varying lymphoid organs have been implicated by different investigators. See refs 3, 4 for reviews.

The most thorough stem cell studies were done before the existence of B and T cells was recognized. In addition, they also usually used marrow as a stem cell source. Since marrow is now known to be a good B-cell source (20), new B cells might arise either from more primitive progenitors or from self-renewal. These facts must be kept in mind when interpreting the older studies.

IDENTIFICATION OF THE STEM CELL

If one gives a mouse a radiation dose of 1,000 rads, it will die of complete hemopoietic collapse in about 2 weeks. Because of radiation-induced chromosome damage, hemopoietic precursor cells will die when they attempt to divide in the process

of differentiating into new hemopoietic cells.

The death of the mouse can be prevented by the transplantation of isogeneic bone marrow. Ford et al. (8) were the first to show that it is the transplanted bone marrow that repopulates the irradiated host and that a true chimera is produced. Their studies made use of the T6 chromosome marker, a chromosomal abnormality present in all dividing cells of a particular CBA mouse substrain. They found that irradiated CBA mice transplanted with T6-CBA bone marrow cells survived the irradiation and at later times had T6 marked cells in their bone marrow, thymus, spleen, lymph node and Peyer's patches (7).

Clearly, bone marrow contains stem cells capable of repopulating the hemopoietic system. The data imply it may also contain stem cells capable of repopulating the immune system; the radiation dose used by Ford et al. (8) was sufficiently large to sterilize the dividing cells in the antigen-sensitive unit (13), in particular B cells. However, it is now known that marrow is a good source of B cells (20) so that new B cells could also arise from self-renewal of B cells in the graft. Micklem and co-workers (18) extended the earlier T6 studies of Ford et al. to show that bone marrow (but not thymus, lymph node or thoracic duct lymph) contains stem cells capable of repopulating both the myeloid and lymphoid systems.

It is difficult from studies of this nature to deduce whether there are one or several different stem-cell populations and what relationship exists between the different T6 cells found in the chimera: All cells in the transplanted bone marrow have the T6 marker irrespective of how closely related they might be; the T6 marker can be seen only in metaphase cells so that only a small fraction of the cells examined can be definitely assigned to the donor; there is no direct assay for the stem cell(s) involved; and the only correlation with cell function is anatomical location. All of these problems have been considered, with more or less success, by later workers.

One of the most powerful tools for the study of stem cells has been the spleen colony assay of Till and Mc Culloch (33). Colonies are found in the spleens of lethally irradiated mice transplanted with syngeneic bone marrow. Each of these colonies is comprised of the descendants of a single hemopoietic stem cell (2, 38): immature erythrocytes, immature granulocytes, megakaryocytes, additional stem cells, and other cells that cannot be identified. The number of colonies observed can be used to obtain a quantitative estimate of the number of stem cells present in the cell suspension transplanted (32, 34).

Trentin et al. (36) combined the T6 marker technique and the spleen colony technique to show that the hemopoietic stem cell may also be a lymphoid stem cell. They injected lethally irradiated CBA mice with CBA-T6 bone marrow, collected the ensuing spleen colonies, and used pools of several colonies to repopulate lethally irradiated secondary recipients. In some cases, marrow and spleen from these secondary mice were used to repopulate lethally irradiated tertiary recipients. Secondary and tertiary recipients surviving more than 30 days mounted immune responses equivalent to those of appropriate control mice when immunized against several different antigens. Most secondary and tertiary recipients had the T6 marker in 100% of mitotic hemopoietic and lymphoid cells. They concluded that the hemopoietic stem cell may also be the lymphoid stem cell.

Three criticisms may be made of this study. First, the T6 marker is not unique to the hemopoietic stem cell so that the cell repopulating the lymphoid system, even if T6 marked, may merely be present as a contaminant in the spleen colonies selected for transplantation. Second, because of the low frequency of mitotic cells in lymph node, only a very small proportion of the cells were shown to contain the marker. Third, the identification of the T6 marker in lymphoid cells is based on anatomical correlation rather than a direct demonstration of the T6 marker in a functional lymphoid cell. Even if the marker is in lymphoid cells, it is not clear whether it is in B cells, T cells or both.

The first of these objections was overcome in the studies of Wu and colleagues (38, 39). These studies depend on some special properties of the W/W^v mouse (26). It has a genetically determined anemia that can be cured by transplantation of coisogeneic +/+ bone marrow. Before cure, the marrow of these mice will not form splenic colonies; after, it will. It is not necessary to irradiate the recipient and a very small number of transplanted bone marrow cells can cure the anemia. Wu et al. (38) transplanted W/W^v mice with sublethally irradiated +/+ bone marrow at a dilution such that each recipient should receive only one surviving stem cell and at a radiation dose such that this stem cell is likely to show some radiation-induced chromosome damage. Approximately 2 months later, the thymus or marrow of each recipient was examined for chromosomally marked cells. If markers were found, the marrow was transplanted into coisogeneic +/+ or W/+ secondary recipients and the resulting spleen colonies scored for the chromosome marker. Essentially all colonies contained the marker, and typically, more than 95% of the metaphases scored in each colony had the unique marker chromosome. In each case, the marker seen in the spleen colonies was identical to that seen in the marrow inoculum and different from all other markers induced. The clonal origin of the marked cells was thus ensured. The small, unmarked dividing cell population usually seen presumably represents unrelated cells that have been trapped in the colony by chance. By direct correlation with the morphology of the cells in the colonies, these experiments proved conclusively that stem cells, granulocytes and red cells must be members of the same clone.

Wu and co-workers (39) next extended their studies to test whether the hemopoietic stem cell may also be a stem cell for the lymphoid system. Direct correlation with the morphology of the cells in the colonies is not possible because neither morphologically identifiable lymphoid cells nor cells capable of specifically binding antigen (40) are seen in spleen colonies. This observation does not rule out the possibility that they are produced there. Lymphoid cells may either migrate from the colony before they become morphologically recognizable as such or might take longer to mature than the time in which the colony is sufficiently discrete for analysis (about 14 days). To test the hypothesis that the myeloid and lymphoid systems have a common stem cell, W/Wᵛ mice were transplanted with irradiated +/+ marrow as described above. After 2–6 months, the thymuses of these animals were examined for marked cells. In 8 of 51 animals, a high proportion (56–88%) of thymocyte metaphases carried a marker unique to that mouse. The same marker was also always found in the bone marrow of the animal and in a proportion of spleen colonies derived from

that marrow. Only one of the mice (one left for 6 months before examination, in contrast to 2–3 months for the rest) showed marked cells in lymph node. They hypothesized that it might take considerable time for peripheral lymphoid organs to be repopulated in their unirradiated mice, in contrast to the case in the irradiated mouse (18). In another experiment, marked marrow from a W/Wᵛ mouse was transplanted into irradiated +/+ or W/+ mice to form spleen colonies which in turn were pooled and transplanted into irradiated +/+ mice. One month later, the animals were immunized with sheep erythrocytes and their lymph nodes examined for both antibody-producing cells and chromosome markers. All animals contained chromosomally marked cells in their lymph nodes. The highest percentage, 67%, was in the animal with the largest immune response. They concluded that it is probable that cells of the hemopoietic and immune systems are derived from the same stem cell.

The major limitation of these studies is that the chromosome marker was not demonstrated directly in cells of known lymphoid function. Since essentially all dividing cells in thymus carry the θ antigen (see e.g., 27), it is reasonable to conclude that the hemopoietic stem cell and the stem cell for at least some mature T cells are members of the same clone. In mouse lymph node, one typically finds that 80% of the lymphoid cells are T cells with the remainder being all (or mostly) B cells (25). Thus, the studies of Wu et al. provide no definitive evidence concerning the origin of B cells. Even if one assumes all the marked cells seen in lymph node to be lymphoid the data are consistent with them all being T cells.

A similar conclusion can be reached

from a study of Nowell and co-workers (21). They gave rats near-lethal doses of X-rays and allowed them to recover. They then looked for (and found) the same radiation-induced abnormal karyotype in spleen colonies derived from the marrow, and both mixed lymphocyte cultures and phytohemagglutinin (PHA) cultures set up using peripheral blood leukocytes. The percent abnormal karyotypes seen in culture was always small (less than 7%) and it cannot be definitely excluded that these marked karyotypes were in nonlymphoid cells. In any case, the lymphoid cells responding in these types of cultures are thought to be T cells (12).

Cell separation studies using velocity sedimentation in the earth's gravitational field have established that B cells can develop from a progenitor population, not merely through self-renewal. These studies are also consistent with the ultimate progenitor being the hemopoietic stem cell. This is most clearly shown in the studies of Lafleur et al. (14, 16), based on earlier work defining the sedimentation profiles of the hemopoietic stem cell (37) and the B cell (20). This work will be discussed in detail later.

The study of Edwards and colleagues (5) was a direct attempt to investigate the relationship between B cells and hemopoietic stem cells. They adapted with some modification the technique of Wu and co-workers (38) for repopulating W/W^v mice with the progeny of a single stem cell bearing a unique radiation-induced chromosome marker. To overcome the difficulty of both examining the karyotype and demonstrating lymphoid function in the same cell, they chose to look for the marker in a lymphoid population which they could obtain in sufficient purity that independent measurements of karyotype and function

could unambiguously assign an abnormal karyotype to a cell class of known function. The cell class chosen was the rosette-forming cell in clonally repopulated mice undergoing a secondary immune response to sheep erythrocytes. When rosettes were formed in spleen cell suspensions and a velocity sedimentation separation performed, a fraction could be found in which 70% of the objects (single cells, cell clumps, rosettes) were in fact lymphoid rosettes and 90% of the metaphase cells were in these rosettes. Up to 80% of these metaphases contained the unique radiation-induced chromosome marker, the same marker as seen when spleen colonies derived from the marrow of these mice were examined. They concluded that rosette-forming cells are in the same clone as the hemopoietic stem cell.

The main weakness of this work lies in its failure to distinguish whether the rosette-forming cells examined are in the B- or T-cell lineage. It is now widely recognized that both can form rosettes, although under the experimental conditions of Edwards et al. (5) it is very likely that T rosettes dissociated during the cell separation process (6). Thus, with some reservation, one can conclude that B cells, as well as T cells, are in the same clone as the hemopoietic stem cell.

As pointed out by several authors (5, 21, 36), in those experiments in

TABLE 1. Absolute frequency estimates (per 10^3 nucleated cells)

	CFU[a]	PB[b]	B₂[b]
Marrow	0.5	13	140
Spleen	0.1	32	500
Lymph node	<0.001	<2	250

[a] Colony-forming units, estimated from ref 17, assuming $f = 0.2$.   [b] From ref 15.

which the B- and/or T-cell population is replaced by one or at most a few stem cells, it appears that all possible specificities in both the B- and T-cell populations are regenerated. This strongly implies that the stem cell is not specificity restricted and that specificity is acquired at some point along the development pathway to B and T lymphocytes.

DEVELOPMENT OF B CELLS FROM STEM CELLS

Figure 1 and Tables 1 and 2 summarize what is known about the stem-cell to B-cell development pathway based on the work of Lafleur et al. (14–16), who studied the development of B cells responding against sheep erythrocytes in mice. The rationale of this series of experiments was rather different than that of the experiments described in the preceding section. Instead of following the development pathway forward from

TABLE 2. Features distinguishing stationary cell populations in B-cell differentiation

	CFU	PB	B_2
Surface Ig present	(No)[a]	Yes	Yes
Can initiate response	No	No	Yes
Modal sedimentation velocity (mm/hr)	3.9	~5	3.0

[a] Probably no receptors present. But see ref 16.

the stem cell, they followed it backwards from the B cell.

When bone marrow is transplanted into lethally irradiated mice, at least 12 days elapse before immunization with an antigen such as sheep erythrocytes produces a detectable response (35). The marrow contains B cells. Thus, as one might expect, and as was shown by Gregory and Lajtha (10), the long lag results from the slow recovery of T cells. When velocity sedimentation cell separation is used to prepare a pool of marrow

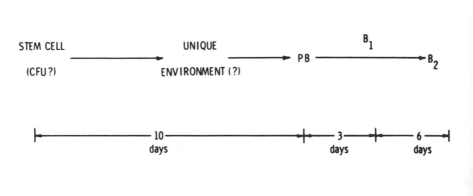

Figure 1. A possible model of the B-cell differentiation pathway. See text.

cells free of B cells but containing more rapidly sedimenting cells ("stem-cell pool"), identical recovery kinetics are obtained (14). Apparently T-cell regeneration is still limiting the recovery. If large numbers of thymus cells are added, either with the stem-cell pool or at the time of immunization, some activity can be seen within 3 days of transplantation. Apparently, new B cells arise very rapidly from some precursor population. Lafleur and co-workers (14) were able to develop a linear assay for this precursor (PB cell) based on the immune response obtained when one immunizes 7 days after transplantation of the marrow stem-cell pool mixed with thymus cells. This assay was used to measure the sedimentation profile of the PB cell. It has a modal sedimentation velocity of about 5 mm/hr and a shape consistent with a population of cells primarily not in cell cycle (19).

It should be noted that the actual quantity measured in the PB-cell assay is the number of antibody-producing cells produced. It is assumed that all B cells of the appropriate specificity existing at the time of immunization will be induced into development and that the number of progeny of each will be the same. When a cell separation is performed, the number of new B cells seen in any fraction will be related to the number of B-cell progenitors in that fraction that have had time to differentiate into B cells. If PB cells of differing sedimentation velocity produce differing numbers of B cells this procedure will distort the actual shape of the PB profile. The standard PB-cell assay was a 7-day interval between transplantation and immunization. This interval appears to detect a homogeneous population with the properties described below. If a much longer time interval is used, both the number of fractions showing activity

and the activity per fraction increase. This observation suggests that one is beginning to detect progenitors more primitive than PB cells. These more primitive progenitors dominate the profile of active cells because the more primitive the precursor, the more progeny (antibody-producing cells) per precursor.

When the sedimentation profile of cells in marrow with surface Ig was measured (15), there was a peak at 3 mm/hr, corresponding to B cells, and a long shoulder extending out beyond 5 mm/hr. The shoulder is assumed to represent PB cells and perhaps also intermediates between PB and B cells. This correlation was strengthened by sedimentation studies of lymph node and spleen cells. PB-cell activity was seen in spleen, but not lymph node. Ig-bearing cells were seen in the PB-cell region of spleen, but not lymph node. The relative numbers of B cells to PB cells in marrow, spleen, and lymph node as assessed either by transplantation activity or relative numbers of Ig-bearing cells are similar. Estimates of the frequencies of the B cell, PB cell and CFU (spleen colony-forming unit or hemopoietic stem cell) are given in Table 1.

Sedimentation analysis shows clearly that the PB cell and the CFU are not identical but does not exclude the possibility that PB cells are a subpopulation of CFU or are descended from CFU. Lafleur et al. (16) favor the latter. They found that if immunization were delayed 2 weeks after transplantation of the marrow stem-cell pool, substantially more activity was obtained and the profile of the cell population giving rise to the activity was very similar to the CFU profile. Both PB and B cells were destroyed by an anti-IgM serum which did not affect CFU. Limiting dilution analysis suggested that PB cells were already specificity restricted

(15) whereas, as discussed in the previous section, the ultimate stem cell is thought not to be.

PB cells might be thought of as a reserve population of committed B-cell precursors. They can be stimulated into differentiation and proliferation to produce functional B cells within 3–4 days. On the other hand, it would appear to take at least 13 days to produce functional B cells from the stem cell. More definitive data have been obtained on this point by Yung and colleagues (40). They measured the time required to produce both antigen-binding cells and immunocompetent cells against *Salmonella* antigens and against sheep erythrocytes on transplantation of a single spleen colony derived from a stem cell in fetal mouse liver. Antigen-binding cells specific for *S. adelaide* H antigen did not appear until 18–20 days after transplantation; cells specific for sheep erythrocytes required a longer period, 30–33 days. Test of immunocompetence with these two antigens showed similar results: Antibody production to bacterial antigens began between 19 and 26 days while the response to sheep erythrocytes occurred after 34 days. These results are similar to those of Silverstein et al. who observed that responses to different antigens occur at different times in the development of fetal lambs (28).

The development of PB cells into B cells is probably complex. Defining as B cells those cells that can be initiated into developing into antibody-producing cells, Lafleur et al. (15) found that B cells that have just been produced from PB cells are much larger than the B cells found in normal marrow. Their data are consistent with it taking 9–14 days for these large B cells to proliferate and differentiate into "normal" B cells. They designate the

"transitional" B cell as a B_1 cell and the "normal" B cell as a B_2 cell.

Strober and Dilley (30, 31) have data in rats which they explain with a model consistent with assuming varying degrees of differentiation down the PB $\rightarrow B_1 \rightarrow B_2$ pathway depending upon the degree of previous exposure of the animal to the antigen.

Osmond and Nossal (22, 23) have studied the density of surface Ig on small lymphocytes in murine marrow, spleen and lymph node by radioautographic measurements of antiglobulin binding over a broad range of concentrations. As the ^{125}I-antiglobulin concentration was increased, the percentage of labeled lymphocytes in spleen and lymph node reached well-defined plateaus. However, marrow lymphocytes continued to be labeled with much higher concentrations of antiglobulin than those required for maximum labeling of cells in spleen and lymph node. This result suggests that marrow lymphocytes have a broad range in receptor density, with about one half bearing no detectable Ig. Combining ^{131}I-antiglobulin measurements with in vivo uptake of ^{3}H TdR, they concluded that the Ig-bearing lymphocytes were not themselves proliferating but arose from proliferating precursors. Non-Ig-bearing lymphocytes were the first to show ^{3}H label, and within 2 days, 90% were labeled. Ig-bearing cells showed rapid linear increase in numbers labeled after a lag of 1.5 days; high avidity Ig-labeling cells were delayed a further 0.5 days. They concluded that B cells arise from a non-Ig-bearing lymphocyte-like precursor.

Superficially, these data appear incompatible with those of Lafleur et al., who found PB cells in high frequency in spleen as well as bone marrow and found that PB cells could be inactivated with anti-Ig sera. In a subsequent study (D. G. Osmond, H. von

Boehmer and R. G. Miller, in preparation) the antiglobulin serum of Osmond and Nossal showed a sedimentation profile of Ig-bearing cells in marrow similar to that seen by Lafleur et al. The labeled cells in the PB-cell region were morphologically identified as small lymphocytes and would have been scored as Ig-bearing noncycling small lymphocytes in the studies of Osmond and Nossal. It may be that the Ig receptors are largely lost in the B_1 transitional phase (when the cells are actively cycling) and that these B_1 transitional cells are the B-cell precursor lymphocyte population studied by Osmond and Nossal.

A particularly puzzling problem in the differentiation of B cells from stem cells in mammals is whether a unique lymphoid environment, analogous to the bursa of Fabricius in birds, is required. Both the bone marrow (1) and the gut-associated lymphoid tissue (3) have been suggested as sites for B-cell differentiation. However, no direct evidence exists to support the requirement for either site.

We have recently (unpublished data) attempted to investigate the role of the bone marrow environment.

On injection, ^{89}Sr is incorporated into bone. There, it emits a low energy electron that makes the bone marrow a hostile environment for differentiation. The bone shields other tissues from this low energy radiation (9). Mice were pretreated with ^{89}Sr, exposed to lethal whole-body irradiation, and then given the B cell or stem cell fraction isolated from bone marrow. The ability of B cells, PB cells, and stem cells to differentiate in these recipients is summarized in Table 3. B cells function normally. The activity of PB cells and earlier precursors (assayed by immunization 15–30 days after grafting precursors) is slightly depressed. However, this suppression probably represents circulation of cells through the marrow rather than the differentiation of cells in that site. If the marrow was essential for differentiation in the same way that the thymus is for T lymphocytes, the suppression should have been much greater. Measurement of the colony-forming cells in marrow illustrates that the marrow cavity in the ^{89}Sr-treated recipients was lethal to cells residing there. Thirty days after transplantation the marrow of the ^{89}Sr-treated group contained only 4% of the CFU found in the control group. We conclude that it is unlikely that the bone marrow plays an essential role in the differentiation of B lymphocytes.

CONCLUSION

One sees that very little is known about the B-cell development pathway. The stem cell may have been identified and something is known about the terminal stages of the development pathway. However, the stages between the stem cell and the PB cell are completely unknown. The stage that is perhaps the most interesting of all, the stage in which specificity is acquired, is presumably somewhere in this region.

TABLE 3. Effect of marrow ablation on B-cell development

Cell type	Relative activity in ^{89}Sr-recipient, %
B cell[a]	79
PB cell[a]	29
Early precursor (27 d)[a]	60
CFU (marrow—33 d)[b]	4.9
CFU (spleen—33d)[c]	240

[a] Antibody-producing cells per spleen in ^{89}Sr-treated recipients relative to untreated controls.
[b] Colony-forming units (CFU) per femur in ^{89}Sr-treated recipients relative to untreated controls.
[c] CFU per spleen in ^{89}Sr-treated recipients relative to untreated controls.

Since the topic of this symposium is aging, we would like to conclude by indicating how an understanding of B-cell differentiation may be related to the aging problem. What is known about cellular deficiencies in the age-related decline of the immune system has been reviewed recently (11). Briefly, it is well established that both humoral and cellular immunity decline markedly with age once an animal has passed adolescence. For humoral immunity, it is known that the decline is primarily due to intrinsic changes in the immunocompetent cell population required to initiate the response. Thus, in the humoral immune response of mice to a particulate antigen such as sheep erythrocytes, a response that requires the presence of both immunocompetent B and T lymphocytes for its initiation, both lymphocyte populations undergo marked changes with age. In particular, the number of B cells in BC3F$_1$ mice 30–35 months old was estimated to be reduced about 3.5-fold, the proliferative capacity of each of these B cells was reduced 5- to 10-fold, and their ability to interact with T cells and/or antigen may also be reduced (24). The precise nature of these B-cell defects is unknown but it is reasonable to assume that a more detailed knowledge of the B-cell development pathway might be of some help in understanding them. Thus, for example, the known decline in the colony-forming ability of marrow cells subjected to serial transplantation into irradiated mice (17, 29) may play a role.

REFERENCES

1. ABDOU, N. I., AND N. L. ABDOU. *Science* 175: 446, 1972.
2. BECKER, A. J., E. A. McCULLOCH AND J. E. TILL. *Nature* 197: 452, 1963.
3. COOPER, M. D., AND A. R. LAWTON. In: *Contemporary Topics in Immunobiology*, edited by M. G. Hanna, Jr. New York: Plenum, 1972, vol. 1, p. 49.
4. COOPER, M. D., A. R. LAWTON AND P. W. KINCADE. In: *Contemporary Topics in Immunobiology*, edited by M. G. Hanna, Jr. New York: Plenum, 1972, vol. 1, p. 33.
5. EDWARDS, G. E., R. G. MILLER AND R. A. PHILLIPS. *J. Immunol.* 105: 719, 1970.
6. ELLIOTT, B. E., AND J. S. HASKILL. *European J. Immunol.* 3: 68, 1973.
7. EVANS, E. P., D. A. OGDEN, C. E. FORD AND H. S. MICKLEM. *Nature* 216: 36, 1967.
8. FORD, C. E., J. L. HAMERTON, D. W. H. BARNES AND J. F. LOUTIT. *Nature* 177: 452, 1956.
9. FRIED, W., C. W. GURNEY AND M. SWATEK. *Radiation Res.* 24: 50, 1966.
10. GREGORY, C. J., AND L. G. LAJTHA. *Intern. J. Radiation Biol.* 17: 117, 1970.
11. HEIDRICK, M. L. AND T. MAKINODAN. *Gerontologia* 18: 305, 1972.
12. JANOSSY, G., AND M. F. GREAVES. *Clin. Exptl. Immunol.* 10: 525, 1972.
13. KENNEDY, J. C., J. E. TILL, L. SIMINOVITCH AND E. A. McCULLOCH. *J. Immunol.* 94: 715, 1965.
14. LAFLEUR, L., R. G. MILLER AND R. A. PHILLIPS. *J. Exptl. Med.* 135: 1363, 1972.
15. LAFLEUR, L., R. G. MILLER AND R. A. PHILLIPS. *J. Exptl. Med.* 137: 954, 1973.
16. LAFLEUR, L., B. J. UNDERDOWN, R. G. MILLER AND R. A. PHILLIPS. *Ser. Haematol.* 5: 50, 1972.
17. METCALF, D., AND M. A. S. MOORE. In: *Haemopoietic Cells*, edited by A. Neuberger and E. L. Tatum. Amsterdam: North-Holland, 1971, vol. 24.
18. MICKLEM, H. S., C. E. FORD, E. P. EVANS AND J. GRAY. *Proc. Roy. Soc. London Ser. B* 165: 78, 1966.
19. MILLER, R. G. In: *Techniques in Biophysics and Cell Biology*, edited by R. Pain and B. Smith. London: Wiley, 1973, vol. 1, p. 87.
20. MILLER, R. G., AND R. A. PHILLIPS. *Proc. Soc. Exptl. Biol. Med.* 135: 63, 1970.
21. NOWELL, P. C., B. E. HIRSCH, D. H. FOX AND D. B. WILSON. *J. Cellular Physiol.* 75: 151, 1970.
22. OSMOND, D. G., AND G. J. V. NOSSAL. *Cellular Immunol.* 13: 117, 1974.
23. OSMOND, D. G., AND G. J. V. NOSSAL. *Cellular Immunol.* 13: 132, 1974.

24. PRICE, G. B., AND T. MAKINODAN. *J. Immunol.* 108: 403, 1972.
25. RAFF, M. C. *Transplant. Rev.* 6: 52, 1971.
26. RUSSELL, E. S. In: *Methodology in Mammalian Genetics*, edited by W. J. Burdette. San Francisco: Holden-Day, 1963, p. 217.
27. SHORTMAN, K., AND H. JACKSON. *Cellular Immunol.* 12: 230, 1974.
28. SILVERSTEIN, A. M., C. J. PARSHALL, JR. AND J. W. UHR. *Science* 154: 1675, 1966.
29. SIMINOVITCH, L., J. E. TILL AND E. A. McCULLOCH. *J. Cellular Comp. Physiol.* 64: 23, 1964.
30. STROBER, S., AND J. DILLEY. *J. Exptl. Med.* 137: 1275, 1973.
31. STROBER, S., AND J. DILLEY. *J. Exptl. Med.* 138: 1331, 1973.
32. TILL, J. E. *Ser. Haematol.* 5: 5, 1972.
33. TILL, J. E., AND E. A. McCULLOCH. *Radiation Res.* 14: 213, 1961.
34. TILL, J. E., AND E. A. McCULLOCH. *Ser. Haematol.* 5: 15, 1972.
35. TILL, J. E., E. A. McCULLOCH, R. A. PHILLIPS AND L. SIMINOVITCH. *Cold Spring Harbor Symp. Quant. Biol.* 32: 461, 1967.
36. TRENTIN, J., N. WOLF, V. CHENG, W. FAHLBERG, D. WEISS AND R. BONHAG. *J. Immunol.* 98: 1326, 1967.
37. WORTON, R. G., E. A. McCULLOCH AND J. E. TILL. *J. Cellular Physiol.* 74: 171, 1969.
38. WU, A. M., J. F. TILL, L. SIMINOVITCH AND E. A. McCULLOCH. *J. Cellular Physiol.* 69: 177, 1967.
39. WU, A. M., J. E. TILL, L. SIMINOVITCH AND E. A. McCULLOCH. *J. Exptl. Med.* 127: 455, 1968.
40. YUNG, L. L. L., T. C. WYN-EVANS AND E. DIENER. *European J. Immunol.* 3: 224, 1973.

Ontogeny of B-lymphocyte function with respect to the heterogeneity of antibody affinity[1,2]

GREGORY W. SISKIND[3] AND EDMOND A. GOIDL

*Division of Allergy and Immunology, Department of Medicine
Cornell University Medical College, New York, New York 10021*

ABSTRACT

Neonatal liver or adult spleen was used as a source of B-lymphocytes in reconstituting lethally irradiated, syngeneic mice. Recipients were all given excess adult, syngeneic thymus cells and were immunized with dinitrophenylated bovine gamma globulin. The distribution of avidities of plaque-forming cells produced by immunized recipients of neonatal liver was highly restricted in comparison with animals reconstituted with adult spleen indicating a restriction of B-lymphocyte heterogeneity in the neonatal mouse.—SISKIND, G. W. AND E. A. GOIDL. Ontogeny of B-lymphocyte function with respect to the heterogeneity of antibody affinity. *Federation Proc.* 34: 151–152, 1975.

Antibody is generally highly heterogeneous with respect to its affinity for the antigenic determinant (3, 6–8). This heterogeneity presumably represents the formation of a number of distinct antibody molecules differing in the amino acid sequence of their hypervariable regions It is generally assumed that individual B lymphocytes secrete a homogeneous antibody product (5) and that the heterogeneity of serum antibody reflects a corresponding heterogeneity of antibody-forming B lymphocytes. We were interested in studying the ontogeny of the ability to generate a heterogeneous immune response such as is characteristic of

[1] From Session V, *Development and Aging in Organ Systems*, of the FASEB Conference on *Biology of Development and Aging*, presented at the 58th Annual Meeting of the Federation of American Societies for Experimental Biology, Atlantic City, N.J., April 11, 1974.

[2] Supported in part by research grant AM-13701 from the Public Health Service.

[3] Career Scientist of the Health Research Council of the City of New York under Investigatorship I-593.

adult animals. In order to study ontogeny of B lymphocytes with regard to such a function it is necessary to avoid other control mechanisms that might influence the expression of the functional capacity of the B-lymphocyte population. Studies on the immune response of immature animals appeared inadequate to approach this question. Factors other than the capabilities of the B lymphocytes could well impose restrictions on the immune response of immature animals.

It was therefore decided to employ a cell transfer system in which neonatal or fetal tissues would be transferred to lethally irradiated (800 R) syngeneic (LAF$_1$) mice. All recipients received excess (1×10^8) adult, syngeneic thymus cells so that T-lymphocyte function would not limit their response, and were immunized by the intraperitoneal injection of 500 μg 2,4-dinitrophenylated bovine gamma globulin (DNP-BGG) in complete Freund's adjuvant. Assays for direct and indirect anti-DNP plaque-forming cells (PFC) in the spleen were carried out by the Kennedy-Axelrad monolayer method (4) using sheep red blood cells coated with DNP-ovalbumin by the chromic chloride technique (2). The distribution of plaque-forming cells with respect to the avidity of the antibody they produce was determined from the concentration dependence of hapten inhibition of plaque formation (1).

It was necessary to validate the experimental system by showing that the selection for high affinity antibody synthesis occurs in a similar manner, with similar heterogeneity, in the cell transfer system as in normal animals. In both normal mice and irradiated recipients of adult spleen and thymus cells there was a progressive increase in the high avidity plaque-forming cells and an increase in heterogeneity with time after immunization. Maxi-

mum affinity and heterogeneity were observed at 3 weeks after immunization. The reconstituted animals differed from normal mice only in showing a slightly slower development of the immune response with a somewhat reduced peak response. In addition, the direct plaque-forming cell response in the reconstituted animals was more prolonged, and showed a definite progressive increase in avidity with time after immunization in the cell transfer recipients.

Irradiated animals reconstituted with 10^8 thymus cells plus a single neonatal (within 24 hours of birth) liver produced an immune response the magnitude of which was comparable to that produced by irradiated mice reconstituted with one-half of an adult spleen. However, in 22 out of 24 recipients of neonatal liver the response was clearly more restricted with respect to heterogeneity of affinity than the response of irradiated animals reconstituted with cells from one-half of an adult spleen. In 9 of 24 recipients of neonatal livers a very marked restriction in heterogeneity was apparent. Twenty recipients of one-half individual adult spleens produced highly heterogeneous responses with the exception of two animals which showed slightly restricted heterogeneity. Five animals reconstituted with 5×10^7 pooled adult spleen cells plus 1×10^8 thymus cells and five recipients of 3×10^7 pooled adult bone marrow cells plus 1×10^8 thymus cells all produced highly heterogeneous responses. The recipients of neonatal liver generally had only low avidity plaque-forming cells. However, 3 of the 24 recipients of neonatal liver had plaque-forming cells of high avidity but of restricted heterogeneity.

Spleens from 1-week-old mice when transferred into irradiated animals yield responses comparable to that of neonatal liver. Recipients of spleens from 2-week-old animals, in contrast, behaved like recipients of adult spleen.

Tissues from neonatal donors are essentially in a "germfree" environment until used in the transfer studies. It was possible that exposure to normal bacterial flora is important in differentiation of the capacity to produce a heterogeneous immune response. "Germfree" BALB/c mice immunized with DNP-bovine gamma globulin produced a heterogeneous immune response indistinguishable from that of conventionally reared animals. Thus, the restricted heterogeneity of the response generated by B cells from neonatal donors cannot be ascribed to the germfree state of the donor mice.

The results thus suggest that B lymphocytes present in neonatal mice are restricted with respect to the spectrum of different anti-DNP antibodies that they are capable of synthesizing. The use of a cell transfer system and excess adult T lymphocytes makes it improbable that other controls (e.g., T-lymphocyte function or antigen "processing") are involved

in the observed restriction in heterogeneity. The mechanisms for the progressive expansion of the animal's capacity to make a spectrum of different anti-DNP antibodies is not clear. The data presented are consistent either with a somatic mutation mechanism for generation of antibody diversity or with a germ-line theory of antibody diversity in which different germ-line genes come to be expressed at different times, presumably in a random order.

REFERENCES

1. ANDERSSON, B., *J. Exptl. Med.* 132: 77, 1970.
2. JANDL, J. H., AND R. L. SIMMONS. *Brit. J. Haematol.* 3: 19, 1957.
3. KARUSH, F. *Advan. Immunol.* 2: 1, 1962.
4. KENNEDY, J. C., AND M. A. AXELRAD. *Immunology* 20: 253, 1971.
5. KLINMAN, N. R. *Immunochemistry* 6: 757, 1969.
6. SISKIND, G. W., AND B. BENACERRAF. *Advan. Immunol.* 10: 1, 1969.
7. WERBLIN, T. P., Y. T. KIM, F. QUAGLIATA AND G. W. SISKIND. *Immunology* 24: 477, 1973.
8. WERBLIN, T. P., AND G. W. SISKIND. *Transplant. Rev.* 8. 104, 1972.

Effects of aging on the differentiation and proliferation potentials of cells of the immune system[1]

T. MAKINODAN AND W. H. ADLER

Laboratory of Cellular and Comparative Physiology
Gerontology Research Center, National Institute of Child Health
and Human Development, National Institutes of Health
Bethesda, and the Baltimore City Hospitals
Baltimore, Maryland 21224

ABSTRACT

An attempt has been made here to show that the immune system can begin to decline in function shortly after an individual reaches maturity. The decline is due in part to changes in the environment of the cells but primarily to changes in the precursor cells of the system. This is reflected in their inability to proliferate and possibly differentiate efficiently. These findings show that the immune system can serve as an excellent model to study how aging can perturb the process of cells undergoing proliferation and differentiation.— MAKINODAN, T. AND W. H. ADLER. Effects of aging on the differtiation and proliferation potentials of cells of the immune system. *Federation Proc.* 34: 153–158, 1975.

Until recently few investigators have studied the immune systems of aging individuals, and their approach has been primarily phenomenological, relating immune activities with diseases (42, 53). However, now more investigators are studying the immune systems of aging individuals, and most of them are examining how aging affects the differentiation process of cells of the immune system. The initial findings have been most encouraging (25).

They suggest that indeed aging can influence the differentiation potential of certain cells of the immune system and consequently alter the functional activities of the system. If so, the

[1] From Session V, *Development and Aging in Organ Systems*, of the FASEB Conference on *Biology of Development and Aging*, presented at the 58th Annual Meeting of the Federation of American Societies for Experimental Biology, Atlantic City, N.J., April 11, 1974.

immune system may be the choice model system to study how aging can affect cells with potentials to differentiate and proliferate. There are many compelling reasons for this view, and some of these are listed in Table 1.

In this presentation we wish to address ourselves briefly to *a*) what is currently known regarding the effects of aging on immune activities at the individual and cellular levels, and *b*) what major problems are confronting us. Our discussion will focus more on the humoral or B-cell immune system than on the cell-mediated or T-cell immune system simply because the former system has been more amenable to quantitative evaluation at the cellular level (see below).

EFFECTS OF AGING ON THE B-CELL IMMUNE SYSTEM

Age-related pattern of change in activity

In general, B-cell immune activities decline as one ages and variation in immune activities between individuals increases with age (15, 33, 34, 36,

TABLE 1. The advantages of studying the immune system as an attractive model for the cellular aging process

1) Functional activities of the immune system generally decline as one ages

2) Knowledge of the system at the cellular, molecular, genetic, developmental and phylogenetic levels is as comprehensive if not more so, than most physiological systems affected by aging

3) The system is amenable to cellular and molecular scrutiny and therefore offers a great promise for its successful manipulation

4) Prevention or reversal of the decline in immune activities may modulate the severity of age-related immunodeficiency diseases which are disruptive of many physiological functions

49, 52, 54). Figure 1 shows the effect of age on B-cell immune activity of the human and mouse. For comparison, the life-span of both species has been adjusted in terms of fractions of a mean life expectancy (human: 70 years = 1.0; long-lived mouse: 30 months = 1.0) (33, 34). By doing so, it can be seen that the age-related pattern of rise and decline in antibody synthesis in the human is remarkably similar to that in the mouse. Moreover, the onset of decline in these B-cell immune indexes occurs shortly after the thymus begins to involute, the serum thymosin level begins to decline (4, 16) and long before age-related immunodeficiency diseases (autoimmune diseases, certain types of cancer, certain types of bacterial and fungal-induced diseases) are manifested (45, 53, 55), although there may not be a function of declining humoral immune activity.

It should not be surprising that there have been exceptions to the "rule"; i.e., reports showing no decline with age in any functional activities (14, 29, 48). These exceptions may rise from several sources.[2] In any event, they may prove to be highly advantageous, for they may offer us an insight as to how to successfully replenish the immune systems of individuals manifesting declining activities.

---

[2] Differences in the life expectancy of sub-populations within species; in the type, dose and schedule of injections of antigens; in type of immune-response assays; in the manner of analyzing the data statistically; in the source of tissue being sampled and the sampling size, especially since variation between individuals increases with age; etc. In view of these considerations, the exceptions may be more apparent than real.

Nature of the decline with age in immune activities

The decline with age in B-cell immune activities can be due to *a*) changes in the environment of cells of the immune system, *b*) changes in the cells, or *c*) both. This problem was approached by assessing the antibody synthesizing activities of spleen cells from young and old mice in young and old recipient mice rendering themselves immunologically inert (3, 41). The activity of spleen cells should vary depending on which of the three causes is responsible for the decline (see Table 2). Table 2 summarizes the expected or predicted results one would obtain in this experimental model depending on the cause of the loss of activity. The experimental results revealed that both factors were involved, but that only 10% of the decline can

TABLE 2. Cell transfer approach to resolve the role cellular and environmental changes play in the decline with age in immune activity[a]

Cause of decline in activity	Donors of cell	Recipients	
		young	old
Cellular	Young	High	High
	Old	Low	Low
Environmental	Young	High	Low
	Old	High	Low
Both	Young	High	Low
	Old	Low	Low

[a] A fixed number of donor spleen cells is injected with an optimum dose of antigen into X-rayed syngeneic recipients and the peak response is assessed subsequently.

be accounted for by changes in the environment of the cells and 90% of the decline to changes in the old cell population (41).

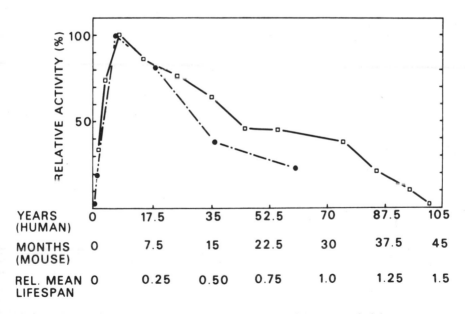

YEARS (HUMAN)

MONTHS (MOUSE)

REL. MEAN LIFESPAN

Figure 1. Effect of age on serum agglutinin titers in the human and mouse. □ natural serum anti-A isoagglutinin titers in humans (52); ● peak serum agglutinin response to sheep red blood cell stimulation by intact mice (34).

Cellular environmental changes

We believe that there are at least two factors responsible for environmental changes. One is noncellular and systemic. This factor(s) was detected by assessing the B-cell immune activity of spleen cells of young mice in immunologically inert young and old recipient mice (41). Fixed numbers of spleen cells were cultured in either the spleen or the peritoneal cavity of recipient mice. A difference in activity was observed between young and old recipients, but not between sites of culture and, moreover, the difference in activity between old and young recipients was twofold for either site. A comparable twofold difference in activity was also observed when bone marrow cells were assessed for their stem-cell activity in the spleens of young and old recipient mice (9).

At present we do not know what the factor(s) is. It could be either deleterious to or essential for cells of the immune system, or there could be too much or too little of it.

There is another age-related change that can be localized in the spleen of aging mice (41). It is not known if this change is reflective of noncellular factor(s) and/or non-antigen-responsive cells. In any event, it can be seen to interfere with the antigen-sensitive cell's maximal response to limiting doses of antigen. As shown in Fig. 2, this is reflected by the difference in slopes of the log antigen dose–log immune response regression curves of young ($\sim$2.7) and old mice ($\sim$1.3) and 10 times more antigen is needed to maximally stimulate old mice (10^7 sheep erythrocytes) than young mice (10^6 sheep erythrocytes). In contrast, the dose of antigen required to maximally stimulate dispersed spleen cells from young and old mice in vitro is the same (Halsall, unpublished data). Along with this observation is the finding that the dose-response line slope is different in the old and young mice. These findings suggest that changes are taking place in the spleen with age that are preventing limiting amounts of antigen from stimulating the antigen-sensitive cells effectively.

One possible explanation for this phenomenon is that antigens when administered to old mice become coated with a factor(s), causing them to become trapped in areas of the spleen that are not easily accessible to antigen-sensitive cells and that can be dislodged when the cells are dispersed mechanically. This may explain why antigens localize poorly in the follicles (31, 36) and germinal centers are absent in old mice (32). If so, this phenomenon may have a bearing on immune surveillance, for it implies that the ability of individuals to "sense" antigens, especially "weak" antigens, can decline with age without any appreciable loss of number and activity of antigen-sensitive cells.

Another explanation is that it reflects cellular changes. If so, macrophages would be the likely candidate,

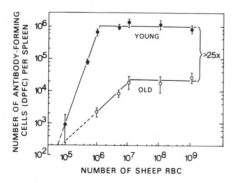

Figure 2. Effect of antigen dose on peak antibody response of young and old mice. Vertical bars indicate 95% confidence limits. (From (41).)

and we can offer two reasons. *1*) Perkins (40) and, more recently, Heidrick (23) have reported that the phagocytic activities of individual macrophages are unaltered or even enhanced with age. This implies that with age macrophages with po tentials to destroy antigens can compete with antigen-sensitive cells more effectively. *2*) Macrophages in the spleen, unlike those in the peritoneal cavity, should be extremely susceptible to shearing damage when spleen cells are dispersed manually, for many of them possess extensive dendritic processes (39). This can account for the lack of difference in the antigen dose to maximally stimulate dispersed spleen cells of young and old mice in vitro. It might also account for the problems in quantitation of macrophage numbers in a whole spleen population, since quantitation usually relies on some functional ability rather than a distinct morphologic entity.

Cellular changes

Three types of cellular changes that could cause a decline in measurable immune function are *a*) an absolute decrease in the number of functionally competent cells through death, *b*) a relative decrease in their number due to an increase in the number of incompetent, "suppressor" type cells, and/or *c*) a decrease in functional ability of existing cells, either decreases in division potential, or a decreased ability to interact with antigen or other cells.

To illustrate certain facets of these possibilities, it would be useful to review models of cellular differentiation in terms of compartment and triangle (Christmas tree) models (Figs. 3 and 4).

The compartment model emphasizes the importance of relative and absolute cell numbers at each stage

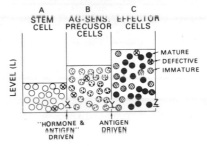

LEVEL OF COMPARTMENT (L) PER UNIT TIME (T)

$$a) \frac{dL_A}{dT} = f\left[GT, -\frac{dX}{dT} - \frac{dF_A}{dT}\right]$$

$$b) \frac{dL_B}{dT} = f\left[\frac{dX}{dT} - \frac{dY}{dT} - \frac{dF_B}{dT}, GT(?)\right]$$

$$c) \frac{dL_C}{dT} = f\left[\frac{dY}{dT} - \frac{dZ}{dT} - \frac{dF_C}{dT}, GT\right]$$

where:

GT, generation time; F, functional impairment ; X, differentiation of A to B cells; Y, differentiation of B to C cells; Z, cell death.

Figure 3. A three-compartment model of cellular differentiation in an immune response.

of "competence" or differentiation. The triangle model brings in the concept of cell division and its importance in determining the eventual size of a clone of cells.

As demonstrated in Fig. 4B and 4C, a defect in cell division or in differentiation can result in population changes in the absolute number of functional cells or in the functional capacity of cells, either due to a lack of immunocompetent cells or an increase of nonimmunologically reacting but possibly specific antigen-recognizing "competing" cells.

Both models use the concept that stem (S) cells are the primordial cells of the immune system. These cells can be influenced to differentiate to a more functional state and are classified as thymic-derived T cells, bone marrow-derived B cells or accessory A cells (macrophages). T and B cells are able to interact specifically with antigen while A cells and S cells probably do not. B and T cells are able to further differentiate in the presence of antigen and A cells by proliferation and transformation into functional effector cells; e.g., either synthesizing antibody or participating in delayed hypersensitivity mechanisms.

With the overall view of a "perfect," "normal" functioning immune system, we can begin to approach the separate problems that can help to explain the changes seen in immunologic capability with the aging process.

Physical properties of the cellular populations found in splenic tissues. Mouse spleen weight remains relatively constant, or increases slightly between 6 months and 2 years of age in long-lived mice reared in a relatively clean housing condition (33, 34). After 2 years of age the tumor incidence increases and spleen tumors

can markedly affect weight and cellularity. The number of viable cells per unit wet, nontumor-containing, spleen weight remains relatively constant or decreases only slightly, suggesting that with age either the average cell size or the frequency of fragile cells (cells that are extremely susceptible to injury when dispersed manually) is increasing slightly. Our preliminary studies (unpublished) on spleen cells of 6- and 24-months-old mice measuring cell size distribution and frequency of fragile cells suggest that the latter possibility is more likely. Density distribution analysis (20, and Makinodan, unpublished), using Ficoll and bovine serum albumin (BSA) discontinuous gradients, shows that the frequency of less dense cells (ρ, 1.06–1.08) increases at the expense of the more dense cells (ρ, 1.10–1.12). Figure 5 shows the difference in BSA density

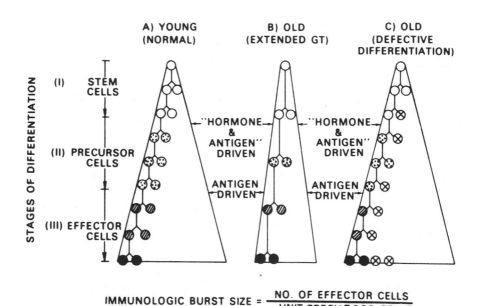

Figure 4. Triangle models of cellular differentiation in an immune response. ⊗ defective cell.

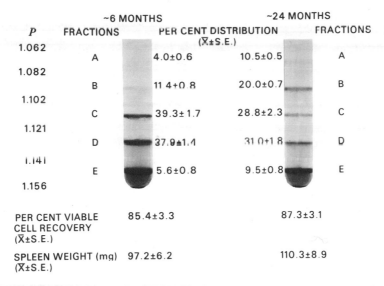

P	~6 MONTHS FRACTIONS	PER CENT DISTRIBUTION ($\bar{X}\pm$S.E.)		~24 MONTHS FRACTIONS
1.062				
	A	4.0±0.6	10.5±0.5	A
1.082				
	B	11.4±0.8	20.0±0.7	B
1.102				
	C	39.3±1.7	28.8±2.3	C
1.121				
	D	37.9±1.4	31.0±1.8	D
1.141				
	E	5.6±0.8	9.5±0.8	E
1.156				

PER CENT VIABLE CELL RECOVERY ($\bar{X}\pm$S.E.)	85.4±3.3	87.3±3.1
SPLEEN WEIGHT (mg) ($\bar{X}\pm$S.E.)	97.2±6.2	110.3±8.9

Figure 5. Density distribution of spleen cells of young and old BC3F₁ mice. Sample size per group, 6–12.

profile between spleen cells of approximately 6 and 24 months old, long-lived $BC3F_1$ mice (mean life-span, 30 months; maximum life-span, 47 months). This finding of density shift in population can also be seen in young mice that are immunized with red cells or allogeneic lymphocytes, or in mice that are bearing a tumor. However, in the above cases, the spleen cell number has also increased whereas in the 24-month-old normal mice this is not the case.

Stem (S) cells. Studies of the age effects on S cells have been limited primarily to the mouse. In the bone marrow, where the bulk of S cells reside (~90%), the concentration declines gradually with age after adulthood (9, 11, 12), but, as the concentration declines, the total cellularity increases proportionately (9). Therefore, the total number of S cells remains relatively constant throughout life (9, 11). These studies show that S cells can

self-replicate throughout the natural life-span of the mouse without exhausting themselves, unlike passaged stem cells (22, 30, 46).

There is no evidence to indicate that the hematopoietic ability of S cells declines with age (22). However, their ability to generate lymphatic cells may be affected, at least kinetically, as judged by their impaired ability to reconstitute X-rayed young syngeneic recipients (41) and by their impaired ability to generate B cells in thymectomized X-rayed young syngeneic recipients (13). Their ability to recover from fractionated sublethal doses of X-rays and generate hematopoietic colonies also seems to be impaired (10). These studies, although limited in number and scope, when taken together, indicate that certain functional properties of S cells have been affected by aging. It would seem fruitful to resolve whether the altered functional properties are due primarily to a slowing down with age of their proliferative rate, as the above studies suggest to us, and whether the alterations are permanent or reversible.

Accessory (A) cells. The A cells participate in both B- and T-cell immune responses in a nonspecific manner, are relatively radioresistant, adhere to glass and plastics, do not give rise to functional effector cells and phagocytize opsonized particles effectively (26, 37, 43, 44). Because they generally confront the antigens before antigenic-specific T and B cells do, any defect in them could result in a decreased immune response without any appreciable decline in number or function of T and B cells. Accordingly, peritoneal A cells from young and old mice were assessed for their functional capacities. The results showed that the phagocytic activity of A cells of old mice was equal to, if not better than, that of young mice (40). Measurements of the activity of three hydrolytic enzymes showed an increase with age (23). Finally, it was found that the ability of A cells to initiate antibody response in vivo and in vitro is also unaffected by aging (25).

B cells. The B cell population representation in the spleen does not seem to change appreciably with age. Thus, for example, the number of B cells in the spleen of disease-free, long-lived, old mice is about the same as that in the spleen of young mice. This is based on the number of cells bearing immunoglobulin receptors and cells susceptible to anti-B-cell reagent (2, 35, 50). Of course, subpopulations of B cells may fluctuate, depending on their susceptibility to various regulatory forces, including antigenic loads, associated with the aging process. Support of this view comes from studies showing shifts in the serum concentration of im-

munoglobulin classes in aging humans (7, 18, 19, 28) and a slight decline in the number of B cells responsive to an antigen in mice (41).

T cells participating in B-cell immune responses. Studies on age-related changes in T cells participating in B-cell immune responses have been minimal. This is due primarily to our lack of understanding how these cells function. We know that in general a few will enhance a response and many will suppress it. We do not know whether or not there exist two distinct subpopulations of regulator T cells or one population of regulator T cells with the potential to enhance or suppress a B-cell immune response, depending on their relative number. In any event, recent studies showed that with age the relative number of T cells participating in a B-cell immune response decreases in short-lived, autoimmune-prone mice (21) and increases slightly in a long-lived mouse (41). The former observation could account for the emergence of autoantibodies in aging short-lived mice. Because excessive numbers of regulator T cells tend to interfere with the response of B cells to antigenic stimulation, the latter observation could account for the apparent decline in the number of functional B-cell units, which will be discussed subsequently.

Immunocompetent unit of precursor cells and immunological burst size. In a typical immune response an antigen-specific precursor cell rarely responds to antigenic stimulation in absence of other cells. This view is based on frequency response and dose–response relationship studies of limiting numbers of cells (6, 8, 17, 38). That is, unlike a cancer cell or a bacterium with a high "culture efficiency," an immunocompetent unit is made up of two or more cells (T–A, B–A, T–A–B, etc.), and the number of each cell type can vary from one to many (17). Obviously, one of the cell types making up an immunocompetent unit is limiting because it is either few in numbers or there is a factor(s) in the cellular environmental milieu that is suppressing it from participating in the union.

To investigate what role the immunocompetent unit plays in the decline with age in B-cell immune activities, it was assessed by the limiting dilution method. The results revealed that it too declines, but its decline is responsible for only a fraction of the decline in B-cell immune activities in the whole animal. For example, in a study of the anti-sheep erythrocyte response in situ (41), a 50-fold difference in response per spleen was observed between young and old mice, but only a five fold difference in the number of immunocompetent units per spleen. This would mean that the immunological burst size (number of effector progeny cells per unit number of immunocompetent units), a quantitative index of differentiation, has declined with age by 10-fold (see Table 3).

Another interesting observation

in this series of studies was that the relative decline with age in the number of immunocompetent units responsive to sheep erythrocytes was greater than that of the individual cell types making up the immunocompetent unit (41). This would suggest that the number or proportion of cells with the ability to interfere with antigen-sensitive B cells in their response to antigenic stimulation is increasing with age. Consistent with this view is the observation that the relative number of T cells participating in the response of B cells to sheep erythrocytes increases with age.

These results demonstrate that the differentiating cells of the B-cell immune system are highly vulnerable to the deleterious effects of the aging process.

EFFECTS OF AGING ON THE T-CELL IMMUNE SYSTEM

Complexity of the system

The quantitation of the T-cell immune system is a difficult task and, as such, the T-cell immune system is usually "measured" in qualitative terms. The same set of hypotheses used to define, describe, and examine

TABLE 3. Quantitative evaluation of the differentiation process of spleen cells of young and old BC3F$_1$ mice in response to sheep RBC stimulation in situ

	A		B		C	
Relative age of mice, months	Response, DPFC/spleen, $\times 10^{-6}$	Ratio of $\frac{young}{old}$	I.U. per spleen $\times 10^{-3}$	Ratio of $\frac{young}{old}$	I.B.S per spleen, A/B $\times 10^{-3}$	Ratio of $\frac{young}{old}$
Young, 3–4	1.0		1.0		1.0	
		50		5		10
Old, 30–35	0.02		0.2		0.1	

Abbreviations: DPFC, direct plaque antibody-forming cells; I.U., immunocompetent unit; I.B.S., immunological burst size. Values presented are average; for detail see ref 41, p. 403.

the humoral immune system can be turned to the examination of the cellular immune system. The examination can be divided into two areas, in vivo measurements and in vitro performance indexes.

It is in the in vivo studies that the greatest difficulty lies. Briefly, the problem is that the usual measure of cellular immunity is a delayed hypersensitivity skin test; however, not all animals will demonstrate an easily described skin reaction. The reaction is poorly quantifiable even when manifest, and the antigens needed to induce delayed hypersensitivity must be carefully chosen and, in general, are difficult to use in human studies. Therefore, the study of T-cell function has more and more moved over into the area of using various in vitro culture techniques. One of the most widely used techniques to study T-cell function is the short-term culture of various lymphoid tissues. By stimulating the T cells with various specific mitogens or alloantigens (51), it is possible to determine the proliferative capacity of the various T lymphocytes found in those tissues. The actual population representation of T cells in various tissues can be quantitated by relying on the finding 1) that mouse T cells carry on their surface an antigen (Thy-1; θ) that can be detected by using appropriate antisera (5), and 2) human T cells will rosette in the presence of sheep erythrocytes (27). By quantitating the T cells and examining a "functional" characteristic, i.e., proliferative ability, it is possible to do studies on humans and animals totally in vitro and to qualitate and quantitate various age-related changes.

Nature of the decline in activity with age

The results overall would seen to suggest that the primary age-related effect on the T-cell immune system would be a defect in T-cell proliferative capacity. This conclusion is based on the following data. 1) The total lymphocyte cell number in the mouse spleen remains constant with age; furthermore the percent of cells carrying the T-cell antigen marker, theta, remains constant with age (Makinodan, unpublished data). However, the proliferative response of these T cells to the mitogens, PHA, Concanavalin A, or to the stimulatory effects of allogeneic cells in the so-called mixed lymphocyte culture all decrease markedly with age (2, 47). Correlative evidence of a proliferative defect can be found in the studies of Heidrick (24) in which a marked decrease of the cyclic nucleotide, guanosine monophosphate, concentration is found in the lymphoid cells from aged mice. This compound has been shown to increase when a lymphocyte is stimulated by mitogens and, as such, this decrease with age correlates well with the lack of mitogenic response.

Perhaps the most intriguing facet of these data is the appreciation of the temporal relationship of aging and decreased T-cell functions, i.e., the fall-off in certain T-cell functions occurs very early in the life of the mouse. In the long-lived hybrids it occurs later than in the shorter-lived A, C57 or CBA strains. Therefore, if one were to look for aging causative factors, one might need to consider the T cell involved in cell-mediated immunity and B-cell humoral immunity.

An experiment that demonstrates the difference in the age effects on the T-cell system and the supposed B-cell system is one in which the PHA, Con-A, and lipopolysaccharide (endotoxin) mitogenic effects on spleen cells were assayed in different ages of mice. Endotoxin mitogenic responsiveness is thought to be a

B-cell function in that immunoglobulin coated, antibody-forming cell precursors, bone marrow-derived cells,
are considered to be the responsive
population. Therefore lipopolysaccharide responsiveness is possibly a
measure of B-cell proliferative ability.
When the BC3F$_1$ spleen cells are
examined for lipopolysaccharide responsiveness, it can be seen that at
24 months of age, when both PHA
and Con-A responses are about at
the level of 10% of the 3-month
level, the lipopolysaccharide response
is about at the 90% level (Fig. 6).

Possible significance

Speculations can be made as to what
the presence of an "unbalanced" immune system may mean, but until
further studies can be designed to
determine the environment–host relationship in which the host is a
T-cell deficient, B-cell normal individual, the speculations remain as
such. It may be that many of the
age-related immune phenomena,
such as auto-antibody, immune complex disease and tumorogenesis, may
be results of this imbalance.

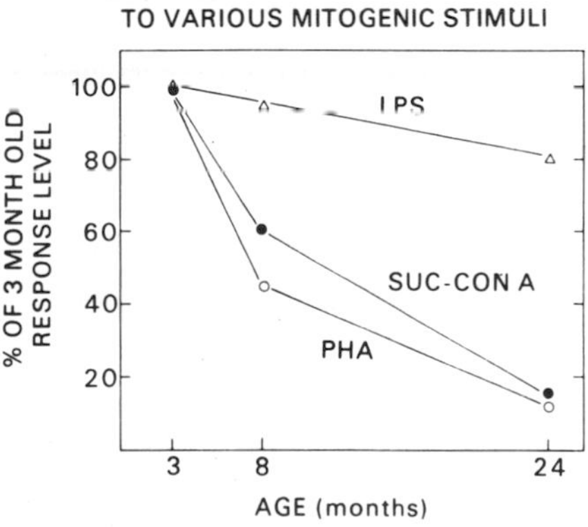

CONCLUDING REMARKS

An attempt has been made here to
show that the immune system can
begin to decline in function shortly
after an individual reaches maturity.
The decline is due in part to changes
in the environment of the cells but
primarily to changes in the precursor
cells of the system. This is reflected
in their ability to proliferate and
possibly differentiate efficiently.
These findings show that the immune
system can serve as an excellent model
to study how aging can perturb the
process of cells undergoing proliferation and differentiation.

We believe that in future studies
some of us should address ourselves
to a) the nature of altered activity
of immune cells, i.e., whether it
reflects alterations of genetic information or alterations of regulation; b) the
nature of loss of certain precursor
cells late in life, i.e., whether the
loss is due to switching on of a
self-destructive gene or whether they
are being killed by autoaggressive
cells; and c) the consequence of
replenishing deteriorating immune
systems of aged individuals.

TO VARIOUS MITOGENIC STIMULI

Figure 6. In vitro response of BC3F$_1$ spleen
cells from mice of different ages to various
mitogenic stimuli. Sample size per group,
6–11. Comparisons of responsiveness are
based on the comparative levels of tritiated
thymidine incorporation in 72-hour cultures
of spleen cells with the labeled thymidine
being present for the last 18 hours of culture.

REFERENCES

1. ADLER, W. H. An autoimmune theory
of aging. In: *Theoretical Aspects of Aging*,
edited by M. Rockstein. New York:
Academic, 1974, p. 33–42.
2. ADLER, W. H., T. TAKIGUCHI AND R. T.
SMITH. *J. Immunol.* 107: 1357, 1971.
3. ALBRIGHT, J. F., AND T. MAKINODAN.
J. Cellular Physiol. 67 (Suppl. 1): 185,
1966.
4. BACH, J. F., M. DARDENNE AND J. C.
SALOMON. *Clin. Exptl. Immunol.* 14: 247,
1973.

5. BOYSE, E. A., L. J. OLD AND E. STOCK-
   ERT. *Ann. N.Y. Acad. Sci.* 99: 574, 1962.
6. BROWN, R. A., T. MAKINODAN AND J. F.
   ALBRIGHT. *Nature* 210: 1383, 1966.
7. BUCKLEY, C. E., AND F. C. DORSEY.
   J. Immunol. 105: 964, 1970.
8. CELADA, F. *J. Exptl. Med.* 125: 199, 1967.
9. CHEN, M. G. *J. Cellular Physiol.* 78: 225,
   1971.
10. CHEN, M. G. *Proc. Soc. Exptl. Biol. Med.*
    145: 1181, 1974.
11. COGGLE, J. E., AND C. PROUKAKIS. *Geronto-
    logia* 16: 25, 1970.
12. DAVIS, M. L., A. C. UPTON AND L. C.
    SATTERFIELD. *Proc. Soc. Exptl. Biol. Med.*
    137: 1452, 1971.
13. FARRAR, J. J. *J. Immunol.* 112: 1613, 1974.
14. FULK, R. V., D. S. FEDSON, M. A. HUBER,
    J. R. FITZPATRICK AND J. A. KASEL.
    J. Immunol. 104: 8, 1970.
15. FURAHATA, T., AND M. EGUCHI. *Proc.
    Japan Acad.* 31: 55, 1955.
16. GOLDSTEIN, A. L., J. A. HOOPER, R. S.
    SCHULOF, G. A. COHEN, G. B. THUR-
    MAN, M. C. MCDANIEL, A. WHITE AND
    M. DARDENNE. *Federation Proc.* 33: 2053,
    1974.
17. GROVES, D. L., W. E. LEVER AND* T.
    MAKINODAN. *J. Immunol.* 104: 148, 1970.
18. HAFERKAMP, O., D. SCHLETTWEIN-
    GSELL, H. G. SCHWICK AND K. STORIKO.
    Gerontologia 12: 30, 1966.
19. HALLGREN, H. M., C. E. BUCKLEY, V. A.
    GILBERTSON AND E. J. YUNIS. *J. Im-
    munol.* 111: 1101, 1973.
20. HALSALL, M. H., M. L. HEIDRICK, J. W.
    DEITCHMAN AND T. MAKINODAN. *Ger-
    ontologist* 13: 46, 1973.
21. HARDIN, J. A., T. M. CHUSEO AND A. D.
    STEINBERG. *J. Immunol.* 111: 650, 1973.
22. HARRISON, D. E. *Proc. Natl. Acad. Sci.
    U.S.* 70: 3184, 1973.
23. HEIDRICK, M. L. *Gerontologist* 12: 28, 1972.
24. HEIDRICK, M. L. *J. Cell Biol.* 57: 139, 1973.
25. HEIDRICK, M. L., AND T. MAKINODAN.
    Gerontologia 18: 305, 1972.
26. HOFFMAN, M. *Immunology* 18: 791, 1970.
27. JONDAL, M., G. HOLM AND H. WIGZELL.
    J. Exptl. Med. 136: 207, 1972.
28. KALFF, M. W. *Clin. Chim. Acta* 28: 277,
    1970.
29. KISHIMOTO, S., I. TSUYUGUCHI AND Y.
    YAMAMURA. *Clin. Exptl. Immunol.* 5: 525,
    1969.

30. LAJTHA, L. J., AND R. SCHOFIELD. *Advan.
    Gerontol. Res.* 3: 131, 1971.
31. LEGGE, J. S., AND C. M. AUSTIN. *Australian
    J. Exptl. Biol. Med. Sci.* 46: 361, 1968.
32. MAKINODAN, T., F. CHINO, W. E. LEVER
    AND B. S. BREWEN. *J. Gerontol.* 26:
    515, 1971.
33. MAKINODAN, T., AND W. J. PETERSON.
    J. Immunol. 93: 886, 1964.
34. MAKINODAN, T., AND W. J. PETERSON.
    Develop. Biol. 14: 96, 1966.
35. MATHIES, M., L. LIPPS, G. S. SMITH AND
    R. L. WALFORD. *J. Gerontol.* 28: 425,
    1973.
36. METCALF, D., R. MOULDS AND B. PIKE.
    Clin. Exptl. Immunol. 2: 109, 1966.
37. MOSIER, D. E. *Science* 158: 1573, 1967.
38. MOSIER, D. E., AND L. W. COPPLESON.
    Proc. Natl. Acad. Sci. U.S. 61: 542, 1968.
39. NOSSAL, G. J. V., G. L. ADA AND C. M.
    AUSTIN. *Australian J. Exptl. Biol. Med.
    Sci.* 42: 311, 1964.
40. PERKINS, E. H. *J. Reticuloendothel. Soc.*
    9: 642, 1971.
41. PRICE, G. B., AND T. MAKINODAN. *J.
    Immunol.* 108: 403; 413, 1972.
42. RAM, J. S. *J. Gerontol.* 22: 92, 1967.
43. ROSEMAN, J. *Science* 165: 1125, 1969.
44. SHORTMAN, K., AND J. PALMER. *Cellular
    Immunol.* 2: 399, 1971.
45. SIGEL, M. M., AND R. A. GOOD. *Tol-
    erance, Autoimmunity and Aging.* Spring-
    field, Ill.: Thomas, 1972, 181 p.
46. SIMINOVITCH, L., J. E. TILL AND E. A.
    MCCULLOCH. *J. Cellular Comp. Physiol.*
    64: 23, 1964.
47. SMITH, R. T. *Transplant. Rev.* 11: 178, 1972.
48. SOLOMONOVA, K., AND S. VIZEV. *Z.
    Immunitaetsforsch.* 146: 81, 1973.
49. SOMERS, H., AND W. J. KUHINS. *Proc.
    Soc. Exptl. Biol. Med.* 141: 1104, 1972.
50. STUTMAN, O. *J. Immunol.* 109: 602, 1972.
51. TAKIGUCHI, T., W. H. ADLER AND R. T.
    SMITH. *J. Exptl. Med.* 133: 63, 1971.
52. THOMSEN, O., AND K. KETTEL. *Z. Im-
    munitaetsforsch.* 63: 67, 1929.
53. WALFORD, R. L. *The Immunologic Theory
    of Aging.* Copenhagen, Munksgaard,
    1969, 248 p.
54. WIGZELL, H., AND J. STJERNSWÄRD. *J.
    Natl. Cancer Inst.* 37: 513, 1966.
55. YUNIS, E. J., G. FERNANDES AND O.
    STUTMAN. *J. Clin. Pathol.* 56: 280, 1971.

Age-related changes, including synergy and suppression, in the mixed lymphocyte reaction in long-lived mice[1,2]

MARIA GERBASE-DeLIMA, PAT MEREDITH
AND ROY L. WALFORD
Department of Pathology, UCLA School of Medicine
Los Angeles, California 90024

ABSTRACT

The mixed lymphocyte culture reaction represents the in vitro counterpart of the recognition phase of the graft-versus-host reaction, and of allograft rejection. The mixed lymphocyte culture reactivities of lymph node and spleen cells from all strains of mice studied, including long-lived strains, and of thymus cells from most strains show a striking decline with advanced age. Furthermore, studies of "synergy" between subpopulations of T cells in the mixed lymphocyte culture reaction suggest that the cells of the recirculating lymphoid pool (T$_0$ cells) in particular display a functional decline. Finally, spleen cells from old mice of appropriate strains inhibit or suppress the mixed lymphocyte culture reactivity of lymph node or spleen cells from young mice.—GERBASE-DeLIMA, M., P. MEREDITH AND R. L. WALFORD. Age-related changes, including synergy and suppression, in the mixed lymphocyte reaction in long-lived mice. *Federation Proc.* 34: 159–161, 1975.

The immune system undergoes a remarkable series of changes with advancing age (16, 18). These include a marked falloff in the antibody response to thymic-dependent antigens (8) and a later occurring, less marked decrease in response to thymic-independent antigens (4). The responses of mouse spleen cells

[1] From Session V, *Development and Aging in Organ Systems*, of the FASEB Conference on *Biology of Development and Aging*, presented at the 58th Annual Meeting of the Federation of American Societies for Experimental Biology, Atlantic City, N.J., April 11, 1974.

[2] This study was supported by Public Health Service Grants CA12788 and HD00534.

Abbreviations: MLC, mixed lymphocyte culture; GVH, graft-versus-host.

269

to stimulation by mitogens such as PHA, pokeweed, con-A, bacterial lipopolysaccharide, and PPD all show a rather striking decline with advanced age (4, 9). Classical cellular immune reactions also show an age-related decline. Spleen cells from old mice display a reduced ability to elicit graft-versus-host reactions (10). The cell mediated lymphocytotoxic reaction (target cell lysis) also declines with age in old mice (5), as does the ability of old mice to reject transplanted tumor cells (11).

MIXED LYMPHOCYTE CULTURE REACTION

The mixed lymphocyte culture (MLC)-reaction probably represents the in vitro counterpart of the recognition phase of the graft-versus-host (GVH) reaction, and of allograft rejection. Representing a purely thymic-dependent function, it is one of the most useful and clearcut systems for studying age-related changes in cellular immunity. Our basic technique has been described in detail elsewhere (12, 14). In our present method the responding cells at various cell concentrations are incubated with a constant number (8 $\times$ 10^5) of mitomycin-C treated allogeneic cells for 48 hours at 37 C in a total volume of 0.2 ml in a humidified atmosphere. Then 3 μCi of [^{3}H]thymidine are added to each suspension and the incubation continued another 18 hours. The reaction is stopped by chilling to 4 C and a harvesting procedure carried out employing a multiple automated sample harvester. Counting of radioactivity is done by liquid scintillation techniques. Control values of syngeneic combinations are subtracted from experimental (allogeneic) values. All tests are done in quadruplicate and means and standard errors computed.

We have measured age-related changes in the MLC-reaction of responding spleen cells from C57BL/6J mice (7); spleen, lymph node and thymus cells from (C57BL/6 $\times$ 129)F$_1$-hybrid mice (13); and recently of lymphoid populations from (LP $\times$ 129)F$_1$-hybrid and BALB/cJ and ICR mice. The spleen and lymph node cells from all strains studied showed a decline in MLC-reactivity with age, down to 25% or less of the response of cells from young animals. (By "age" or "old" we refer to animals at or beyond the 50% survival point of the particular strain.) The MLC-reactivities of thymus cells of C57BL/6J, BALB/cJ and ICR mice also decline progressively with age. In (C57BL/6J $\times$ 129)F$_1$-hybrid mice, however, the thymus cells sometimes showed decreased reactivity with age, at other times a considerable increase in reactivity—possibly due to individual and age-related variations in the proportion of immature to mature cells in the thymus in this stain. Figure 1 gives a comparison of mixed lymphocyte reactivities of responding lymph node, spleen, and thymus cells from 4- and 24-month-old BALB/cJ mice.

SYNERGY

Cantor and Asofsky (1, 2) presented evidence for the synergistic interaction of two thymus-dependent lymphoid populations in the GVH response. One cell type (T$_2$ cells) was obtained from the recirculating lymphoid pool, and the second (T$_1$ cells) was found particularly in thymus and spleen. The GVH response obtained by injecting a mixture of these cell populations was greater than could be expected from summing the individual responses. Similar interactions among T-cell subsets have been demonstrated by several groups of investigators using the MLC-reaction (3, 12, 14) and the cell-mediated cytotoxic reaction (15). We have shown that essentially all the phenomena displayed by T-cell subpopulations interacting in the GVH response, as documented by Cantor and Asofsky (1, 2), can be duplicated in vitro with the MLC-reaction (12). For optimum synergy both populations must be allogeneic to the stimulator cells, pretreatment of either population with mitomycin-C abolishes synergy, anti-theta serum abolishes both MLC-responding and MLC-synergizing activities of cells, both T-cell subpopulations are present in the spleen and display different migratory patterns when injected into irradiated mice—one population going to spleens and the other to lymph nodes.

The effects of age of the donor animals on synergy between responding thymus and lymph node, and thymus and spleen cells from 3-, 18-, and 30-month-old (C57BL/6J × 129)F_1-hybrid mice are shown in Fig. 2. The values are expressed here in percent of the "expected" values. Thus, a mixture of thymus and lymph node cells from young mice gave an approximately 600% "observed" response compared to the "expected" response ("expected" = the sum of the reactivities of the individual responding cell populations incubated separately with stimulator cells). When lymph node cells from middle-aged and old mice were incubated with young thymus cells, the degree of synergy declined progressively. On the other hand, when thymus cells from increasingly old

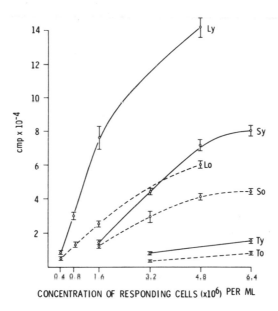

CONCENTRATION OF RESPONDING CELLS (x10⁶) PER ML

Figure 1. [³H]thymidine uptake in cpm of lymph node, spleen, and thymus cells from 4- and 24-month-old BALB/cJ mice plotted against the concentration of responding cells in the one-way MLC-reaction. L = lymph node, S = spleen, T = thymus; lowercase y = young, o = old. Each point represents the mean value of quadriplicate samples, the vertical bars represent 2 standard errors.

animals were incubated with lymph-oid cells from young partners, the young thymus cells gave greater synergy than either middle-aged or old cells but no appreciable difference was observed between thymocytes from middle-aged compared to old animals. When young responding thymus cells were incubated with either young or old responding spleen cells in this strain, synergy was obtained with young but not with old spleen cells (Fig. 2). By contrast, young or old thymus cells synergized about equally well with young spleen cells (Fig. 2).

Our studies of the MLC-reaction and synergy in relation to age have led us to conclude that so far as cellular immune function is concerned, it is particularly the T_2-like cell populations that suffer a functional decline. Attempts at immunologic rejuvenation by injection of cells from young into older animals might have best chance of success if T_2-cell-rich populations are employed.

SUPPRESSION

An age-related appearance or increase of cells in mouse spleen that inhibited the proliferation of spleen cells stimulated with mitogens was reported by Halsall et al. (6). In Fig. 3 we present studies with 7- and 34-month-old $(129 \times LP)F_1$-hybrid mice which suggest that the MLC-response may be suppressed by spleen cells from old mice. The "observed" values, obtained when two responding cell populations were mixed and incubated with a stimulating population, were compared with the "expected" values. In this strain combination we observed no synergy between young lymph node and young spleen cell populations, i.e., the observed values were approximately the same as the expected values (Fig. 3). However, when young lymph node cells were incubated with old spleen cells, the observed values were considerably lower than the expected values. This is quite the reverse of

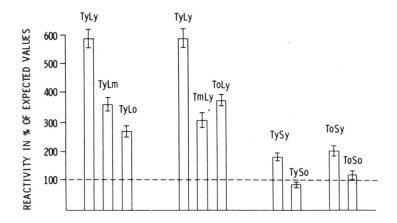

Figure 2. MLC-reactivities ("synergy") of various thymus–lymph node cell and thymus–spleen cell combinations from 3-, 18-, and 30-month-old (C57BL/6J $\times$ 129)F₁-hybrid mice, expressed in percent of the "expected" value. Ratio of numbers of thymus to lymph node or spleen cells was 4 to 1 in all cases. Lowercase m = middle-aged, other designations as in Figure 1. Each column represents the mean value of 6 separate experiments.

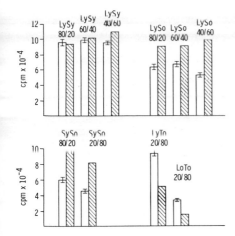

Figure 3. [³H]thymidine uptake in cpm of various mixtures, in the ratios given, of lymph node and spleen cells, young and old spleen cells, and lymph node and thymus cells from 7- and 34-month-old (129/J × LP)F₁-hybrid mice in the one-way MLC-reaction. □ = observed values, ▩ = expected values.

synergy. Furthermore, when a mixture of young and old spleen cells was incubated with stimulator cells, the overall MLC-reaction was also less than the expected value. By contrast, when either young or old lymph node cells were incubated with either young (not shown) or old thymus cells, a substantial amount of synergy was noted (Fig. 3).

The above findings are again somewhat strain specific. For example, when young and old spleen cells from C57BL/10J mice were incubated together with stimulator cells, or old spleen cells with young lymph node cells, neither synergy nor suppression was found. When spleen cells from 4-month-old and 28-month-old (BALB/cJ × C57BL/6J)F₁-hybrid mice were incubated together with stimulator cells, a substantial degree of suppression was obtained. We also noted suppression when spleen cells

from 12- and 24-month-old ICR mice (an outbred strain) were incubated together as responding cells versus a mixture of stimulator cells from CBA, DBA/2J, and C57BL/6J mice. Thus, in three of four strain combinations tested, we have found evidence of a population of cells in the spleens of old mice which suppress the mixed lymphocyte reaction

We wish to acknowledge the technical assistance of Mr. Jerry Jacobson and Ms. Rosalie Hooper.

REFERENCES

1. CANTOR, H., AND R. ASOFSKY. *J. Exptl. Med.* 131: 235, 1970.

2. CANTOR, H., AND R. ASOFSKY. *J. Exptl. Med.* 135: 764, 1972.

3. COHEN, D., AND M. L. HOWE. *Proc. Natl. Acad. Sci. U.S.* 70: 2707, 1973.

4. GERBASE-DELIMA, M., J. WILKINSON, G. S. SMITH, AND R. L. WALFORD. *J. Gerontol.* 29: 261, 1974.

5. GOODMAN, S. A., AND T. MAKINODAN. *J. Immunol.* In press.

6. HALSALL, M. H., M. L. HEIDRICK, J. W. DEITCHMAN AND T. MAKINODAN. *Gerontologist* 13: 46, 1973.

7. KONEN, T. G., G. S. SMITH AND R. L. WALFORD. *J. Immunol.* 110: 1216, 1973.

8. MAKINODAN, T., E. H. PERKINS AND M. G. CHEN. *Advan. Gerontol. Res.* 3: 171, 1971.

9. MATHIES, M., L. LIPPS, G. S. SMITH AND R. L. WALFORD. *J. Gerontol.* 28: 425, 1973.

10. PETERSON, W. F. *Gerontologist* 12: 30, 1972.

11. TELLER, M. N. In: *Tolerance, Autoimmunity and Aging*, edited by L. Gitman, M. Bunch and M. Rockstein. Springfield, Ill.: Thomas, 1972, pp. 18–32.

12. TITTOR, W., M. GERBASE-DELIMA AND R. L. WALFORD. *J. Exptl. Med.*

13. TITTOR, W., M. GERBASE-DELIMA AND R. L. WALFORD. *J. Immunol.* (submitted).

14. TITTOR, W., AND R. L. WALFORD. *Nature* 247: 371, 1974.

15. WAGNER, H. *J. Exptl. Med.* 138: 1379, 1973.

16. WALFORD, R. L. *The Immunologic Theory of Aging.* Copenhagen: Munksgaard, 1969.

17. WALFORD, R. L. *Federation Proc.* 33: 2020, 1974.
18. YUNIS, E. J., G. FERNANDES, J. SMITH, O. STUTMAN AND R. A. GOOD. In: *Microenvironmental Aspects of Immunity.* New York: Plenum, 1972, p. 301–306.

Panel discussion on T-cell heterogeneity

Participants:
Richard Asofsky, *NIH*, Chairman; Donald Mosier, *NIH*
Guy Bonnard, *NIH*; Robert Tigelaar, *NIH*
Harvey Cantor, *Children's Cancer Research Foundation, Boston*
Richard Gershon, *Yale University School of Medicine*
and Irving Weissman, *Stanford University*

The lymphoid system consists of precursors of antibody forming cells (B cells) and their progeny plasma cells, cells which differentiate under the influence of the thymus (T cells), phagocytic cells (monocytes and macrophages), and perhaps other cells with ill-defined functions.

Diversity among antibody forming cells was discussed very briefly, because its existence is so well established. Such cells are derived from B-cell precursors, and are terminal cells in a pathway of differentiation that ultimately displays remarkable heterogeneity. Antibody forming cells, with almost no exception, each synthesize and elaborate large amounts of a single immunoglobulin product. In man, the immunoglobulin in each such cell consists of only one of eight possible classes of heavy chain, and only one of two possible classes of light chain. The same is true in experimental animals. Evidence in rabbits shows that each cell synthesizes only one of several allelic forms (allotypes) of both light and heavy chains. Each cell synthesizes only one specificity of antibody. There is also considerable evidence that precursor B cells show such specialization, for example, each B cell expresses only one allotype. There are a minimum of 16 combinations of light and heavy chains in plasma cells in man, and perhaps that much diversity among B cells.

B cells, plasma cells, and their immunoglobulin products have been relatively easy to study, since these products were easy to isolate and to characterize both in their normal form and as myeloma proteins. All stages of B-cell differentiation could be examined with highly specific antisera to immunoglobulins using immunofluorescent and radiolabeling methods, among others. The task in examining T cells is far more difficult. These cells contain little if any immunoglobulin, and many, if not all T-cell functions are mediated by products that are poorly defined, and have not been obtained in sufficient amounts for chemical characterization. Studies of T cells, therefore, consist of an examination of the function of populations of cells. At least three such functions of T cells have been defined in in vitro tests: *1*) rapid cell division on exposure to antigen; *2*) the release of macrophage inhibiting factor (MIF), a soluble material which prevents macrophage migration; and *3*) specific lysis of cells to which the population has been immunized. None of these effects is the exclusive property of T cells, and the participation of such cells must be explicitly demonstrated. In vivo, primary allograft rejection, graft-versus-host (GVH) reactions, and delayed skin hypersensitivity are primarily functions of T cells. It has also been shown that T cells modulate the differentiation of B cells. In addition to the well studied "helper" T cells, which assist or make possible the differentiation of B cells, there exists a phenomenon of T-cell mediated suppression of this differentiation.

The first evidence of T-cell heterogeneity came from studies of GVH reactions. It was shown that the reactivities of cells from different tissues fell on one of a family of parallel lines when reactivity was plotted as a function of the cell inoculum. Reactivities were therefore commensurable; e.g., peripheral lymph node cells were 15 times as active as thymocytes in one assay. Mixtures of these two populations resulted in reactions two or more times greater than expected by adding reactivities. One population seemed to amplify the activity of the other. This work was done in mice, and both populations were sensitive to lysis with an alloantiserum specific for T cells, anti-thy-1.2. Similar synergy was demonstrated in several laboratories using in vitro assays. Mixtures of cells display such synergy in proliferation assays and in the development of cytotoxic lymphocytes. Two possibilities for synergism were discussed, neither of which has been excluded: *1*) there are at least two kinds of T cell, an amplifier and a cell which inflicts immunologic injury; or *2*) both cells represent different stages in a single path of maturation, at some stages of which T cells have amplifying properties that are lacking at others.

Detailed studies of the generation of cytotoxic lymphocytes in vitro both in man and in mice indicate that synergy may be a consequence of antigenic diversity. Lymphocytes from allogeneic animals or people may differ at the major histocompatibility complex at either well-defined, serologically determined (SD) specificities, or at less well-defined closely linked specificities which simulate proliferation (LD specificities). Rare instances exist of LD differences only; no cytotoxic lymphocytes are generated, despite the stimulation of proliferation. Similar instances can be found of SD differences only; neither proliferation nor the generation of cytotoxic lymphocytes results. Cells differing from stimulating cells at both LD and SD generate cytotoxic lymphocytes. The requirement for two specificities has been demonstrated by mixing cells that differ from stimulating cells at SD only with those that differ at LD only. In this "3-way" mixture, cytotoxic lymphocytes are generated, despite the fact that neither population is capable of such generation alone.

Experimental evidence has been obtained showing both physiological and physical differences in two effector functions of T cells, the capacity to release MIF, and the capacity to lyse target cells. In mice immunized with allogeneic cells intraperitoneally *1*) cytotoxic activity was confined to the spleen, while MIF activity was found in both spleen and lymph node; *2*) reconstitution of heavily irradiated mice with immunized spleen cells resulted in a very similar distribution of these activities; and *3*) velocity sedimentation of immune spleen cells at $1 \times g$ showed different profiles of activity for MIF and cytotoxicity. Fractions were obtained that were very enriched for one activity with respect to the other.

Experiments were described showing suppressor activity for T cells. A commonly used protocol for obtaining cells that augment the activity of B cells (helpers) can be altered by administering very large doses of antigen. A population of T cells so obtained suppresses the activity of B cells even in the presence of helpers. Similar active suppresion can be demonstrated in GVH reactions measured by in vivo proliferation. If thymocytes are given to irradiated allogeneic hosts, proliferation of donor cells occurs in spleen and lymph node, which reaches an early maximum, then declines. If spleens are removed early from these hosts, high and sustained proliferation is seen in lymph node. Reversion to a normal pattern can be obtained by reinoculating cells from the spleens that had been removed.

The panel agreed that there was no conclusive evidence concerning T-cell heterogeneity, but that there was much circumstantial evidence for functional heterogeneity among these cells. Diversity in the lymphoid system is expressed in the specialized diversification of cell function, exemplified best by the differentiation into T and B cells and by the high degree of specialization in the progeny of B cells. Similar specialization among T cells should come as no surprise.

Development and aging at the molecular level

H. N. MUNRO

Physiological Chemistry Laboratories
Department of Nutrition and Food Science
Massachusetts Institute of Technology
Cambridge, Massachusetts 02139

The poet Wordsworth tells us that "the Child is father of the Man," an aphorism fittingly descriptive of the continuum of growth, development and aging in which each part of the sequence is a prelude to the next stage. In this Interdisciplinary Symposium in the series on development and aging, we examine molecular and biochemical mechanisms involved in these processes at two important periods of the life of the mammal. First, changes in metabolic control are discussed in relation to the perinatal period. Second, molecular and biochemical changes are examined during the terminal period of the natural life-span of the mammal. The data gathered at these two periods of life serve to illustrate that control mechanisms encoded in the genome of the fertilized ovum continue to undergo change throughout the whole life-span of the organism.

A period of rapid metabolic change occurs around the time of birth of the mammal. The perinatal period involves a transition from an environment of uniform temperature and constant nutrient supply through the umbilical vein to one of variable temperature and intermittent food supply through the alimentary tract. The responses of intermediary metabolism during this transition have been extensively documented and are well represented in this symposium. It should be pointed out, however, that the perinatal period causes changes in metabolism additional to those of carbohydrate, fat and protein. In this introduction to the symposium, I shall deal briefly with changes in iron and copper metabolism during the perinatal period. These studies are reviewed in detail elsewhere (7) and illustrate *a*) how the distribution of these two minerals changes during this short fraction of the life-span of the animal, *b*) how the chemical structure of proteins associated with storage of these minerals alters, and *c*) how several processes in their perinatal metabolism are coordinated so that the storage forms of these minerals are made available to the neonatal animal at a time when the animal is nutritionally dependent on milk, which is notoriously poor in iron and copper.

277

Study of iron transfer from mother to fetus shows that the major deposition of fetal iron occurs late in pregnancy, much of it in the form of ferritin in the liver (6). Figure 1 illustrates the rapid accumulation of ferritin iron in rat liver during the last 4 days of gestation. After birth, this stored iron is extensively raided during the suckling period, in order to make hemoglobin and other iron-containing compounds of metabolic importance. The ferritin deposited before birth and removed during suckling differs structurally from ferritin found in adult liver since it has an apoferritin shell that is dis-

tinct although chemically related to adult ferritin, and is thus a fetal-type isoferritin. This can be demonstrated by their different electrophoresis mobilities on acrylamide gels. If a large dose of iron is given to the rat towards the end of the suckling period, much new ferritin is quickly deposited in the liver; this ferritin is electrophoretically of the adult type (Table 1). Thus a change in ferritin isoprotein expression occurs in the liver during the perinatal period.

Copper metabolism follows a somewhat similar pattern, with deposition occurring in the liver just prior to

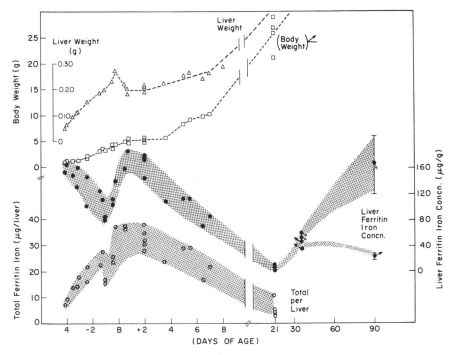

Figure 1. Changes in rat liver ferritin iron before and after birth. The upper two curves show perinatal changes in liver weight and body weight for comparison with curves for ferritin iron concentration (●) and total ferritin iron per liver (○). Age is given in days relative to birth (B). Note that the data for ferritin iron concentration after weaning are divided into male and female values. The shaded area depicts the limits of the experimental values. (Reproduced with permission from Linder et al. (7).)

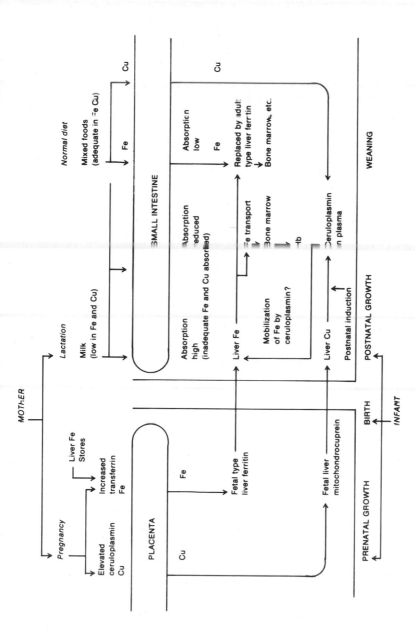

Figure 2. Schematic presentation of iron and copper metabolism in the terminal stages of pregnancy, in lactation and after weaning. (Reproduced with permission from Linder et al. (7).)

TABLE 1. Effect of iron induction on the amount and species of ferritin in the liver of the infant rat[a]

Age of rat before/after birth	Total liver ferritin, μg Fe/ organ	Relative migration rate
Adult rat		1.00
−4 to +1 days	35	1.10[b]
+20 to +21 days	5	1.13[b]
Same, iron injected (10 mg Fe for 24 hours)	280	1.04

[a] Data are taken from Linder et al. (6) and represent mean values for ferritin iron and R_f of migration of ferritin extracted from livers of rats at the ages shown, with or without prior injection of iron as Imferon. The R_fs of migration were recalculated to give values relative to the R_f of control adult liver ferritin which was always run simultaneously with experimental samples. The differences between values for ferritin iron concentration are significant at the 0.01 level.   [b] Significantly different from other two values ($P < 0.01$).

birth in the form of a fetal copper-storage protein, mitochondrocuprein, that diminishes in amount after birth as the copper is transferred from the liver to the plasma protein ceruloplasmin (7). There is evidence that the formation of ceruloplasmin at this time is in some way involved in mobilization of iron from the liver. The coordinated nature of these and other changes occurring in iron and copper metabolism during the perinatal period is shown diagrammatically in Fig. 2. Thus perinatal iron and copper metabolism involve substitution of adult for fetal mechanisms analogous to changes occurring in other metabolic systems at this time.

In the adult, changes caused by aging result in much less dramatic metabolic alterations, so that significant changes generally require observation over long periods of time. From the age of 25 onwards, adults show a progressive loss of lean body mass as measured by the ^{40}K content of the body (2) and a steady erosion of physiological performance (9). The loss of cells and the reduction in the amounts of individual proteins within the cells imply an imbalance between protein synthesis and breakdown, so that the intracellular level is not maintained. There is some evidence (10) that the capacity of the liver to maintain the normal level of albumin in the blood is impaired in elderly people, because the response of the synthetic machinery to hypoalbuminemia is sluggish. In animal models, Adelman (1) has shown a progressive lengthening of the time required for enzyme adaptation to hormonal stimuli, and has analyzed the underlying causes. Changes in hormone receptor properties (8) and in the characteristics of nuclear proteins (5) represent other age-related alterations in mechanisms regulating cell responses. The well-known diminution in muscle power with aging may similarly be correlated with the changes in sodium and potassium flux (3) and in myosin properties (4) reported in this symposium. Further work is certainly needed to probe the molecular and biochemical basis of the aging process.

REFERENCES

1. ADELMAN, R. C. Federation Proc. 34: 179, 1975.

2. FORBES, G. B., AND J. C. REINA. Metabolism 19: 653, 1970.

3. GOLDBERG, P. B., S. I. BASKIN AND J. ROBERTS. Federation Proc. 34: 188, 1975.

4. KALDOR, G., AND B. K. MIN. Federation Proc. 34: 191, 1975.

5. LIEW, C. C., AND A. G. GORNALL. Federation Proc. 34: 186, 1975.

6. LINDER, M. C., J. R. MOOR, L. E. SCOTT AND H. N. MUNRO. Biochem. J. 129: 455, 1972.

7. LINDER, M. C., AND H. N. MUNRO. *Enzyme* 15: 111, 1973.

8. ROTH, G. S. *Federation Proc.* 34: 183, 1975.

9. SHOCK, N. W. In: *Nutrition in Old Age,* edited by L. A. Carlson. Uppsala: Almqvist & Wiksell.

10. YAN, S. H. Y., AND J. J. FRANKS. *J. Lab. Clin. Med.* 72: 449, 1968.

Hormonal regulation of hepatic P-enolpyruvate carboxykinase (GTP) during development[1,2]

RICHARD W. HANSON,[3] LEA RESHEF AND JOHN BALLARD

Fels Research Institute and Department of Biochemistry
Temple University School of Medicine, Philadelphia
Pennsylvania 19140; Department of Biochemistry
Hebrew University-Hadassah Medical School
Jerusalem, Israel; and the CSIRO, Division
of Nutritional Biochemistry, Adelaide, Australia

ABSTRACT

Hepatic gluconeogenesis in the rat does not begin until birth. The enzyme P-enolpyruvate carboxykinase appears initially at birth and is the final enzyme in the gluconeogenic sequence to develop. The appearance of this enzyme in the cytosol of rat liver is caused by the stimulation of enzyme synthesis, probably due directly to an increase in the hepatic concentration of cAMP. Enzyme degradation does not begin until 36 hours after birth. Studies with fetal rats in utero have shown that dibutyryl cAMP or glucagon will stimulate P-enolpyruvate carboxykinase synthesis and that this effect can be blocked by insulin. Insulin is known to depress the synthesis of P-enolpyruvate carboxykinase in adult rat liver and in Reuber H-35 liver cells in culture. The glucocorticoids are without effect on the synthesis of the enzyme in fetal rat liver. Work by Girard et al. (*J. Clin. Invest.* 52: 3190, 1973) has established that the molar ratio of insulin to glucagon drops from 10 immediately after birth, to 1 after one hour. This is due to both a rise in glucagon and a fall in insulin concentrations at birth. These studies, together with our work on the synthesis of P-enolpyruvate carboxykinase, indicate that the sharp drop in the concentration of insulin may relieve the normal inhibition of enzyme synthesis. This would allow the initial stimulation of enzyme synthesis by the glucagon-mediated rise in the concentration of cAMP.—HANSON, R. W., L. RESHEF AND J. BALLARD. Hormonal regulation of hepatic P-enolpyruvate carboxykinase (GTP) during development. *Federation Proc.* 34: 166–171, 1975.

[1] From Session VI, *Development and Aging at the Molecular Level*, of the FASEB Conference on *Biology of Development and Aging*, presented at the 58th Annual Meeting of the Federation of American Societies for Experimental Biology, Atlantic City, N.J., April 11, 1974.

[2] This work was supported in part by grants AM-11279, HD-05874, CA-10916 and AM-16009 from the National Institutes of Health.

[3] Recipient of a Career Development Award, K4-AM-15365 from the Public Health Service.

P-enolpyruvate carboxykinase = phosphoenolpyruvate carboxykinase (GTP), (EC 4.1.1.34); cAMP = adenosine-3'-5'-monophosphate; dibutyryl cAMP = N^6,O^2-dibutyryl cAMP.

In the life-span of animals there are periods when metabolic processes are altered in response to stimuli of various types. One of the most dramatic of these periods is at birth when the newborn passes from the fetal environment, which is characterized by a dependence on maternal regulation of substrate supply, to a condition after birth where the availability of important substrates for the various metabolic pathways becomes subject to external, environmental factors. This transition is from a state of consistent metabolite supply to one in which the metabolic machinery must have flexibility to withstand periods of starvation, dietary imbalances, and the like, while still providing for the basic energetic and biosynthetic needs of the total organism. The birth transition may also provide a valuable tool for studies of the hormonal regulation of enzyme concentrations. One hepatic enzyme associated with gluconeogenesis, P-enolpyruvate carboxykinase, appears initially at birth (3). It may be possible to determine experimentally the basic mechanisms that cause the appearance of these enzymes, and to reconstruct the sequential series of events that will lead to the full metabolic capacity of the liver. In this review we will focus on the development of hepatic gluconeogenesis in the rat, with special emphasis on the key enzyme P-enolpyruvate carboxykinase.

DEVELOPMENT OF GLUCONEOGENESIS

The ability to synthesize glucose from precursors such as lactate, alanine and glycerol is absent in the fetal rat liver (4). This process develops immediately after birth and allows the rat to maintain its blood glucose concentration within narrowly defined limits. Yeung and Oliver (30) have reported that the blood glucose levels drop from 71 mg per 100 ml of blood just before delivery to 14 mg by 2 hours. After 5 hours the blood glucose concentration is 60 mg per 100 ml, indicating a rapid correction of these low blood glucose levels. The rise in the concentration of blood glucose is due to the breakdown of the abundant store of liver glycogen and to the initial appearance at this time of hepatic gluconeogenesis (4, 30).

There are two major factors that are known to account for the development of gluconeogenesis in the neonate. Philippidis and Ballard (17) noted that the oxidation–reduction state of the hepatic cytosol, as measured by the NAD/NADH ratio, went from 40 in the fetus to 700 in the newborn. This marked shift toward oxidation is one of the primary events contributing to the net flux of precursor carbon to glucose. A second and equally important factor is the initial appearance of the enzyme P-enolpyruvate carboxykinase. Of all the specific gluconeogenic enzymes, P-enolpyruvate carboxykinase is absent in fetal rat liver, and its activity rises in parallel with the capacity of the neonatal liver to synthesize glucose (Fig. 1). The premature delivery of the animals, as early as 2 days prior to term, will also cause the appearance of P-enolpyruvate carboxykinase (32). The initial development of the enzyme is, therefore, clearly linked to the birth process. The questions that are immediately posed from these studies are what factors regulate the initial development of P-enolpyruvate carboxykinase and how are these processes triggered at birth?

DEVELOPMENT OF HEPATIC P-ENOLPYRUVATE CARBOXYKINASE

A number of hormones are known to alter the activity of P-enolpyruvate carboxykinase in *adult* liver. Lardy and his colleagues (7, 16, 20) were the first to demonstrate clearly the complexity of the hormonal interactions regulating the steady-state levels of the enzyme. Glucagon (30), norepinephrine (22), epinephrine (20, 30), thyroxine (15) and cAMP (31) all increase the activity of the enzyme, whereas insulin (25) de-

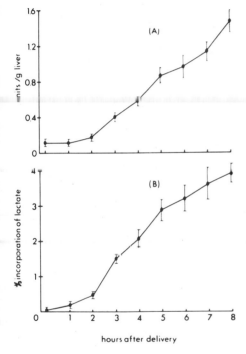

Figure 1. The time course of the development of P-enolpyruvate carboxykinase and gluconeogenesis from lactate in rat liver at birth. *A)* Fetal rats (21 days gestation) were delivered and the activity of P-enolpyruvate carboxykinase measured as outlined in ref 3. *B)* The incorporation of lactate was measured by the injection of 1 μCi of [3-^{14}C] lactate intraperitoneally into newborn rats. The radioactivity incorporated into glycogen and blood glucose was determined after 15 min by procedures given in detail in ref 1. Values, ± SEM, are expressed as a percentage of the injected dose of lactate.

TABLE 1. Lack of effect of glucocorticoids on the activity of fetal rat liver P-enolpyruvate carboxykinase

Treatment			Enzyme activity, mU/g liver
Control (0.9% NaCl)			35
Dibutyryl cAMP	0.2	μmole	751
Dibytyryl cAMP + triamcinolone	0.2 2	μmole mg	615
Triamcinolone	1 2 5	mg mg mg	65 31 46
Hydrocortisone	0.5 1 2	mg mg mg	15 15 17

Fetal rats, 21 days gestation, were injected in utero with the compounds listed. After 6 hours the animals were delivered and the activity of the enzyme measured in liver cytosol (100,000 × g, 30 min) as reported previously (3). One unit of activity is the amount of enzyme that catalyzes the fixation of one μmole of $^{14}CO_2$ per min at 37 C.

creases its activity. The glucocorticoids administered in vivo have a more complicated action since they have been reported to both increase hepatic P-enolpyruvate carboxykinase (7) and decrease the activity of the enzyme in the livers of adrenalectomized rats (21).

In studies with fetal rats, Yeung and Oliver (30) noted that the injection of epinephrine, norepinephrine, glucagon, or dibutyryl cAMP all induced hepatic P-enolpyruvate carboxykinase in utero. The induction of the enzyme caused by premature delivery could also be blocked by the administration, in utero, of glucose, galactose and fructose (30) or by the injection of insulin (31). Triamcinolone or hydrocortisone (32) were ineffective in inducing the enzyme in fetal rat liver (Table 1). Thus, dibutyryl cAMP or hormones capable of increasing the intracellular concentration of cAMP all induce the premature appearance of P-enolpyruvate carboxykinase in the livers of fetal rats; and insulin or compounds that cause insulin secretion can block the development of the enzyme.

The mechanisms by which these hormones act to alter the activity of hepatic P-enolpyruvate carboxykinase have been investigated. Two general approaches to this aspect of the problem have been used. The first of these employs inhibitors of specific steps in the synthesis of enzyme protein. Actinomycin D, which blocks DNA-dependent RNA synthesis, was shown to inhibit the induction of P-enolpyruvate carboxykinase at birth when injected into the fetal animals in utero. Inhibitors such as cycloheximide and puromycin, which act at the translational level, also prevent the appearance of enzyme activity (30). These studies provide suggestive evidence that the birth process stimulates de novo synthesis of hepatic P-enolpyruvate carboxykinase. Since the action of inhibitors is seldom specific to a single site of action, it is necessary to use a second approach, a direct measurement of enzyme synthesis and degradation, to determine the mechanisms responsible for the rapid development of the enzyme.

METHODS FOR THE STUDY OF ENZYME TURNOVER

The methods used in studies of enzyme synthesis and degradation were introduced by Schimke and his associates (23, 24) and by Kenney (13, 14). They involve the isolation of the enzyme being studied from a cytosol fraction of a specific tissue by immunoprecipitation with an antibody prepared against the enzyme. This technique allows the pulse labeling of the enzyme with an amino acid (leucine is the most widely used) and quantitation by measuring the radioactivity in the immunoprecipitate. Usually the radioactivity in the enzyme is expressed as a percentage of that in cytosol protein isolated from the same tissue, to give a relative rate of synthesis of the enzyme. This procedure affords great specificity, but the antibody to be used must be carefully evaluated to avoid nonspecific cross-reactions with other proteins. Until recently, it was customary to test the specificity of the antibody by analysis of Ouchterlony double-diffusion patterns, and most studies published using these techniques include a photograph of an Ouchterlony pattern. Recently, Silpananta and Goodridge (26) suggested the use of sodium dodecyl sulfate–polyacrylamide gel electrophoresis as an additional method to assess the specificity of the antibody. This procedure is now widely used, since its high degree of resolution allows an accurate measurement of the radioactive proteins in an immunoprecipitate. An antigen–antibody precipitate of P-enolpyruvate carboxykinase isolated from liver cytosol of a rat injected with [³H]leucine and subjected to electrophoresis is shown in Fig. 2. The absorbancy at 280 mμ indicates the presence of three major protein peaks. The protein in fractions 16–20 is the heavy chain of the antibody, while fractions 30–34 contain the light chain. P-enolpyruvate carboxykinase with a molecular weight of 73,000 (2) is in fractions 12–14 and is the only protein labeled. A second precipitation ($AgAb_2$) is carried out using the supernatant from the first precipitation, but with purified P-enolpyruvate carboxykinase added. Negligible levels of radioactivity were found after electrophoresis. From experiments of this type we have concluded that our antibody against rat liver cytosol P-enolpyruvate carboxykinase is specific for that enzyme and can be used to determine accurately the synthesis rate of the enzyme in vivo. Complete details of the purification of the enzyme (2) and the preparation and specificity of the antibody have been published (12, 19).

In the experiments presented in

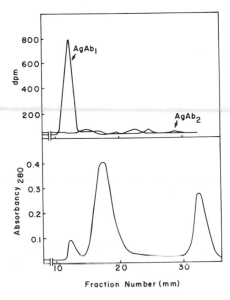

Figure 2. The separation of radioactive P-enolpyruvate carboxykinase from rat liver cytosol after the separation with antibody. Adult rats were injected with 100 μCi [³H] leucine and after 40 min the livers were removed and homogenized. The enzyme in the cytosol (100,000 × g, 30 min) was precipitated with specific goat antibody by the methods outlined in ref 12. The antigen–antibody precipitate was then dissociated by heating in 2% SDS, 2% dithiothreitol in 0.01 M phosphate buffer, pH 7.0. Electrophoresis was for 16 hours. Complete details of the preparation of the gels are provided in ref 12. After electrophoresis the gels were scanned at 280 mμ, then extruded in 1 mm sections for the determination of radioactivity. A second antigen–antibody precipitate was also included (AgAb₂).

this review, the fetal rats in utero were injected intraperitoneally with [4,5-³H]L-leucine (30–40 Ci/mmole) and killed after 40 min. The liver was removed, homogenized in 4 volumes of 0.25 M sucrose, and a 100,000 × g (30 min) cytosol fraction prepared. For studies of enzyme degradation, nonradioactive leucine (5 μmole/fetal rat) was injected after 40 min and the labeling in the enzyme determined at the appropriate time using the antibody technique (see refs 10, 12, 19 for detailed procedures).

HORMONAL CONTROL OF P-ENOLPYRUVATE CARBOXYKINASE DEVELOPMENT

Glucagon and dibutyryl cAMP

At birth the synthesis of the enzyme increases from negligible levels to a rate of 2.4% of the cytosol proteins (Fig. 3). This increase was not due to the activation of a preexisting apoenzyme since we could demonstrate no reactivity with our antibody prior to delivery (19). This agrees with the studies of Yeung and Oliver (30) with actinomycin D and clearly indicates that de novo enzyme synthesis accounts for the rapid increase of the enzyme at birth. Degradation of hepatic P-enolpyruvate carboxykinase could not be demonstrated over the first 36 hours. After this time enzyme degradation began, with an average half-time of 12 hours.

To study further the hormonal regulators responsible for this increase in hepatic P-enolpyruvate carboxykinase synthesis, it is convenient to use fetal rats in utero. If either glucagon or dibutyryl cAMP is administered, the activity of the enzyme increases rapidly, with a peak at about 6 hours. By 25 hours the activity has returned to normal low levels

(Fig. 4). This increased activity is due to a stimulation of the rate of enzyme synthesis by cAMP (Fig. 5), which occurs in the absence of any measurable degradation over the first 9 hours after the administration of dibutyryl cAMP. It thus seems established that the capacity for enzyme degradation exists in the fetal rat liver, but the enzyme protein is not degraded during the period of initial protein synthesis.

Philippidis and Ballard (18) demonstrated that the injection of glu-

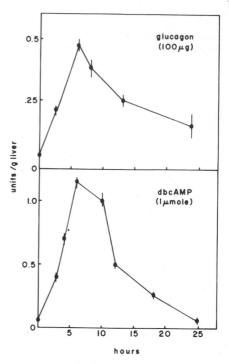

Figure 4. The effect of glucagon and dibutyryl cAMP on the activity of hepatic P-enolpyruvate carboxykinase in fetal rats in utero. Fetal rats, 21 days in utero, were injected with glucagon or dibutyryl cAMP at the concentrations indicated in the figure. The enzyme was assayed at the times shown. (See ref 10 for details).

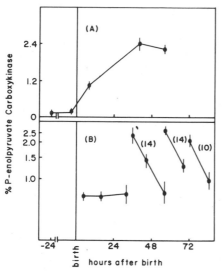

Figure 3. The rate of synthesis and degradation of hepatic P-enolpyruvate carboxykinase in the neonatal rat. *A)* The rate of synthesis in the liver of rats 21 days in utero and after delivery was measured using the antibody procedures outlined in Fig. 2. The rate of enzyme synthesis was expressed as a percentage of the synthesis rate of cytosol proteins. *B)* Enzyme degradation was measured by injecting 3 μCi of [¹⁴C] leucine into fetal or newborn rats, followed by an injection of nonradioactive leucine (6 μmoles/rat) and the animals were killed at the times indicated in the figure. The isolation of the enzyme using the antibody was given in detail in refs 10, 12, 19.

cagon into 21-day fetal rats in utero increased the activity of P-enolpyruvate carboxykinase. Subsequently, it was noted (10) that either glucagon or dibutyryl cAMP can induce the synthesis of this enzyme as early as 15 days in utero (0.9 g body weight). The pattern of induction of P-enolpyruvate carboxykinase, therefore, differs from tyrosine aminotransferase since the former enzyme can be stimulated by both glucagon and cAMP at a relatively early stage of development whereas tyrosine aminotransferase cannot be induced

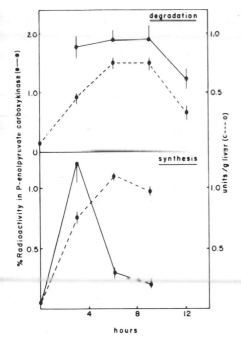

Figure 5. The synthesis and degradation of hepatic P-enolpyruvate carboxykinase in fetal rats injected with dibutyryl cAMP in utero. Fetal rats, 21 days gestation, were injected in utero with 1 μmole of dibutyryl cAMP and the rates of synthesis and degradation measured as outlined in Fig. 3. The animals were not delivered but remained in utero during the 12-hour experimental period. For details see ref 10.

by glucagon before day 20 of gestation (9). A number of reports (5, 6, 11) have established the presence of adenylate cyclase in the livers of fetal rats 4 days before birth. However, Butcher and Potter (6) noted that glucagon did not increase the hepatic levels of cAMP to the extent expected on the basis of the response of adenylate cyclase to hormone administration. This result was not due to an elevation in phosphodiesterase activity, since the rate of cAMP breakdown remains unchanged dur-

ing the 4-day period immediately before birth (6). An alternative explanation may be a lower glucagon affinity for, or a lower content of, hormone receptor protein in fetal rat liver. This point, as well as the developmental pattern of adenylate cyclase prior to 4 days before birth, remains to be clearly established.

Insulin

Insulin is known to prevent the initial appearance of hepatic P-enolpyruvate carboxykinase if injected into rats prior to delivery (31). This hormone will also partially inhibit the increase in enzyme activity if injected together with dibutyryl cAMP into fetal rats in utero (Fig. 6). Tilghman et al. (28) reported that insulin will decrease the rate of P-enolpyruvate carboxykinase synthesis in the liver of diabetic adult rats. This decrease, termed "deinduction," was rapid, having a half-time of about 40 min. It was suggested that the mRNA for P-enolpyruvate carboxykinase was turning over at a rapid rate due to a mechanism as yet poorly understood (28).

In order to simplify the number of possible interactions of insulin on the liver cell, we have measured its effect on P-enolpyruvate carboxykinase in the Reuber H-35 hepatoma cell in culture. In these studies we have demonstrated that insulin in the absence of glucose will block the induction of the enzyme normally caused by dibutyryl cAMP and will decrease the rate of enzyme synthesis in cell cultures already stimulated by dibutyryl cAMP (Gunn, Tilghman and Hanson, unpublished results). It is thus established that insulin can act directly on the liver cell to decrease the rate of enzyme synthesis and it is probable that this effect explains the observation of Yeung and Oliver (31) that insulin or compounds that cause insulin secretion will block the induction of P-enolpyruvate carboxykinase.

Glucocorticoids

The glucocorticoids are the other group of hormones that have been reported to increase the activity of hepatic P-enolpyruvate carboxykinase (29). However, triamcinolone, at concentrations capable of inducing tyrosine aminotransferase, had no effect on P-enolpyruvate carboxykinase in fetal rat liver. This is illustrated

in Table 1, in which the effects of both triamcinolone and hydrocortisone at a variety of concentrations are reported. The fetal rats were 21 days in utero and were capable of responding to administered dibutyryl cAMP but not to the glucocorticoids. These same compounds will stimulate the activity by increasing the synthesis rate of the enzyme in Reuber H-35 cells (28). The reason for the difference between cultured liver cells and the fetal liver with respect to P-enolpyruvate carboxykinase induction by glucocorticoids is not known.

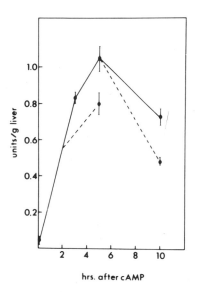

Figure 6. The effect of insulin on the induction in utero of rat liver P-enolpyruvate carboxykinase by dibutyryl cAMP. Fetal rats, 21 days gestation, were injected in utero with 1 μmole of dibutyryl cAMP followed by 0.5 units of insulin in 0.1 ml of 0.9% NaCl. Some animals (solid lines) were injected only with dibutyryl cAMP. Insulin was injected at 2 hours and the animals delivered 3 hours later, or at 6 hours and the animals delivered 5 hours later. The dashed lines represent the activity of P-enolpyruvate carboxykinase in insulin-treated animals and the values are the mean ± SEM for five litters.

MECHANISMS THAT REGULATE P-ENOLPYRUVATE CARBOXYKINASE SYNTHESIS

The fetal rat liver can act as an excellent model for studies of the mechanisms that regulate the synthesis of P-enolpyruvate carboxykinase. Since the enzyme is absent before birth, processes such as the transcription of DNA, mRNA processing and translation of specific template for P-enolpyruvate carboxykinase probably occur at birth. Such a condition would be useful in determining the mechanism by which various hormones act on enzyme synthesis. We have demonstrated that the synthesis of P-enolpyruvate carboxykinase in the fetal rat liver can be blocked by the administration of a transcriptional inhibitor, actinomycin D (10). This compound will also block the premature synthesis of the enzyme by dibutyryl cAMP injected in utero. These findings suggest that cAMP stimulates the formation of mRNA for enzyme synthesis. Wicks and McKibbin (29), using Reuber H-35 cells in culture, have suggested that dibutyryl cAMP is acting at the translational level, since actinomycin D did not prevent the induction of the enzyme by dibutyryl cAMP. Since inhibitors have variable

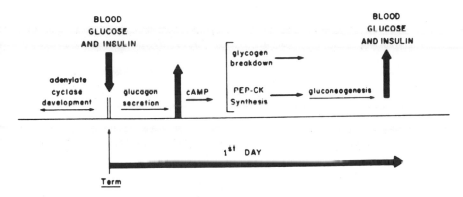

Figure 7. Factors that regulate the levels of hepatic gluconeogenesis in the neonatal rat.

effects and are dependent on many factors, such as time of exposure and concentration, they offer an equivocal basis for a complete understanding of the possible site of hormone action. In fetal liver, however, P-enolpyruvate carboxykinase is absent and its synthesis is stimulated by dibutyryl cAMP. It is difficult to understand how cAMP can act by increasing the translation rate of existing mRNA under conditions where the enzyme is absent in the liver since this would require mRNA for the enzyme to be present but not translated prior to birth. Alternatively some other hormone, either alone or in combination with cAMP, might be responsible for enzyme synthesis at birth. However, such a possibility should be tested directly by the isolation and translation in vitro of P-enolpyruvate carboxykinase mRNA.

PHYSIOLOGICAL ASPECTS OF THE REGULATION OF P-ENOLPYRUVATE CARBOXYKINASE AT BIRTH

On the basis of the information available it is possible to construct a model to explain the hormonal regulation of hepatic P-enolpyruvate carboxykinase in rat liver at birth. The two major regulatory factors are cAMP, increased in concentration within the liver cell by glucagon; and insulin. The concentration of glucagon in fetal rat serum (21 days gestation) is 270 pg per ml as compared to 560 in the mother (8). Insulin concentrations, on the other hand, are 8.0 ng per ml in the fetus and only 0.92 in the mother. At birth the concentration of glucagon rises about threefold whereas the levels of insulin drop to about 1 ng per ml within 2 hours after delivery. The molar ratio of insulin to glucagon therefore changes from about 10 in the fetus just before delivery, to approximately 1 in the newborn. These important observations come from the work of Girard et al. (8) and, when considered together with our data on the effects of both insulin and glucagon on the synthesis of hepatic P-enolpyruvate carboxykinase, provide an insight into the hormonal regulation of the enzyme.

Since the concentration of glucagon in the fetus is relatively high (30% of the newborn) and the levels of cAMP are also close to those observed in the animals immediately after birth, it would appear that some enzyme should be synthesized in the fetal rat liver. The reason that there are negligible levels of P-enolpyruvate carboxykinase in fetal rat liver is probably due to the depressive effect of the high concentration of insulin in the fetus. The drop in blood glucose associated with birth triggers the increase in glucagon and therefore cAMP and causes a sharp decline in the concentration of insulin. This fall in insulin releases the inhibition of P-enolpyruvate carboxykinase synthesis, with a resultant initiation of enzyme synthesis.

We can construct a sequence of events that, on the basis of the available experimental information, accounts for the initial changes in the regulation of blood glucose noted at birth (Fig. 7). The primary stimulus for this process is the cessation of the maternal blood supply which results in a rapid fall in the concentration of glucose in the blood of neonatal rat (4, 29). Snell and Walker (27) have demonstrated that the rate of glucose utilization is also diminished dramatically at about 2 hours after delivery. However, the limited supply of blood glucose is rapidly depleted and is replenished by glycogenolysis and hepatic gluconeogenesis. The net result of these changes in blood glucose is an immediate drop in the concentration of insulin and a rise in glucagon levels. During the last 7 days of development the activity of adenylate cyclase steadily rises (11) so that the liver is "competent" to respond to hormones such as glucagon that stimulate the synthesis of cAMP. Glycogen breakdown is an important factor in the return of the blood glucose concentration back to normal levels. However, the hormonal maintenance of blood glucose depends on hepatic gluconeogenesis and the initial appearance of P-enolpyruvate carboxykinase at birth completes the gluconeogenesis sequence. The rise in cAMP and decline in insulin are the primary triggers for the initial synthesis of the enzyme, which occurs in the absence of enzyme degradation (19). The resultant of these effects is the return of blood glucose levels to normal. The regulation of hepatic gluconeogenesis and P-enolpyruvate carboxykinase are then subject to the dietary and hormonal stimuli that determine their appropriate levels.

The authors are indebted to Dr. Sidney Weinhouse for his generous support and encouragement during these studies.

REFERENCES

1. BALLARD, F. J. *Biochem. J.* 121: 196, 1971.
2. BALLARD, F. J., AND R. W. HANSON. *J. Biol. Chem.* 244: 5625, 1969.
3. BALLARD, F. J., AND R. W. HANSON. *Biochem. J.* 104: 866, 1967.
4. BALLARD, F. J., AND I. T. OLIVER. *Biochem. Biophys. Acta* 71: 578, 1963.
5. BAR, H. P., AND P. HAHN. *Can. J. Biochem.* 49: 85, 1971.
6. BUTCHER, F. R., AND V. R. POTTER. *Cancer Res.* 32: 2141, 1972.
7. FOSTER, D. O., H. A. LARDY, P. D. RAY AND J. B. JOHNSTON. *Biochemistry* 6: 2120, 1967.
8. GIRARD, J. R., G. S. CUENDET, E. B. MARLISS, A. KERVRAN, M. RIEUTORT AND R. ASSAN. *J. Clin. Invest.* 52: 3190, 1973.
9. GREENGARD, O. *Science* 163: 891, 1969.
10. HANSON, R. W., L. FISHER, F. J. BALLARD AND L. RESHEF. *Enzyme* 15: 97, 1974.
11. HOMMES, F. A., AND A. BEERE. *Biochim. Biophys. Acta* 237: 296, 1971.
12. HOPGOOD, M. F., F. J. BALLARD, L. RESHEF AND R. W. HANSON. *Biochem. J.* 134: 445, 1973.
13. KENNEY, F. T. *J. Biol. Chem.* 237: 3495, 1962.
14. KENNEY, F. T. *J. Biol. Chem.* 242: 4367, 1967.
15. NAGAI, K., AND H. NAKAGAWA. *J. Biochem., Tokyo* 71: 125, 1972.
16. NORDLIE, R. C., AND H. A. LARDY. *Biochem. Z.* 338: 356, 1963.
17. PHILIPPIDIS, H., AND F. J. BALLARD. *Biochem. J.* 113: 651, 1969.
18. PHILIPPIDIS, H. A., AND F. J. BALLARD. *Biochem. J.* 120: 385, 1970.
19. PHILIPPIDIS, H., R. W. HANSON, L. RESHEF, M. HOPGOOD AND F. J. BALLARD. *Biochem. J.* 126: 1127, 1972.

20. RAY, P. D., D. O. FOSTER AND H. A. LARDY. *J. Biol. Chem.* 241: 3904, 1966.

21. RESHEF, L., F. J. BALLARD AND R. W. HANSON. *J. Biol. Chem.* 244: 5577, 1969.

22. RESHEF, L., AND R. W. HANSON. *Biochem. J.* 127: 809, 1972.

23. SCHIMKE, R. T. *J. Biol. Chem.* 239: 3808, 1964.

24. SCHIMKE, R. T., E. W. SWEENY AND C. M. BERLIN. *J. Biol. Chem.* 240: 322, 1965.

25. SHRAGO, E., J. W. YOUNG AND H. A. LARDY. *Science* 158: 1527, 1967.

26. SILPANANTA, P., AND A. G. GOODRIDGE. *J. Biol. Chem.* 246: 5754, 1971.

27. SNELL, K., AND W. WALKER. *Biochem. J.* 132: 739, 1973.

28. TILGHMAN, S. M., R. W. HANSON, L. RESHEF, M. F. HOPGOOD AND F. J. BALLARD. *Proc. Natl. Acad. Sci. U.S.* 71: 1304, 1974.

29. WICKS, W. D., AND J. B. McKIBBIN. *Biochem. Biophys. Res. Commun.* 48: 205, 1972.

30. YEUNG, D., AND I. T. OLIVER. *Biochem. J.* 108: 325, 1968.

31. YEUNG, D., AND I. T. OLIVER. *Biochemistry* 7: 3231, 1968.

32. YEUNG, D., R. S. STANLEY AND I. T. OLIVER. *Biochem. J.* 105: 1219, 1967.

Pre- and postnatal enzyme capacity for drug metabolite production[1]

JAMES R. GILLETTE AND BITTEN STRIPP

Laboratory of Chemical Pharmacology
National Heart and Lung Institute
National Institutes of Health
Bethesda, Maryland 20014

ABSTRACT

Most lipid-soluble foreign compounds including drugs, insecticides and many environmental pollutants are metabolized in animals by cytochrome P-450 enzymes in the endoplasmic reticulum of liver. These enzymes are virtually absent in fetuses of laboratory animals, but their activities increase to adult levels within 3–8 weeks after birth. In human fetuses, the enzymes appear during the first half of pregnancy, and their activities during gestation reach about one third of those found in adults. The species differences in fetal activities apparently parallel the differences in the development of liver endoplasmic reticulum. In laboratory animals, the rough-surfaced reticulum does not develop until 4 days before birth and the smooth-surfaced reticulum develops only after birth. In man, however, the rough-surfaced form appears at about 7 to 9 weeks of gestation, whereas the smooth-surfaced form appears at about the 3rd month of pregnancy. Despite the early development of these enzymes in humans, they probably play only a minor role in limiting the accumulation of most foreign compounds in human fetuses. Nevertheless, they may play an important role in drug-induced toxicities, particularly those that are mediated through the formation of chemically reactive metabolites—GILLETTE, J. R. AND B. STRIPP. Pre- and postnatal enzyme capacity for drug metabolite production. *Federation Proc.* 34: 172–178, 1975.

Although some drugs are eliminated from the body largely unchanged, most are converted to a wide variety of metabolites before they are excreted into urine, bile or the breath. Those drugs that have been designed to resemble normal body substances are usually metabolized by the same enzymes that metabolize the substances they are de-

[1] From Session VI, *Development and Aging at the Molecular Level*, of the FASEB Conference on *Biology of Development and Aging*, presented at the 58th Annual Meeting of the Federation of American Societies for Experimental Biology, Atlantic City, N.J., April 11, 1974.

signed to mimic. But most drugs have no endogenous counterpart and thus are metabolized by nonspecific enzymes.

Several years ago, Williams (78) pointed out that the reactions by which most drugs are metabolized could be classified according to two phases. Phase I includes those reactions that either convert one functional group into another (as in the oxidation of alcohol to acetaldehyde and acetic acid), or introduce polar groups into nonpolar compounds (as in the hydroxylation of aromatic compounds, the reduction of nitro compounds and the hydrolysis of esters). Phase II includes those reactions that conjugate polar groups with glucuronate, sulfate, glycine, glutamine, glutathione, or methyl groups.

Most of the oxidative Phase I reactions occur in liver endoplasmic reticulum and are catalyzed by mixed-function oxidases consisting of NADPH-cytochrome c reductase and carbon monoxide sensitive hemoproteins, collectively called cytochrome P-450 (21). The reactions catalyzed by these cytochrome P-450-dependent mixed-function oxidases include such diverse reactions as the hydroxylation of unsaturated and saturated hydrocarbon groups, the oxidative dealkylation of tertiary and secondary amines, the oxidative cleavage of alkyl-aryl ethers, the sulfoxidation of thio ethers, the epoxidation of unsaturated hydrocarbon groups, and the N-hydroxylation of aryl amines and acetylated aryl amines. Indeed, the versatility of these enzymes is unique in the field of biochemistry.

In the current view of the mechanisms of these enzymes, equivalent amounts of drug, oxygen and NADPH are utilized during the oxidative reaction. The drug substrates combine with the oxidized form of cytochrome P-450 to form complexes that are reduced by an electron from NADPH cytochrome c reductase. Until recently, it was generally accepted that the reduced cytochrome P-450 substrate complexes then reacted with oxygen to form oxygenated complexes that then accept a second electron to form "activated oxygen" complexes (21, 25). But the evidence now suggests that in mammalian systems the reduced cytochrome P-450 substrate complexes can accept the second electron before they react with oxygen (3). The source of the second electron has also been debated in the past (4). But it now appears that it can originate either from NADPH by way of NADPH cytochrome c reductase or from NADH by way of NADH cytochrome b_5 reductase and cytochrome b_5, which are also present in liver microsomes (6). However the "activated oxygen" cytochrome P-450–substrate complexes may be formed, they rearrange to form oxidized cytochrome P-450 and oxidized products.

Various substrates and inhibitors combine with the oxidized form of cytochrome P-450 and thereby cause small but significant changes in its absorbance spectrum (25, 59, 68). Some substances, such as hexobarbital, aminopyrine and ethylmorphine, cause a decrease in the spectrum at about 417 nm and an increase at about 391 nm; such substances are called Type I compounds. Other substances, such as nicotinamide and aniline, cause a decrease in the spectrum at about 418 nm and an increase at about 423 nm and are called Type II compounds. Still other substances cause both kinds of spectral changes and some cause an intensification of the maximum at about 417 nm. Because of the complexities of these spectral changes and because several endogenous substances including steroids and fatty acids can also alter the absorbance spectrum of cytochrome P-450, the interpretation of the apparent affinity constants and maximal values for the spectral changes is frequently difficult, if not impossible. Nevertheless, it is usually found that Type I compounds are metabolized more rapidly than Type II compounds because the oxidized cytochrome P 450 complexes with Type I compounds are reduced by NADPH more rapidly than are those with Type II compounds (20).

The cytochrome P-450 enzyme systems can be inhibited in several different ways (28). For example, various substances can combine reversibly with the oxidized form of cytochrome P-450 and thereby competitively inhibit the metabolism of a given substrate (45). Other substances, such as piperonyl butoxide, are converted to a metabolite that combines with cytochrome P-450 in a way that prevents the conversion of reduced cytochrome P-450 to its oxygenated form (18). In addition, some electron acceptors, such as cytochrome c and menadione, can inhibit the metabolism of drugs by competing with cytochrome P-450 for the electrons from NADPH cytochrome c reductase (21, 25, 28). In fact, there is evidence that cytochrome b_5-mediated reactions in liver microsomes may also inhibit drug metabolism by channeling the electrons of NADPH cytochrome c reductase away from cytochrome P-450 (9, 76). In accord with this view the rate of drug metabolism may sometimes be greater in the presence of both NADH and NADPH than the sum of the rates in the presence of NADH or NADPH alone. The activities of the cytochrome P-450 enzymes may also be impaired by the prior administration of large doses of certain cations such as Co^{2+} which inhibit ferrochelatase and thereby lead to a decrease in the synthesis of cytochrome P-450 heme (73) or by the prior administration of carbon tetrachloride (5, 70) or certain allylic compounds (11, 42) which lead to the destruction of cytochrome P-450.

Repetitive administration of a wide variety of substances can accelerate drug metabolism by increasing the activity of cytochrome P 450 systems in liver (6, 7). Indeed, more than 200 substances, including barbiturates, polycyclic hydrocarbons, steroids, polychlorinated insecticides, and even the aromatic oils found in wood chips used in animal bedding, enhance the metabolism of drugs by the cytochrome P-450 systems. These substances, however, increase the activity of the enzyme systems in different ways. Pretreatment of animals with phenobarbital causes increases in the amounts of both cytochrome P-450 and NADPH cytochrome c reductase, whereas pretreatment of rats with spironolactone causes very little change in the amount of cytochrome P-450 but increases the activity of NADPH cytochrome c reductase (25). By contrast, pretreatment of animals with 3-methylcholanthrene results in the formation of a variant of cytochrome P-450, called cytochrome P-448, but has little or no effect on the activity of NADPH cytochrome c reductase (25). Not only does the absorbance spectrum of the carbon monoxide complex of this variant differ from that of the normal kind of cytochrome P-450, but the substrate specificity of the variant differs markedly from that of the normal form. Thus, pretreatment of animals with 3-methylcholanthrene results in marked increases in the metabolism of substances, such as the hydroxylation of 3,4-benzpyrene, but has little or no effect on others, such as the hydroxylation of hexobarbital and the N-demethylation of ethylmorphine.

PERINATAL DEVELOPMENT OF CYTOCHROME P 450 ENZYME SYSTEMS

Initial studies on the metabolism of drugs by neonates of various animal species, including rat (13), guinea pig (38), rabbit (17), hamster (53), and swine (71), suggested that the cytochrome P-450 enzymes were either barely detectable or absent at birth. Accordingly, the concentration of cytochrome P-450 and the activity of NADPH cytochrome c reductase are considerably lower in neonatal animals than in adults. Moreover, the formation of glucuronides of several drugs by UDPglucuronosyltransferase (ED 2.4.1.17) in hepatic endoplasmic reticulum is also slower in neonatal animals than in adults (34, 35), but the relative rates of glucuronidation are higher than the relative activities of the cytochrome P-450 systems.

Recent studies utilizing sensitive analytical methods have shown presence of cytochrome P-450 in animal fetuses during the last third phase of pregnancy (26, 75). For example, in our studies we have found that hepatic microsomes from rabbit fetuses ranging in age from 2–10 days before birth could oxidize 3,4-benzpyrene, chlorcyclizine, and testosterone (26). Although the rates of oxidation were highly variable, the mean values of the rates were about 1% of those obtained with liver microsomes from their mothers (Table 1). In similar experiments, Kuenzig et al. (40) found that liver microsomes from guinea pig fetuses obtained 10–20 days before term could hydroxylate 3,4-benzpyrene and N-demethylate p-chloro-N-methylaniline at about 1% of the rate of liver microsomes from their mothers. But they also found that the activity of the enzymes catalyzing these reactions were increased about five fold

TABLE 1. In vitro metabolic activity in fetal and maternal liver of rabbits[a] during the last third phase of pregnancy[b]

Substrate	Rate of metabolism, picomol/mg microsomal protein per hour	
	fetal	maternal
3,4-Benzpyrene	168–174	10,000–12,000
^{14}C-Testosterone	1,200–7,800	264,000–330,000
^{14}C-Chlorcyclizine	1,200	77,000
^{14}C-Nitrofurazone	2,100–10,000	3,000–5,820

[a] Livers from fetuses in one pregnant rabbit were pooled: values represent the range obtained from 1–3 separate experiments. [b] B. Stripp, R. Menard and J. Gillette, unpublished results.

during the last 10 days of pregnancy.

Because the activities of the cytochrome P-450 enzyme systems in laboratory animals are low, it was assumed for many years that human fetuses would also metabolize drugs very slowly. However, liver microsomes from human fetuses are not only able to metabolize such substrates as testosterone (12, 43), laurate (79), desmethylimipramine (64), ethylmorphine (60), aniline (60), aminopyrine (79), chlorpromazine (58), hexobarbital (58) and p-nitroanisole (60) but the rates of metabolism per gram of liver of many of these substrates are about 30–50% of those of human adults (56). Moreover, it is generally accepted that the liver represents about 4–5% of the fetal weight but only about 2% of the adult weight; thus the activities of these enzymes per body weight of the fetus may approach those of human adults. By contrast, however, the activity of 3,4-benzpyrene hydroxylase in liver microsomes from human fetuses is only about 2.5% of that from adults, a value which is similar to that found with other animal species (56).

Since cytochrome P-450 enzymes are also present in several extra-hepatic tissues of adult animals, it seemed possible that these enzymes might play an important role in the metabolism of drugs in fetuses. However, neither cytochrome P-450 nor the O-demethylation of p-nitroanisole have been detected in lung, kidney and intestinal mucosa from fetal swine (72). By contrast, in human fetal tissues, the oxidation of chlorpromazine, and the reduction of p-nitrobenzoic acid, occurred in kidney and small intestine (57) and the N-demethylation of N-methylaniline in small intestine, kidney and adrenals (54). Moreover, the hydroxylation of 3,4-benzpyrene occurs more rapidly in human fetal adrenal than in liver (39). Since fetal adrenal plays an important role in steroidogenesis during pregnancy (74) it seems possible that adrenal tissue may possess unique oxidative metabolic activity during fetal life.

It is noteworthy that noncytochrome P-450-dependent enzymes that catalyze the hydrolysis of procaine are about equally active in lung, liver, kidney and intestinal mucosa from fetal swine and that the activities are between 25 and 100% of those found in the tissues in adult swine (72). Similarly, the 9,000 × g supernatant of fetal liver from rabbits reduces nitrofurazone about as rapidly as do livers from adults (Table 1).

After parturition the rates of drug metabolism by liver cytochrome P-450 systems increase until they reach adult levels within 3–8 weeks. However, the sequence of development depends not only on the animal species but also on the substrate and the pathway of metabolism. For example, in rabbits the rates of metabolism of aminopyrine, benzphetamine and 3,4-benzpyrene reach about 10–25% of the adult levels by the end of the first week after birth and approach adult levels within a month (16). Similarly, the activity of p-nitroanisole in swine is about one-half the adult level at about 1 week after birth and attains adult levels at about 2 weeks of age (72). In guinea pigs, however, the metabolism of 3,4-benzpyrene, p-chloro-N-methyl aniline and chlorcyclazine reaches a maximum between 3–5 days after birth and then declines to adult levels (Kuenig, personal communication). In male rats, ethylmorphine N-demethylation remains low during the first 2 weeks after birth and then increases markedly between 3 and 4 weeks as the sex difference in drug metabolism that occurs in this animal species becomes manifested (30). By contrast, the hydroxylation of aniline, which occurs at about equal rates in male and female rats, reaches a maximum within the first 2 weeks and then declines to adult levels (30). The relative rates of development of the various enzymes that catalyze the metabolism of testosterone in male rats are especially noteworthy: $16\text{-}\alpha\text{-}$hydroxylation of this steroid remains low during the first 28 days and then increases rapidly, thereafter. Its 6β-hydroxylation increases rapidly during the first week, remains relatively constant until the 49th day and then increases thereafter. By contrast, 7α-hydroxylation reaches a maximum between 7 and 28 days and then declines (8).

In all animal species both the NADPH cytochrome c reductase and the cytochrome P-450 levels increase during the first few weeks after birth. However, the NADPH cytochrome c reductase usually, but not always, develops more rapidly than does the cytochrome P-450 (10, 16, 44). Various attempts have been made to relate changes in the rates of metabolism of various substrates with changes in either the activity of NADPH cytochrome reductase, the rate of cytochrome P-450 reduction, or the concentration of cytochrome P-450. Although some studies have revealed that the rates of drug oxidation are closely related to one or another of these components, most have shown no consistent relationship with any of them (10, 16, 30, 40, 44).

RELATIONSHIPS BETWEEN ENZYME ACTIVITY AND CELLULAR ULTRASTRUCTURE

Since the cytochrome P-450 systems are localized preferentially, although not exclusively, in smooth-surfaced endoplasmic reticulum (15, 22, 31) it is perhaps not surprising that these systems appear in fetuses when the rough-surfaced endoplasmic reticulum develops and that they increase in activity when the smooth-surfaced reticulum develops. In rats, about half of the cells in fetal liver are hemopoietic cells in various forms of development and the other half are small irregularly shaped hepatocytes at 3 to 4 days before birth. The proportion of hemopoietic cells then gradually decreases, and the hepatocytes increase in size until birth. Before parturition, however, the endoplasmic reticulum is almost exclusively the rough-surfaced form. Only after birth does the smooth endoplasmic reticulum begin to develop rapidly. But the process is asynchronous; at any given time, the hepatocytes are in various stages of proliferation of the smooth-surfaced form of the endoplasmic reticulum (41). In man, however, the endoplasmic reticulum appears at a considerably earlier stage of fetal development (80). Even at 7–9 week stage, the endoplasmic reticulum is comprised of short tubules studded with ribosomes. This pattern is markedly changed by the 3rd month at which time the rough-surfaced endoplasmic reticulum becomes organized into parallel cisternae. By contrast, the smooth-surfaced endoplasmic reticulum is absent at 7–9 weeks of age. But in the 3rd month the smooth-surfaced endoplasmic reticulum is considerably developed and extends profusely into the cytoplasm in the form of irregular vesicles.

Many inducers of cytochrome P-450 enzymes not only alter the concentration of cytochrome P-450 in the endoplasmic reticulum, but also promote a proliferation of the smooth-surfaced endoplasmic reticulum (6). The fact that these inducers do not evoke their effects in rabbits prior to 4 days before birth, but can act in neonatal rats (33), raises the possibility that induction either requires the presence of a well-developed endoplasmic reticulum or is modified by the factors that control the normal development of the endoplasmic reticulum. Indeed, if there is a relationship between the normal development of the endoplasmic reticulum and the ability of inducers to increase the activity of cytochrome P-450 enzymes, the inducers may be able to affect the rate of drug metabolism in human fetuses during the last two trimesters even if they do not induce the cytochrome P-450 enzymes in laboratory animals until just prior to birth. In accord with this view, human fetal livers from mothers given phenobarbital tend to metabolize a variety of drugs more rapidly than those from untreated mothers (55).

THEORETICAL ASPECTS OF THE ROLE OF DRUG METABOLISM BY FETAL TISSUES

The finding that liver microsomal enzymes that catalyze the metabolism of drugs develop relatively early in human fetuses has raised the possibility that these enzymes may play an important role in limiting the exposure of human fetuses to foreign compounds. However, until an animal model is found that mimics the development of the human fetal enzymes, it seems unlikely that this possibility can be evaluated experimentally. It may be useful, therefore, to consider various hypothetical situations in order to gain an insight into the relative roles that fetal and maternal enzyme systems play in limiting the exposure of the fetus to various kinds of drugs.

Drugs can cross the placental barrier by a variety of mechanisms, including passive diffusion, pinocytosis, membrane discontinuities, and in some cases by facilitative and active transport systems. For most drugs, however, passive diffusion is the most important of these mechanisms. Indeed, numerous studies have shown that the rate of transport across the placenta is usually related to the proportion of the drug that exists in the maternal blood plasma in its unionized form and to the lipid solubility of the un-ionized drug. Such studies have shown that the concentration of the unbound form of most drugs in fetal plasma usually equilibrates with that in maternal blood very rapidly. Even with compounds as polar as penicillin or as large as insulin, equilibrium between maternal and fetal blood is usually achieved within an hour after their administration to mothers (2).

With compounds that cross the placenta rapidly, the only way that the enzymes in fetal liver can affect the amount of drug entering into the systemic circulation of the fetus is to decrease the concentration of the drug in the umbilical vein as it passes through the fetal liver and enters the fetal hepatic vein. In order to achieve this "first-pass effect," the extraction ratio of the fetal liver (that is the clearance of the drug by the fetal liver divided by the umbilical blood flow rate) would have to be high. But how active would the fetal hepatic enzymes have to be in order to cause a "first-pass effect" in human fetuses? As pointed out in a previous section, the activity of the fetal hepatic cytochrome P-450 enzymes per gram of tissue is only about one-third of that of adults and even when differences in the relative weights of the liver to total body weight are taken into account, the activities per kilogram body weight are similar in fetal and adult humans. Moreover, it is estimated that the hepatic blood flow rates per gram of liver are also similar in fetuses and adults. It thus seems probable that only those lipid-soluble drugs that are rapidly cleared in adults would be rapidly cleared by fetuses. Since a "first-pass effect" occurs in adults with relatively few drugs, such as lidocaine (66), propranolol (69) and nortriptyline (1), it seems likely that the fetal hepatic enzymes play only an insignificant role in protecting the fetus against lipid soluble drugs.

When the extraction ratio of a drug by the livers of adults and fetuses is low and the drugs are able to cross the placenta rapidly, the concentration of the drug in fetal tissues will depend on the sum of the clearances by the maternal and fetal liver. However, the weight of the fetal liver even near term is less than 10% of that of the mother. Thus, even when the activity of the enzyme per body weight of the fetus is similar to that of the mother, the metabolism of such drugs by fetal liver would account for less than 10% of total metabolism and would be expected to affect the fetal tissue levels of the drug to only a trivial extent.

It is evident, therefore, that the

fetal hepatic enzymes can significantly alter the concentration of drugs in tissues only with the drugs that slowly cross the placenta. Even in this situation, however, the clearance of the drug by the fetal liver would have to approach or exceed the sum of the clearances by the placenta and the fetal kidney. But with most drugs equilibrium between maternal and fetal blood is usually achieved within an hour and therefore the drug would have to be metabolized quite rapidly by the fetal hepatic enzymes. Indeed, we have calculated from our previously described model (26) that when the activities of the hepatic enzymes per kilogram body weight are identical in the mother and the fetus, the biological half-life of a drug that distributes with the body water and crosses the placenta rapidly enough to achieve equilibrium within an hour would have to be less than about 3 hours if fetal hepatic enzymes are to have any significant effect on the concentrations of the drug in fetal tissues (unpublished results).

Although single doses of anesthetics are given just before birth, most drugs are given to mothers repeatedly in order to maintain their plasma levels at therapeutically effective concentrations for several days or even weeks. Under these conditions, the plasma levels of the drug in both the mother and the fetus will eventually reach steady states even when the drug crosses the placenta very slowly. If the drug were not metabolized by the fetus, the concentration unbound and un-ionized drug in the fetal plasma would reach values between the lowest and the highest steady-state value found in the mother. However, the fetal hepatic enzymes would be somewhat more effective in reducing the fetal plasma level of the drug under steady-state conditions than they would be after the administration of a single dose of the drug

(unpublished calculations from our previously described model (26)) But still the clearance of the drug by fetal liver enzymes would have to approach or exceed its clearance by the placenta if they are to have any significant effect on the tissue levels of the drug (26).

POSSIBLE ROLES OF FETAL ENZYMES IN DRUG TOXICITY

Although fetal liver enzymes play only an insignificant role in limiting the concentrations of most drugs in fetal tissues, it is still possible that they may exert actions through the formation of drug metabolites. For example, it has been suggested that the drug metabolites may be so polar that they would cross the placental barrier very slowly and therefore would be trapped in the fetus. But the finding that substances as polar as penicillin rapidly cross the placenta (2) suggests that entrapment by this mechanism would occur rarely. Instead, we have suggested that the formation of chemically reactive metabolites by the fetal liver enzymes may be more significant (26).

During the past few years, it has become increasingly evident that the cytochrome P-450 enzyme systems in liver of adult animals can convert chemically inactive compounds to potent arylating or alkylating metabolites that in turn combine covalently with tissue macromolecules and thereby cause a variety of toxicities (23, 24, 27). Indeed, our laboratory has found that the liver necrosis caused by bromobenzene (34, 65), chlorobenzene (65), acetaminophen (36, 48, 49, 70) and furosemide (68) is mediated through the formation of reactive metabolites and that the severity and incidence of the necrosis can be altered by various inducers and inhibitors of the cytochrome P-450 enzymes in liver of adult animals.

Since the activities of the cytochrome P-450 enzymes in liver microsomes usually are considerably lower in rodent fetuses than in their mother, it seems unlikely that halobenzenes or acetaminophen would cause liver necrosis as severely as they would in mothers. In support of this view the in vitro covalent binding of bromobenzene to proteins in homogenates of rabbit fetal liver was less than 10% of that in homogenates of their mother's liver (unpublished results). Moreover, little or no liver necrosis occurs in neonatal rats receiving bromobenzene (50).

The formation of hydroxylamine derivatives, however, can occur in the body by the reduction of nitro compounds as well as by the N-hydroxylation of primary aryl amines and their acetylated derivatives. Some nitro compounds, such as p-nitrobenzoate and chloramphenicol, are reduced anaerobically by cytochrome P-450 systems in liver microsomes, but other nitro compounds are reduced by other enzyme systems (22). For example, recent studies in our laboratory (14, 51) have shown that a series of nitrofuran and nitrothiazole derivatives can be reduced by liver microsomal NADPH cytochrome c reductase or by liver and milk xanthine oxidase.

McCalla et al. (46) recently showed

that nitrofurazone, a topical antibacterial agent that causes the formation of tumors in mammary glands of rats (52), becomes covalently bound to liver proteins when incubated with rat liver homogenates. In addition, we have found that glutathione (GSH) in the homogenates inhibited the covalent binding (26). These findings prompted studies showing that nitrofurazone could deplete the GSH in liver of male mice (26). Even at doses as high as 15 mg per mouse (about 750 mg per kg), however, the liver concentrations of GSH were depleted by only 50%. Thus, it seemed possible that the degree of covalent binding of nitrofurazone metabolites might depend on the concentration of GSH in liver.

Since the reduction of nitrofurazone is catalyzed by xanthine oxidase rather than by cytochrome P-450 in liver, it occurred to us that the covalent binding of nitrofurazone metabolites to proteins in fetal liver might be greater than that of bromobenzene. In fact, as shown in Table 2, the magnitude of covalent binding of nitrofurazone metabolites to proteins in liver of fetal mice was similar to that occurring in their mother's liver at doses above 1.0 mg per mouse. We are still uncertain, however, whether all of the reactive metabolite that is bound by fetal liver protein is formed in the fetal liver or whether most of it is formed in the maternal liver, crosses the placenta, and then becomes covalently bound to the fetal liver protein. Whatever the mechanism for the covalent binding might be our studies illustrate how fetal enzymes might participate in causing fetotoxicities by chemically reactive metabolites that do not escape the tissue in which they are formed. The studies also illustrate how chemicals might cause transplacental carcinogenesis even when they are given long before parturition.

TABLE 2. In vivo binding of ^{14}C-(formyl) nitrofurazone to livers from fetal or adult mice 2–3 days from term

Pretreatment	Source of liver	^{14}C-(Formyl) nitrofurazone
None	Maternal	979 ± 143
None	Fetal	1,035 ± 91

Nitrofurazone: 300 mg/kg i.p. 2 hours before sacrifice. Values are the mean ± SE of four animals, given as picomoles ^{14}C-nitrofurazone equivalents bound/mg protein.

Immediately after parturition the newborn of laboratory animals are particularly sensitive to drugs that act directly on physiological action sites until their liver microsomal enzymes develop. However, they are particularly resistant to compounds that exert toxic effects through the formation of active metabolites. For example, the newborn of rats are less sensitive to the toxic effects of bromobenzene (50) than are their mothers.

On the other hand, the finding of relatively high activities of the cytochrome P-450 enzymes in human fetuses suggests that drugs which exert their actions directly on action sites may be less toxic in neonates of humans than in those of laboratory animals. Nevertheless, there is evidence that the oxidation of at least some drugs is less rapid in newborn children. For example, after the intravenous administration of diazepam, premature newborns had higher and longer lasting blood levels of diazepam than did more fully developed children (19).

However, the enzyme that catalyzes the formation of glucuronides, UDP-glucuronosyltransferase, may be even less developed than are the cytochrome P-450 enzymes in newborn humans. Even though the hepatic cytochrome P-450 enzymes appear in human fetuses at a very early period of gestation, the human fetal liver is unable to catalyze the formation of the glucuronides of p-nitrophenol, 1-naphthol or 4-methylumbelliferone (63). Moreover, clinical studies have revealed that the formation of glucuronides in newborn infants is unusually low. For example, after the administration of diazepam, the glucuronide of N-demethyldiazepam has been isolated from urine of older children but not from that of premature or full-term new-

born infants (19). Moreover, the plasma half-lives of bilirubin (29) and sulfobromphthalein (77), which are converted to glucuronides before they are excreted into urine, are significantly longer in babies up to 30 days of age than they are in 4-month- to 14-year-old children.

If the cytochrome P-450 enzymes that catalyze the oxidation of drugs indeed do develop more rapidly than does UDPglucuronosyltransferase in human neonates, drugs which exert their pharmacologic and toxicologic effects through the formation of chemically reactive or pharmacologically active metabolites may exert greater effects in newborn infants than would be predicted from studies of newborn animals. Clearly, more studies are needed to elucidate changes in the relative importance of Phase I and Phase II reactions during the neonatal development of humans.

REFERENCES

1. ALEXANDERSON, B., O. BORGA AND G. ALVAN. *European J. Clin. Pharmacol.* 5: 181, 1973.
2. ASLING, J. AND E. L. WAY. In: *Fundamentals of Drug Metabolism and Drug Distribution*, edited by B. N. LaDu, H. G. Mandel and E. L. Way. Baltimore: Williams & Wilkins, 1971, p. 88.
3. BALLOU, D. P., C. VEEGER, T. A. VAN DER HOEVEN AND M. J. COON. *FEBS Letters* 38: 337, 1974.
4. BARON, J., A. G. HILDEBRANDT, J. A. PETERSON AND R. W. ESTABROOK. *Drug Metab. Disposition* 1: 129, 1973.
5. CASTRO, J. A., H. SASAME AND J. R. GILLETTE. *Life Sci.* 7: 129, 1968.
6. CONNEY, A. H. *Pharmacol. Rev.* 19: 317, 1967.
7. CONNEY, A. H., AND J. J. BURNS. *Science* 178: 576, 1972.
8. CONNEY, A. H., W. LEVIN, M. JACOBSON AND R. KUNTZMAN. *Clin. Pharmacol. Therap.* 14: 727, 1973.
9. CORREIA, A., AND G. J. MANNERING. *Drug. Metab. Disposition* 1: 139, 1973.
10. DALLNER, G., P. SIEKEVITZ AND G. E. PALADE. *J. Cell Biol.* 30: 97, 1966.
11. DE MATTEIS, F. *Drug Metab. Disposition* 1: 267, 1973.

12. DEMISCH, K., U. AMMEDICK AND W. STAIB. *European J. Biochem.* 8: 284, 1969.

13. ELING, T. E., R. D. HARRISON, B. A. BECKER AND J. R. FOUTS. *J. Pharmacol. Exptl. Therap.* 171: 127, 1970.

14. FELLER, D. R., M. MORITA AND J. R. GILLETTE. *Proc. Soc. Exptl. Biol. Med.* 137: 433, 1971.

15. FOUTS, J. R. *Biochem. Biophys. Res. Commun.* 6: 373, 1961.

16. FOUTS, J. R. In: *Fetal Pharmacology*, edited by L. O. Boreus. New York: Raven, 1973, p. 305.

17. FOUTS, J. R., AND R. H. ADAMSON. *Science* 129: 897, 1959.

18. FRANKLIN, M. R. *Xenobiotica* 1: 181, 1971.

19. GARATTINI, S. Pharmacology-Toxicology Program Symposium, Washington, D.C., May 17–19, 1971.

20. GIGON, P. L., T. E. GRAM AND J. R. GILLETTE. *Mol. Pharmacol.* 5: 109, 1969.

21. GILLETTE, J. R. *Advan. Pharmacol.* 4: 219, 1966.

22. GILLETTE, J. R. In: *Handbook of Experimental Pharmacology* Vol. 28, *Concepts of Biochemical Pharmacology*, Part 2 edited by B. B. Brodie and J. R. Gillette. Berlin, Heidelberg, New York: Springer-Verlag, 1971, p. 349.

23. GILLETTE, J. R. *Biochem. Pharmacol.* 20: 2785, 1974.

24. GILLETTE, J. R. *Biochem. Pharmacol.* 20: 2927, 1974.

25. GILLETTE, J. R., D. C. DAVIS AND H. A. SASAME. *Ann. Rev. Pharmacol.* 12: 57, 1972.

26. GILLETTE, J. R., R. H. MENARD AND B. STRIPP. *Clin. Pharmacol. Therap.* 14: 680, 1973.

27. GILLETTE, J. R., J. R. MITCHELL AND B. B. BRODIE. *Ann. Rev. Pharmacol.* 14: 271, 1974.

28. GILLETTE, J., H. SASAME AND B. STRIPP. *Drug Metab. Disposition* 1: 164, 1973.

29. GLADTKE, E., AND H. RIND. *Monatsschr. Kinderheilk.* 113: 299, 1965.

30. GRAM, T. E., A. M. GUARINO, D. H. SCHROEDER AND J. R. GILLETTE. *Biochem. J.* 113: 681, 1969.

31. GRAM, T. E., L. A. ROGERS AND J. R. FOUTS. *J. Pharmacol. Exptl. Therap.* 155: 479, 1967.

32. GRAM, T. E., D. H. SCHROEDER, D. C. DAVIS, R. L. REAGAN AND A. M. GUARINO. *Biochem. Pharmacol.* 20: 1371, 1971.

33. HART, L. G., R. H. ADAMSON, R. L. DIXON AND J. R. FOUTS. *J. Pharmacol.*

Exptl. Therap. 137: 103, 1962.

34. HARTIALA, K. J. W., AND M. PULKKINEN. *Ann. Med. Exptl. Biol. Fenniae Helsinki* 33: 246, 1955.

35. INSCOE, J. K., AND J. AXELROD. *J. Pharmacol. Exptl. Therap.* 129: 128, 1960.

36. JOLLOW, D. J., J. R. MITCHELL, W. Z. POTTER, D. C. DAVIS, J. R. GILLETTE AND B. B. BRODIE. *J. Pharmacol. Exptl. Therap.* 187: 195, 1973.

37. JOLLOW, D. J., J. R. MITCHELL, N. ZAMPAGLIONE AND J. R. GILLETTE. *Pharmacology* In press.

38. JONDORF, W. R., R. P. MAICKEL AND B. B. BRODIE. *Biochem. Pharmacol.* 1: 352, 1958.

39. JUCHAU, M. R., AND M. G. PEDERSEN. *Life Sci.* 12: 193, 1973.

40. KUENZIG, W., J. J. KAMM, M. BOUBLIK, F. JENKINS AND J. J. BURNS. *J. Pharmacol. Exptl. Therap.* 191: 32, 1974.

41. LESKES, A., P. SIEKEVITZ AND G. E. PALADE. *J. Cell Biol.* 49: 264, 1971.

42. LEVIN, W., M. JACOBSON, E. SERNATINGER AND R. KUNTZMAN. *Drug Metab. Disposition* 1: 275, 1973.

43. LISBONA, B. P., AND J.-C. PLASSE. *Steroids Lipids Res.* 3: 142, 1972.

44. MAC LEOD, S. M., K. W. RENTON AND N. R. EADE. *J. Pharmacol. Exptl. Therap.* 183: 489, 1972.

45. MANNERING, G. J. In: *Handbook of Experimental Pharmacology* Vol. 28, *Concepts in Biochemical Pharmacology*, Part 2, edited by B. B. Brodie and J. R. Gillette. Berlin, Heidelberg, New York: Springer-Verlag, 1971, p. 452.

46. MCCALLA, D. R., A. REVERS AND C. KAISER. *Biochem. Pharmacol.* 20: 3532, 1971.

47. MITCHELL, J. R., D. J. JOLLOW, J. R. GILLETTE AND B. B. BRODIE. *Drug Metab. Disposition* 1: 418, 1973.

48. MITCHELL, J. R., D. J. JOLLOW, W. Z. POTTER, D. C. DAVIS, J. R. GILLETTE AND B. B. BRODIE. *J. Pharmacol. Exptl. Therap.* 187: 185, 1973.

49. MITCHELL, J. R., D. J. JOLLOW, W. Z. POTTER, J. R. GILLETTE AND B. B. BRODIE, *J. Pharmacol. Exptl. Therap.* 187: 211, 1973.

50. MITCHELL, J. R., W. D. REID, B. CHRISTIE, J. MOSKOWITZ, G. KRISHNA AND B. B. BRODIE. *Res. Commun. Chem. Pathol. Pharmacol.* 2: 877, 1971.

51. MORITA, M., D. R. FELLER AND J. R. GILLETTE. *Biochem. Pharmacol.* 20: 217, 1971.

52. MORRIS, J. F., J. M. PRICE, J. J. LALICH AND R. J. STEIN. *Cancer Res.* 29: 2145, 1969.

53. NEBERT, D. W., AND H. V. GELBOIN. *Arch. Biochem. Biophys.* 134: 76, 1969.

54. PELKONEN, O., P. ARVELA AND N. T. KARKI. *Acta Pharmacol. Toxicol.* 30: 385, 1971.

55. PELKONEN, O., P. JOUPPILA AND N. T. KARKI. *Arch. Intern. Pharmacodyn. Ther.* 202: 288, 1973.

56. PELKONEN, O., E. H. KALTIALA, T. K. I. LARMI AND N. T. KARKI. *Clin. Pharmacol. Therap.* In press.

57. PELKONEN, O., M. VORNE, P. JOUPPILA AND N. T. KARKI. *Acta Pharmacol. Toxicol.* 29: 284, 1971.

58. PELKONEN, O., M. VORNE AND N. T. KARKI. *Acta Phys. Scand.* Suppl. 330: 69, 1969.

59. PETERSON, J. A. *Arch. Biochem. Biophys.* 144: 678, 1971.

60. POMP, H., M. SCHNOOR AND K. J. NETTER. *Deut. Med. Wochschr.* 94: 23, 1232, 1969.

61. POTTER, W. Z., D. C. DAVIS, J. R. MITCHELL, D. J. JOLLOW, J. R. GILLETTE AND B. B. BRODIE. *J. Pharmacol. Exptl. Therap.* 187: 202, 1973.

62. RANE, A., AND H. ACKERMAN. *Clin. Pharmacol. Therap.* 13: 663, 1972.

63. RANE, A., F. SJOQVIST AND S. ORRENIUS. *Clin. Pharmacol. Therap.* 14: 666, 1973.

64. RANE, A., C. VON BAHR, S. ORRENIUS AND F. SJOQVIST. In: *Fetal Pharmacology*, edited by L. O. Boreus. New York: Raven, 1973, p. 287.

65. REID, W. D., AND G. KRISHNA. *Exptl. Mol. Pathol.* 18: 80, 1973.

66. ROWLAND, M., P. D. THOMSON, A. GUIOCHAND AND K. L. MELMAN. *Ann. N. Y. Acad. Sci.* 179: 383, 1971.

67. SASAME, H. A., J. R. MITCHELL, S. THORGEIRSSON AND J. R. GILLETTE. *Drug Metab. Disposition* 1: 150, 1973.

68. SCHENKMAN, J. B., D. L. CINTI, P. W. MOLDEUS AND S. ORRENIUS. *Drug Metab. Disposition* 1: 111, 1973.

69. SCHAND, D. G., AND R. E. RANGNO. *Pharmacology* 7: 159, 1972.

70. SMUCKLER, E., F. ARRHENIUS AND T. HULTIN. *Biochem. J.* 103: 55, 1967.

71. SHORT, C. R., AND L. E. DAVIS. *J. Pharmacol. Exptl. Therap.* 174: 185, 1970.

72. SHORT, C. R., M. D. MAINES AND B. A. WESTFALL. *Biol. Neonator.* 21: 54, 1972.

73. TEPHLEY, T. R., C. WEBB, P. TRUSSLER, F. KNIFFEN, E. HASEGAWA AND W. PIPER. *Drug Metab. Disposition* 1: 259, 1973.

74. VILLEE, D. B. *Am. J. Med.* 53: 533, 1972.

75. WELCH, R. M., B. GOMMI, A. P. ALVARES AND A. H. CONNEY. *Cancer Res.* 32: 973, 1972.

76. WEST, S. B., W. LEVIN AND A. Y. H. LU. *Federation Proc.* 33: 587, 1974.

77. WICKMAN, H. M., H. RIND AND E. GLADTKE. *Z. Kinderheilk.* 103: 262, 1968.

78. WILLIAMS, R. T. *Detoxification Mechanisms.* New York: Wiley, 1959.

79. YAFFE, S. J., A. RANE, F. SJOQVIST, L. O. BOREUS AND S. ORRENIUS. *Life Sci.* 9: II, 1189, 1970.

80. ZAMBONI, L. *J. Ultrastruct. Res.* 12: 509, 1965.

Impaired hormonal regulation of enzyme activity during aging[1,2]

RICHARD C. ADELMAN

Fels Research Institute and Department of Biochemistry
Temple University School of Medicine
Philadelphia, Pennsylvania 19140

ABSTRACT

A general feature of all aging populations is the progressively impaired ability to adapt to changes in the surrounding environment. Biochemical expressions of adaptive response include modifications in the rates of enzyme synthesis and degradation, as well as alterations in physiological activity. Therefore, the effects of aging on enzyme adaptation were surveyed in an attempt to explore fundamental biochemical mechanisms in the deterioration of responsiveness. The ability to stimulate adaptive increases in the activity of a large number of enzymes is impaired during aging in a variety of tissues from several different species. The impaired capability for liver enzyme adaptation in a rigorously controlled colony of aging male Sprague-Dawley rats probably reflects alterations in hormonal control mechanisms. The present article reviews and evaluates our interest in understanding the effects of aging on regulation of liver enzyme activity by the hormones, insulin and corticosterone. Specific areas currently under investigation include: *1*) the regulation of their concentrations in blood; *2*) the integrity of their receptor systems in liver; and *3*) effectiveness of the endogenous hormone pools from the viewpoints of the availability of physiological antagonists and the potential for alterations in molecular structure.—ADELMAN, R. C. Impaired hormonal regulation of enzyme activity during aging. *Federation Proc.* 34: 179–182, 1975.

The capability for regulation of enzyme activity is markedly impaired during aging. The significance of this observation lies in the generalized feature of all aging populations that adaptive responsiveness to environmental modification deteriorates as adult members of a population become older. Therefore, comprehension of molecular mechanisms of age-dependent enzyme regulation

[1] From Session VI, *Development and Aging at the Molecular Level*, of the FASEB Conference on *Biology of Development and Aging*, presented at the 58th Annual Meeting of the Federation of American Societies for Experimental Biology, Atlantic City, N.J., April 11, 1974.

[2] Preparation of this manuscript, as well as related experimentation, is supported by research grants HD-04382, HD-05874, CA-12227 and RR-05417 from the National Institutes of Health and IN-88-D from the American Cancer Society.

may provide a unique opportunity to determine the sequence of events that are responsible for a broad spectrum of senescent changes.

This area initially was broached by examining steady-state levels of enzymes during the latter portion of an animal's life-span. There are more than 1,000 publications in which more than 100 different enzyme activities were assayed in several tissues and cell types of a variety of species, ranging from human erythrocytes to homogenates of whole nematodes and houseflies (13). Numerous reviewers attempted to identify trends within specific organs or within related metabolic functions. However, the only reasonable conclusion to emerge from these studies is that aging is not associated with any generalized catastrophic consequences on intracellular steady-state levels of enzymes.

A second approach to the problem of altered enzyme regulation is based on observations of the age-dependent accumulation of aberrantly behaving proteins (13). The most intriguing example of such a phenomenon was reported recently by Gershon and Gershon (15). Their data demonstrate a substantial age-dependent decrease in the ratio of specific catalytic activity to amount of cross-reacting protein when a monospecific antibody is prepared against homogeneous preparations of mouse liver aldolase. The nature of the modification that generates inactive or partially active enzyme molecules during aging has not been identified.

A third approach to this problem concerns the ability to initiate adaptive increases in the tissue levels of enzymes following exposure of experimental animals to a particular stimulus. This phenomenon, known as enzyme adaptation, is impaired during aging in the case of a large number of enzymes from a variety of tissues from several different species, as reviewed previously (1–3, 8). The present article will attempt to evaluate the effects of aging on enzyme adaptation, and will indicate the likely direction of future efforts to comprehend the underlying mechanisms that are responsible for the senescent deterioration in tissue responsiveness.

GENERAL CONSIDERATIONS

The effects of aging on enzyme adaptation are expressed as alterations in magnitude and/or time course of response, although not all adaptations are impaired (3). Patterns of age-dependent enzyme adaptation are susceptible to substantial variation, related to differences in sex, strain, species and conditions of environmental maintenance of experimental animals. This addresses a crucial issue of gerontology; namely, the crying need for rigorous standardization of aging animal colonies. For this reason, and with the generous advice and support of the Adult Development and Aging Branch of the National Institute of Child Health and Human Development, my laboratory now has at its disposal a large colony of aging male Sprague-Dawley rats that are maintained for us commercially, with independent health evaluation. These rats are maintained under environmental conditions as close as possible to constant; even to the extent of providing throughout their lifetime a pasteurized, sterilized diet that is constant with regard both to percent composition and component source. The mean life-span of rats in this colony is approximately 30 months, the maximal life-span approximately 40 months, and pathological lesions still are extremely rare by as late as nearly 24 months (B. J. Cohen and Adelman, ms in preparation).

A typical example of the effects of aging on enzyme adaptation, using this special rat colony, is evident in the response of hepatic glucokinase (E. C. 2.7.1.2) to administration of glucose (4). The activity of this enzyme is markedly increased shortly after intragastric injection of a glucose solution into 2-month-old rats. In contrast, at 24 months of age a great deal more time is required to initiate this enzyme adaptation, whereas the magnitude of response is similar at both ages. The duration of the adaptive latent period increases progressively from 2.5 to 10 hours and is directly proportional to chronological age between 2 and at least 24 months (8). Similar results were obtained for adaptations of two additional liver enzymes, tyrosine aminotransferase (E.C. 2.6.1.5) and microsomal NADPH-cytochrome c reductase (E.C. 1.6.99.3) in response to treatment with ACTH and phenobarbital, respectively (1). Thus, a few years ago this type of observation was proposed as a biochemical method of monitoring the progress of aging (2).

Enzyme adaptation as observed in the liver of intact animals can be subcategorized arbitrarily into three distinct phases. These include: 1) the synthesis and postsynthetic fate of enzyme molecules in liver; 2) the interactions between liver and a variety of circulating hormones whose presence is crucial to many of the enzymes; and 3) the availability and effectiveness of the crucial hormone molecules. The logical issue to resolve first is localization of the origin of a lesion within a specific cell population of a particular tissue. For example delayed adaptation of hepatic enzyme activity may be a consequence of an impairment in the regulation of enzyme synthesis. However, such a modification could originate within the capacity for hepatic gene expression, the binding of a hormone to its hepatic receptor, endocrine gland production of the hormone, neuroendocrinological control of endocrine gland function, and so on. Only following resolution of this issue is it meaningful to pose more fundamental questions at a biochemical level.

HEPATIC CAPABILITY FOR ENZYME ADAPTATION

In order to determine whether or not age-dependent liver enzyme adaptation is a consequence of alterations that are intrinsic to liver, the adaptive capability of newly created liver cells was examined in old rats following partial hepatectomy (1, 2, 6). For glucokinase and microsomal NADPH-cytochrome c reductase, fully regenerated liver retains the patterns of enzyme inducibility characteristic of surgically untreated rats of the same age between 2 and 24 months. Therefore, it was not possible to distinguish between the following two alternative explanations for age-dependent liver enzyme adaptation. 1) Age-dependent modifications might arise from genetic alterations within the liver cell, which are copied during the cell proliferation associated with the regenerative process. 2) The delayed responses might reflect changes of extrahepatic origin.

The impaired ability to initiate at least one liver enzyme adaptation during aging probably is the consequence of a modification in the regulation of de novo enzyme synthesis. The adaptation of microsomal NADPH-cytochrome c reductase in response to treatment with phenobarbital was particularly amenable to such analysis, since the role of enzyme synthesis and degradation had been well-characterized previously by several investigators (e.g., 9). Therefore, rats of different ages were pulse-labeled with radioactive leucine at three distinct times during the course of the enzyme adaptation: *1*) zero time with respect to phenobarbital treatment; *2*) a time at which enzyme activity is increased maximally in young rats, but only slightly in old rats; and *3*) a time at which enzyme activity is increased maximally at both ages (8). The enzyme, cytochrome reductase, was purified to homogeneity from individual rat livers, and specific radioactivity was assessed. The delayed initiation of increased enzyme activity was accompanied by a delayed initiation of increased specific radioactivity. Since age-dependent changes in the leucine pool were not detectable, the delayed enzyme adaptation during aging probably resulted from a delay in the enhanced rate of incorporation of amino acid into enzyme.

It also is evident that the capability of liver to increase the activity of at least certain enzymes, when properly stimulated, does not deteriorate during aging. The general idea of this approach was to inject animals of different ages with hormones that are known to interact directly with liver to increase the activity of specific enzymes. For example, following injections of glucocorticoids, insulin or glucagon, both time course and magnitude of the increase in hepatic tyrosine aminotransferase activity are unaltered during aging of mice and rats (7, 12, 16). Similar results were obtained for the increase in hepatic glucokinase activity following treatment with insulin (7). Therefore, the delays in liver enzyme adaptation during aging probably reflect modifications in hormonal control mechanisms. However, direct in vivo inductions, such as the increase in tyrosine aminotransferase activity following injection of corticosterone, require hormone amounts that are in considerable excess of physiological levels. Thus, it is not yet possible to distinguish between age-dependent modifications in the endogenous supply of hormones and in their biochemical action in liver.

HORMONAL CONTROL OF HEPATIC ENZYME ADAPTATION

Hormonal requirements of glucokinase and tyrosine aminotransferase

Of those enzymes for which impaired adaptability was observed during aging, hormonal regulatory mechanisms are understood only for hepatic glucokinase to any significant degree of detail. It is well recognized that maintenance of glucokinase activity in fed rats is regulated by the availability of circulating insulin (e.g., 7, 10, 20, 21). However, it also is apparent that integrated influence of a broad spectrum of hormones probably is required for complete adaptive responsiveness of this enzyme to glucose (3, 8, 13). For example, the increase in glucokinase activity following administration of glucose to fasted rats is not detectable when fasting is preceded by bilateral adrenalectomy. Whether the apparent requirement for corticosterone is hepatic or pancreatic in nature is not known. Furthermore, both glucagon and epinephrine are highly effective in preventing the glucose-induced recovery of glucokinase activity in fasted rats (18, 24). Since the concentrations of both of these substances are high in the blood of fasted rats, their rates of disappearance from blood following administration of glucose probably determine to a considerable extent the effectiveness of newly secreted insulin.

Similarly, the effect of ACTH on hepatic tyrosine aminotransferase activity probably is exerted through, at least, the combined actions of insulin and corticosterone (7, 8). The requirement for integrity of adrenal function is evident from the inability of ACTH to increase the activity of this enzyme in adrenalectomized rats. In addition, however, the effect of ACTH is inhibited in rats treated simultaneously with insulin anti bodies.

Due to the complex nature of the hormonal interactions that are required for regulation of enzyme activity in liver of intact animals, it seemed appropriate to focus initial efforts on only one or two hormones. The presence of corticosterone and insulin probably is of crucial importance to at least two liver enzymes whose adaptability can deteriorate during aging, i.e., glucokinase and tyrosine aminotransferase. Therefore, it was decided to investigate the effects of aging on the availability to liver and on the effectiveness of these two hormones.

Any one or more of a number of hypothetical modifications in the control of liver function by insulin or corticosterone could account for delayed enzyme adaptation during aging. The most obvious of these, which already are under investigation, include the following. 1) Integrity of the hormone receptor system in liver could be modified. Within the framework of such a possibility are changes in affinity or maximal capacity of binding of hormone to receptor molecule; in the number of available and functional receptor molecules; in the transport of receptor-bound hormone or unknown "second messenger" into the nucleus; and in the subsequent ability to enhance, presumably, transcription or translation. 2) The ability to initiate adaptive increases in the concentration of the crucial hormones per se in blood could be impaired. Such a

lesion might be an immediate consequence either of impaired endocrine gland secretion or an enhanced rate of disappearance of the hormone from blood. 3) The biological effectiveness of the hormones could be reduced. This possibility must be regarded from two entirely different viewpoints. On the one hand, structural modifications might alter potency of the hormone. For example, any impairment in the metabolism of proinsulin would result in the secretion of a protein that is antigenically similar to insulin and that possesses far less hormonal activity (23). Furthermore, age-dependent accumulation of other biosynthetic precursors, posttranslational metabolic products, genetic variants, or even missynthesized protein could produce similar effects. On the other hand, the presence of antagonists could effectively block hormone action, e.g., the effects of epinephrine and glucagon on hepatic response to insulin.

A substantial portion of these experimental approaches currently are in progress. Therefore, the concluding sections of this presentation will summarize briefly the status of the work, and should be considered as preliminary.

Corticosterone

At the present time, the effects of aging on the glucocorticoid receptor system in liver are uncertain. Roth reported (19) that association in vitro of glucocorticoids to their binding proteins in extracts of cytosol from adrenalectomized rats does not change in affinity or maximal capacity beyond 12 months of age. In contrast, Litwack and co-workers (22) observed that glucocorticoid binding capacity decreases during aging when assessed in postmortem samples of human liver. In collaboration with

Litwack's group, the fate of glucocorticoids in hepatic cytoplasm and
nuclei is being correlated with the
induction of tyrosine aminotransferase in rats of different ages.

Unstimulated levels of corticosterone in aorta blood are identical between 2 and 24 months of age
(G. W. Britton, S. Rotenberg, Freeman, Karoly and Adelman, ms submitted). Furthermore, the ability to
produce the hormone in response to
injections of ACTH does not change
beyond 12 months of age. In contrast, the stress of short-term starvation reveals an age-dependent neuroendocrinological lesion which is expressed as: *1*) the reduced ability to
increase corticosterone levels in aorta
blood; and *2*) the inability to increase
hepatic tyrosine aminotransferase
activity.

Insulin

Specific binding of porcine insulin
to purified rat hepatic plasma membranes undergoes no apparent
change in affinity or in maximal capacity beyond 12 months of age (14).
However, interpretation of these data
must await evaluation of the role
of age-dependent changes in liver
cell size, as well as determination of
the relative extent of hormone interaction between molecules of receptor
and insulin-specific protease, each of
which is plasma membrane-bound.

Unstimulated levels of immunoreactive insulin in portal vein blood
of fed or fasted rats decrease pre-
cipitously between 12 and 24 months
of age (14). In contrast, pancreases
of 24-month-old rats are far more
sensitive to administration of glucose in vivo than are younger rats,
and the older animals also are characterized by a tremendous hyper-
insulinemia in response to glucose
(Freeman, Karoly, Britton, E. J.
Masoro, A. I. Kleiner, S. P. Shukla

and Adelman, ms in preparation).
In confirmation of earlier data
(11, 17), administration of glucose
causes two bursts of insulin secretion in 2-month-old rats; one within
a few minutes and another at 1–2
hours. In a manner excitingly analogous to the impaired adaptation of
hepatic glucokinase, the second burst
of insulin secretion is progressively
delayed as our rats age from 2 to
24 months (Freeman et al., ms in
preparation). The relative importance of these two bursts of insulin
secretion to the glucokinase adaptation is not known.

Biological effectiveness of insulin
does not diminish with increasing
age of the rat insulin donor (Freeman et al., ms in preparation). This
was ascertained by isolating pancreatic islets from rats of different
ages, stimulating insulin secretion in
vitro by incubation of the islets with
glucose, and subjecting the freshly
secreted solutions of insulin to simultaneous analysis (double antibody
radioimmunoassay, using purified rat
insulin as a standard; and assessing
the ability to enhance the rate of
oxidation of glucose to CO_2 in isolated rat adipocytes). Biological activity per immunoreactive unit of
insulin is identical between 2 and 24
months.

POTENTIAL SIGNIFICANCE OF THESE STUDIES

Interference with the coordinated
regulation of key enzyme systems,
with associated breakdown of homeostatic mechanisms, is undoubtedly the
underlying cause of many diseases.
The deterioration of enzyme regulation seen in senescent animals is not
yet understood. Nevertheless, a progressively impaired ability to synthesize certain enzymes in response to a
broad spectrum of environmental
alterations probably represents a gen-

eral biochemical expression of aging. Clearly, the increased latent period of adaptation may be the biochemical basis for the increased vulnerability and incidence of certain diseases associated with advanced age. Comprehension of the mechanism of this age-dependent modification may provide an unprecedented opportunity to study the molecular processes of aging.

Elucidation of the mechanisms responsible for at least certain of the age-dependent adaptations referred to above may contribute to the essential understanding of specific pathological states. Two examples, in particular, are most evident. 1) The progressively delayed response by hepatic glucokinase activity to administration of glucose is remarkably similar to the impairment of insulin-dependent tolerance to blood glucose seen in maturity-onset diabetes. 2) The major group of enzymes, of which NADPH-cytochrome c reductase is only one example, the "drug-metabolizing" enzymes of liver endoplasmic reticulum, is involved in the metabolism of chemical carcinogens, other environmental chemicals, drugs, and steroid hormones. Thus, results obtained from this type of research approach may contribute also to the understanding of the age-dependent incidence of certain chemically-induced liver tumors, as well as age-dependent changes in the safety and efficacy of various drugs and hormones.

REFERENCES

1. ADELMAN, R. C. Exptl. Gerontol. 6: 75, 1971.

2. ADELMAN, R. C. Advances in Gerontological Research, edited by B. L. Strehler. New York: Academic, 1972, vol. 4, p. 1.

3. ADELMAN, R. C. Colloquium on Enzyme Induction, edited by D. V. Parke. New York and London: Plenum. In press.

4. ADELMAN, R. C. J. Biol. Chem. 245: 1032, 1970.

5. ADELMAN, R. C. Nature 228: 1095, 1970.

6. ADELMAN, R. C. Biochem. Biophys. Res. Commun. 38: 1149, 1970.

7. ADELMAN, R. C., AND C. FREEMAN. Endocrinology 90: 1551, 1972.

8. ADELMAN, R. C., C. FREEMAN AND B. S. COHEN. Advances in Enzyme Regulation, edited by G. Weber. Oxford and New York: Pergamon, 1972, vol. 10, p. 365.

9. ARIAS, I. M., D. DOYLE AND R. T. SCHIMKE. J. Biol. Chem. 244: 3303, 1969.

10. CAHILL, G. F., JR., J. ASHMORE, A. E. RENOLD AND A. B. HASTINGS. Am. J. Med. 26: 264, 1959.

11. CERASI, E. Acta Endocrinol. 55: 163, 1967.

12. FINCH, C. E., J. R. FOSTER AND A. E. MIRSKY. J. Gen. Physiol. 54: 690, 1969.

13. FREEMAN, C. (Ph.D. Dissertation) Philadelphia: Temple Univ., 1974.

14. FREEMAN, C., K. KAROLY AND R. C. ADELMAN. Biochem. Biophys. Res. Commun. 54: 1573, 1973.

15. GERSHON, H., AND D. GERSHON. Proc. Natl. Acad. Sci. U.S. 70: 909, 1973.

16. GREGERMAN, R. I. Am. J. Physiol. 197: 63, 1959.

17. GRODSKY, G. M., A. A. BATTS, L. L. BENNETT, C. VCELLA, N. B. McWILLIAMS AND D. SMITH. Am. J. Physiol. 205: 638, 1963.

18. NIEMEYER, H., N. PEREZ AND E. RABAJILLE. J. Biol. Chem. 241: 4055, 1966.

19. ROTH, G. S. Endocrinology 94: 82, 1974.

20. RUDERMAN, N. B., AND V. LAURIS. Diabetes 17: 611, 1968.

21. SHARMA, C., R. MANJESHWAR AND S. WEINHOUSE. J. Biol. Chem. 238: 3840, 1963.

22. SINGER, S., H. ITO AND G. LITWACK. Intern. J. Biochem. 4: 569, 1973.

23. STEINER, D. F., AND P. E. OYER. Proc. Natl. Acad. Sci. U.S. 57: 473, 1967.

24. URETA, T., J. RADOJKOVIC AND H. NIEMEYER. J. Biol. Chem. 245: 4819, 1970.

Age-related changes in glucocorticoid binding by rat splenic leukocytes: possible cause of altered adaptive responsiveness[1]

GEORGE S. ROTH

Laboratory of Cellular and Comparative Physiology
Gerontology Research Center
National Institute of Child Health and Human Development
National Institutes of Health, Bethesda, Maryland 20014
and the Baltimore City Hospitals, Baltimore, Maryland 21224

ABSTRACT

Splenic leukocytes of senescent rats (24–26 mo) exhibit a 60% reduction in cortisol-induced inhibition of ^{3}H-uridine uptake when compared to mature adult animals (12–14 mo). The degree of inhibition is directly proportional to cortisol dosage up to 2×10^{-6}M. Specific binding of physiological (nanomolar) concentrations of ^{3}H-cortisol by leukocytic cytosol macromolecules is reduced by over 40% in the older animals. Moreover, Scatchard analyses reveal 60% fewer specific glucocorticoid binding sites in the cytosols of cells from the senescent rats. Such analyses were performed in vitro at 0 C to eliminate metabolism of steroids. In addition, ^{3}H-dexamethasone was used instead of ^{3}H-cortisol to eliminate binding to plasma (or serum) transcortin. Inhibition of ^{3}H-uridine uptake requires specific glucocorticoid binding. The degree of inhibition at varying glucocorticoid dosages is proportional to the amount of specific binding to cytoplasmic macromolecules. Thus, age-related reduction in specific glucocorticoid binding sites may be at least partially responsible for altered responsiveness of splenic leukocytes to these hormones — ROTH, G. S. Age-related changes in glucocorticoid binding by rat splenic leukocytes: possible cause of altered adaptive responsiveness. *Federation Proc.* 34: 183–185, 1975.

Aging animals exhibit an altered ability to respond to certain hormonal stimuli (for a review see 7). Most such responses require interaction of hormones with specific recep-

[1] From Session VI, *Development and Aging at the Molecular Level,* of the FASEB Conference on *Biology of Development and Aging,* presented at the 58th Annual Meeting of the Federation of American Societies for Experimental Biology, Atlantic City, N.J., April 11, 1974.

315

tors. In addition, the degree of response is directly proportional to the amount of hormone binding to receptor (7). A previous survey in this laboratory revealed that the concentrations of specific glucocorticoid

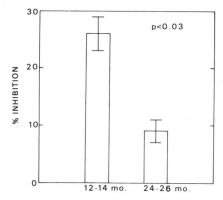

Figure 1. Inhibition of ^{3}H-uridine uptake by 2×10^{-6}M cortisol. Spleens of mature adult (12–14 mo) and old (24–26 mo) virgin male, Wistar rats were teased in RPMI 1640 media containing 20% fetal calf serum at a concentration of about 10^7 leukocytes per/ml. Cultures were divided in half. One part was brought up to 2×10^{-6}M cortisol, the other received phosphate buffered saline (PBS) and served as the control. After 3 hours incubation in 5% CO_2 at 37 C, cells were harvested and resuspended in fresh warm media containing ^{3}H-uridine (specific radioactivity 28Ci/mmole) at a concentration of 1–5 μ Ci/ml. After 30 min additional incubation, cells were again harvested into ice cold PBS. Essentially no loss of leukocytes occurred during the incubations. Contaminating red blood cells were lysed by 15 min exposure to 0.83% ammonium chloride at 0 C. Such treatment removes over 99% of the red cells, while the white cells are recovered quantitatively. The leukocytes were then washed in PBS, collected by centrifugation and lysed in water. Debris was removed by low speed centrifugation and the soluble cellular contents in the supernate were assayed for radioactivity by scintillation counting. Cytosol radioactivity was normalized per milligram of cytosol protein. Histograms represent the mean ± standard error for 3 separate experiments.

binding sites in many rat tissues decrease between adulthood (12–13 mo) and senescence (24–25 mo) (6). It remained to be determined whether such decreased binding is accompanied by decreased biochemical responsiveness to glucocorticoids within the same target cells and tissues. Roth and Adelman (8) have previously made such a correlation with respect to decreased isoproterenol entry into salivary glands and delayed and decreased stimulation of DNA synthesis as rats age. The present report, therefore, attempts to relate decreased responsiveness to glucocorticoids to decreased specific binding in splenic leukocytes of aged male Wistar rats. The use of target cell, rather than target tissue, preparations eliminates possible contributions of extracellular factors within tissue extracts. In addition, age related changes in hormone binding and responsiveness may ultimately be localized at the level of selected cell types.

METHODS AND RESULTS

The ability of glucocorticoids to inhibit substrate entry into lymphoid cells by apparent induction of an inhibitory protein has been well documented (2, 4). In this laboratory, inhibition of ^{3}H-uridine uptake by cultured rat splenic leukocytes following a 3-hour exposure to cortisol is dosage dependent up to 2×10^{-6} M. Figure 1 compares the degree of such inhibition in splenic leukocytes from mature (12–14 mo) and senescent (24–26 mo) male, virgin Wistar rats. Uptake of radioactivity is approximately linear for 30 min when cells are exposed to ^{3}H-uridine following 3 hours previous culturing in the presence or absence of cortisol. Basal levels of uptake are generally slightly lower in the senescent group (data not shown). More important, a 60%

decrease in responsiveness is observed in the cells from the older animals.

Hallahan et al. (2) report that cortisol-induced inhibition of substrate transport into lymphocytes is initially mediated by binding of hormone to specific receptors. Similarly, in this laboratory the degree of ^{3}H-uridine uptake inhibition is directly proportional to the amount of cortisol that enters and specifically binds to cytoplasmic macromolecules in splenic leukocytes. Hallahan et al. (2) also report that at least 10 min exposure to cortisol is required to produce inhibition of substrate entry. Figure 2 compares the amount of specific ^{3}H-cortisol binding by 12- to 14- and 24- to 26-month-old rat splenic leukocytes cultured in the presence of physiological quantities (4×10^{-9} M) of ^{3}H-cortisol for 15 min. Specific uptake of ^{3}H-cortisol and protein per cell is essentially the same in both age groups (data not shown). However, specific binding is reduced more than 40% in the senescent group.

To eliminate the problem of ^{3}H-cortisol metabolism in intact cultured cells, additional binding experiments were performed at 0 C using cell-free cytosols of splenic leukocytes. ^{3}H-Dexamethasone, a fluorinated synthetic analog, was employed instead of cortisol. Dexamethasone does not bind to plasma (or serum) transcortin and, at least in liver, binds only to the true glucocorticoid "receptor" (1).

Kaiser et al. (3) have reported that the binding of glucocorticoids to lymphocytic cytosol macromolecules is not affected by adrenalectomy. Furthermore, Adelman's group has reported that the basal levels of serum corticosterone in intact 12- and 24-month-old rats are comparable (personal communication). However, the possibility remained that endogenous

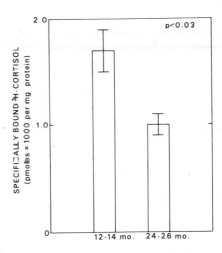

Figure 2. Specific binding of 4 nM ^{3}H-cortisol by cultured spleen cells. Spleen cells from mature and senescent Wistar rats were prepared exactly as in Fig. 1. Cells were then washed in RPMI 1640 media without fetal calf serum, and resuspended in 37 C warm media without serum. ^{3}H-Cortisol (specific radioactivity 80–100 Ci/mmole) was added to a concentration of 4×10^{-9}M. In addition an identical culture containing 2×10^{-5}M unlabeled cortisol was incubated in parallel as a control for nonspecific uptake and binding. After 15 min both cultures were harvested into ice cold PBS. Red cell removal and leukocyte lysis were as described for Fig. 1. Cell lysates were centrifuged at 100,000 × g for 60 min at 4 C to yield cytosol supernates. Unbound ^{3}H-cortisol was removed by adsorption to 2 mg/ml heat activated charcoal. Binding is proportional to cytosol protein concentration, and no appreciable protein is adsorbed to the charcoal under these conditions. Histograms represent the mean ± standard error for individual cell preparations from six individual spleens per age group.

steroids might slightly alter the binding of physiological levels of ^{3}H-glucocorticoids. Therefore, the exact number of specific binding sites was determined by Scatchard analyses (9) using varied concentrations of ^{3}H-dexamethasone. In such analyses the apparent affinity but not the actual determined number of binding sites may be altered by endogenous competing steroids. Scatchard analysis of ^{3}H-dexamethasone binding was performed on cytosols of splenic leukocytes from 12- to 14- and 24- to 26-month-old intact Wistar rats. Cells were lysed in 10^{-2} M Tris buffer, pH 7.4, and centrifuged for 60 min at 100,000 × g. The resultant supernate cytosols were incubated with 5–100 nM ^{3}H-dexamethasone at 0 C for 60–70 min, after which time additional binding is negligible. Identical tubes, containing a 500-fold excess of unlabeled dexamethasone, were run in parallel to corrent for nonspecific binding. Unbound ^{3}H-dexamethasone was removed by adsorption to 5 mg/ml heat activated charcoal. Binding is proportional to cytosol protein concentration, and no appreciable protein is adsorbed to charcoal under these conditions. Figure 3 compares the numbers of

specific dexamethasone binding sites in cytosols of 12- to 14- and 24- to 26-month-old rat splenic leukocytes. An approximately 60% reduction is observed in the senescent group.

DISCUSSION

The data presented here indicate that splenic leukocytes from senescent rats exhibit reductions in biochemical responsiveness, specific binding and numbers of specific binding sites for glucocorticoid hormones when compared to mature adult animals. In fact, at concentrations of glucocorticoid that saturate the specific cytoplasmic binding sites (Figs. 1 and 3), the decrease in responsiveness of the senescent cells is essentially equal to the decrease in the number of these sites. In this and other laboratories, response to hormones requires, and is found to be directly proportional to, the amount of hormone binding to specific receptors (7). Thus the decrease in responsiveness reported here may be at least partially due to the decrease in the number of specific glucocorticoid binding sites in splenic leukocytes of senescent rats.

Important questions which now must be answered include

1) Are the age-associated changes intrinsic to a given splenic leukocyte population, or are they due to an age-related decrease in the proportion of glucocorticoid-responsive cell types?

2) Can such age-related changes in responsiveness be correlated with hormone binding changes in target cells from tissues which do not undergo appreciable cell proliferation or turnover during the lifespan (e.g., neurons, muscle cells, and so on)?

3) If such changes are intrinsic to given target cell populations, what is their cause? Does an "error catastrophe" mechanism such as

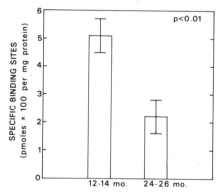

Figure 3. Number of specific dexamethasone binding sites per milligram cytosol protein. Spleen cells from mature and senescent Wistar rats were prepared, and red cells removed as in Fig. 1 and 2. In vitro assessment of the numbers of ^{3}H-dexamethasone binding sites were performed as described in the text. Histograms represent the mean ± standard error for individual cell preparations from six individual spleens per age group.

that proposed by Orgel (5) cause a decrease in the number of functionally active hormone receptors in aged cells, or is there programmed loss of function?

Finally, *4*) can such age-related changes be halted, prevented, or reversed by appropriate biochemical manipulations?

REFERENCES

1. BEATO, M., M. KALIMI AND P. FEIGELSON. *Biochem. Biophys. Res. Comm.* 47: 1464, 1972.

2. HALLAHAN, C., D. YOUNG AND A. MUNCK *J. Biol. Chem.* 248. 2922, 1973.

3. KAISER, N., R. MULHOLLAND AND F. ROSEN. *J. Biol Chem.* 248: 478, 1973.

4. MAKMAN, M. H., B. DVORKIN AND A. WHITE. *Proc. Natl. Acad. Sci. U.S.* 68: 1969, 1971.

5. ORGEL, L. *Proc. Natl. Acad. Sci. U.S.* 49: 517, 1963.

6. ROTH, G. S. *Endocrinology* 94: 82, 1974.

7. ROTH, G. S., AND R. C. ADELMAN. *Exptl. Gerontol.* In press.

8. ROTH, G. S., AND R. C. ADELMAN *J Gerontology* 28: 298, 1973.

9. SCATCHARD, G. *Ann. N.Y. Acad. Sci.* 51: 660, 1949.

Covalent modification of nuclear proteins during aging[1,2]

C. C. LIEW AND A. G. GORNALL

Department of Clinical Biochemistry
Banting Institute, Faculty of Medicine
University of Toronto, Toronto, Canada, M5G 1L5

ABSTRACT

An in vitro assay system has been established to study acetylation and phosphorylation of nuclear proteins from isolated nuclei. Phosphorylation of nuclear proteins reached a peak within 5 min while maximum acetylation occurred about 10 min later. The rate of acetylation of liver nuclear proteins in 15 min incubation was significantly higher in 'old' mice (29 mo) than in 'young' mice (2 mo), while there was no difference in phosphorylation. When nuclear histones were fractionated by polyacrylamide-urea electrophoresis the acetylation of histone F3 was increased in 'old' mice to 129% and F2al to 112% of the values in 'young' mice. Acetylation of phenol-soluble nuclear acidic proteins was increased to 250% and phosphorylation to 138% in 'old' mice as compared to 'young' mice. This increase in covalent modification of acidic proteins was found in two specific fractions when separated by SDS-polyacrylamide gel electrophoresis. By contrast, the labeling of nucleoplasmic proteins, soluble in 0.14 M NaCl, showed no significant difference between the two ages.—LIEW, C. C. AND A. G. GORNALL. Covalent modification of nuclear proteins during aging. *Federation Proc.* 34: 186–187, 1975.

The interaction of nuclear proteins and DNA is believed to be one of the prime regulatory functions in genetic expression (1, 10). Prominent among the theories of aging has been a gradual deterioration of this regulatory process (2, 9, 11, 13). Currently, covalent modification of protein structure by phosphorylation, acetylation and methylation is being viewed as probably playing a significant role in the interaction of protein–protein and protein–nucleotide complexes at both translational and transcriptional levels

[1] From Session VI, *Development and Aging at the Molecular Level*, of the FASEB Conference on *Biology of Development and Aging*, presented at the 58th Annual Meeting of the Federation of American Societies for Experimental Biology, Atlantic City, N.J., April 11, 1974.

[2] Supported by grants from the Medical Research Council of Canada and the Ontario Heart Foundation.

(1, 3, 4, 10). This report provides the first evidence that changes in the co valent modification of nuclear proteins may be involved in the molecular processes of aging.

An in vitro assay system has been established to study acetylation and phosphorylation of nuclear proteins. We have found that nuclei incubated in medium N containing 0.25 M sucrose (5) give much better incorporation of ^{3}H-acetate and ^{32}P into

proteins than other systems tested (unpublished observations). In this medium the phosphorylation of nuclear proteins reached a peak within 5 min while maximum acetylation occurred about 10 min later.

Liver nuclei from 'young' (2 mo) and 'old' (29 mo) mice were incubated with ^{3}H-acetate and $[\gamma$-^{32}P]ATP for periods of 5, 10 and 15 min. Figure 1 shows that while there was no difference in the rate of phosphoryla-

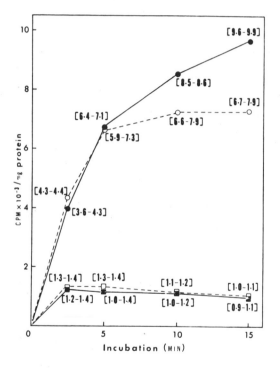

Figure 1. Incorporation of ^{3}H-acetate and ^{32}P into mouse liver nuclear proteins. Mouse liver nuclei were obtained from five animals (C57/6J) aged 2 mo (young) and five aged 29 mo (old). Five μCi of ^{3}H-acetyl-CoA (specific activity 0.52 mCi/mmol) and 50 μCi $[\gamma$-^{32}P]-ATP (sp act 5.7 Ci/mmol) were added to a 1.4 ml nuclear suspension that had been incubated at 37 C for 5 min. Samples were removed at 0, 5, 10 and 15 min. The reaction was terminated by absorbing 50 μl of the nuclear suspension into filter paper strips, followed immediately by immersion in ice-cold 10% TCA and subsequently washing with ethanol and ether as described previously (6). Results represent the mean of two separate experiments. O – – – O and ● — ● represent incorporation of ^{3}H-acetate and □ – – – □ and ■ — ■ the incorporation of ^{32}P into nuclear proteins of 'young' and 'old' mice respectively.

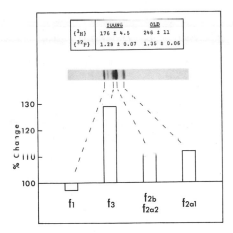

Figure 2. Acetylation and phosphorylation of nucleohistones in vitro. Nuclei from young (2 mo) and old (29 mo) mice were isolated from five animals of each group and incubated for 15 min as described in Fig. 1. Equal amounts (30 μg) of 'young' and 'old' nucleohistones were fractionated by polyacrylamide-urea gel electrophoresis (8). Results show the mean (cpm/μg protein) of three separate experiments, with one standard error, for the whole nucleohistones. The fractionated histones, after determining the specific activity as described previously (7), are expressed as percent changes in acetylation relative to the 'young' mice.

tion of nuclear proteins, the extent of acetylation was greater after 10 min in the older animals. We have made a similar observation (unpublished) in 32-month-old rats.

Liver nuclei from 'young' and 'old' mice were incubated for 15 min with ^{3}H-acetate and [γ-^{32}P]ATP. Total nucleohistones were isolated and found to be more highly acetylated than phosphorylated. As shown in Fig. 2, the rate of acetylation in 'old' mice was approximately 140% of the value in 'young' mice. The histones were separated by polyacrylamide gel electrophoresis into four main fractions. It was found that the rates in 'old' mice averaged 129%

for fraction F3 and for F2al 112% of the values in 'young' animals.

The phenol-soluble nuclear 'acidic' proteins were also examined and the data are shown in Table 1. In 'old' mice the degree of acetylation of these proteins after 15 min was at least twofold greater than in 'young' mice. This increase was found in two specific fractions of the acidic proteins when separated by SDS polyacrylamide gel electrophoresis (ms in preparation). Phosphorylation of nuclear acidic proteins was greater than for histones and in 'old' mice averaged 138% of the value in 'young' animals. By contrast the labeling of nucleoplasmic proteins, soluble in 0.14 M NaCl, showed no significant differences between the two groups.

In summary, it appears that changes in the covalent modification of nuclear proteins occur with aging. This is most notable as an increase in the extent of acetylation of the nuclear acidic proteins. Phosphorylation of the acidic proteins and acetylation of the nucleohistones increase to a lesser degree. We support the view that covalent modification of nuclear proteins is probably involved in the regulation of genetic expression (1, 3, 4, 6). Wulff et al. (14) and others have noted that the

TABLE 1. Acetylation and phosphorylation of nuclear acidic proteins in vitro

Experiments	'Young'	'Old'	Change, %
^{3}H-acetate	8,873	28,344	319
^{32}P	4,630	7,219	156
^{3}H acetate	9,471	17,256	182
^{32}P	5,706	6,813	119

Nuclei isolated from the two groups of mice were incubated as described in Fig. 2. Phenol-soluble nuclear acidic proteins were prepared as described previously (12). Results are expressed as cpm/mg protein. Changes are related to a value of 100% for the 'young' animals.

rate of RNA synthesis is increased in aged mouse and rat liver nuclei. Our results suggest that this increase may be secondary to changes in the covalent modification of nuclear proteins, which in turn may reflect a gradual decline with age in the efficiency of the homeostatic mechanisms that function by regulating expression of the genome.

REFERENCES

1. ALLFREY, V. G. In: *Histones and Nucleohistones*, edited by D. M. P. Phillips. New York and London: Plenum, 1971, p. 241–294.
2. GOLDSTEIN, S. *New Engl. J. Med.* 285: 1120–1129, 1971.
3. GORNALL, A. G., AND C. C. LIEW. *Advan. Enzyme Regul.* 12: 267–285, 1974.
4. HNILICA, L. S. In: *The Structure and Biological Functions of Histones*. Cleveland: Chemical Rubber Co. Press, 1972, p. 79–92.
5. LIEW, C. C., AND A. G. GORNALL. *J. Biol. Chem.* 248: 977–983, 1973.
6. LIEW, C. C., D. SURIA AND A. G. GORNALL. *Endocrinology* 93: 1025–1034, 1973.
7. LUE, P. F., A. G. GORNALL AND C. C. LIEW. *Can. J. Biochem.* 51: 1177–1194, 1973.
8. PANYIM, S., AND R. CHALKLEY. *Arch. Biochem. Biophys.* 130: 337–346, 1969.
9. PRICE, G. B., AND T. MAKINODAN. *Gerontologia* 19: 58–70, 1973.
10. STEIN, G. S., T. C. SPELSBERG AND L. J. KLEINSMITH. *Science* 183: 817–824, 1974.
11. STREHLER, B. *Proc. 9th Intern. Congr. Gerontol.* 2: 33–36, 1972.
12. SURIA, D., AND C. C. LIEW. *Biochem. J.* 137: 355–362, 1974.
13. VON HAHN, V. P. *Advan. Gerontol. Res.* 3: 1–38, 1971.
14. WULFF, V. J., H. V. SAMIS, JR. AND R. S. FALZONE. *Advan. Gerontol. Res.* 2: 37–76, 1970.

Effects of aging on ionic movements of atrial muscle[1,2]

PAULA B. GOLDBERG[3], STEVEN I. BASKIN
AND JAY ROBERTS

Department of Pharmacology
The Medical College of Pennsylvania
Philadelphia, Pennsylvania 19129

ABSTRACT

The effect of age on ion concentrations and fluxes in cardiac muscle was examined. Left atria from rats of 1, 3, 6, 12, 24 and 28 months of age were analyzed for content of total water, sodium and potassium, for ^{14}C-inulin space and for ^{22}Na and ^{42}K influx and efflux rates. Animals of 3 and 24 months of age showed a small but significantly greater water content than those of the other age groups. The inulin space, after a small nonsignificant fall between 1 and 3 mo, increased significantly at 6 mo, then leveled off through 28 mo. Intracellular sodium $(Na)_i$, and potassium $(K)_i$ concentrations were calculated. $(Na)_i$ showed a significant increase from 1 to 3 mo, decreased significantly at 6 mo, and then leveled off. $(K)_i$ exhibited an initial significant decrease from 1 to 3 mo followed at 6 mo by a significant increase which remained unchanged through 28 mo. Trend analyses of the Na influx rates showed that a significant increase with age occurred, except for a decrease at 24 mo. Potassium influx rates remained relatively constant at all ages. Sodium efflux appeared to be multiexponential, with at least two distinct rate constants (k_1 and k_2). Potassium efflux steadily decreased as a function of age. The results are discussed with reference to possible consequences of aging on cardiac physiology and reactivity to pharmacological agents. —GOLDBERG, P. B., S. I. BASKIN AND J. ROBERTS. Effects of aging on ionic movements of atrial muscle. *Federation Proc.* 34: 188–190, 1975.

The effects of aging on excitable membranes, particularly cardiac muscle membrane, have not been studied extensively. Yet it is well known that the aged heart is more prone or susceptible to disease states than is the young heart and that cardiac muscle physiology undergoes profound alterations with age (1, 3, 5, 15, 16). Although the exact mecha-

[1] From Session VI, *Development and Aging at the Molecular Level*, of the FASEB Conference on *Biology of Development and Aging*, presented at the 58th Annual Meeting of the Federation of American Societies for Experimental Biology, Atlantic City, N.J., April 11, 1974.

[2] This work was supported in part by the National Institutes of Health Grant HD 06267.

[3] Supported in part by a fellowship from the Heart Association of Southeastern Pennsylvania.

nisms underlying the reported changes in cardiac activity brought about by senescence are obscure, it would appear likely that they may be linked to changes in electrical activity of, and ionic movements across, the

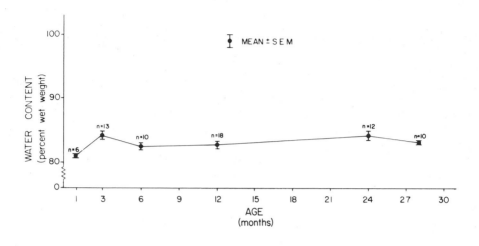

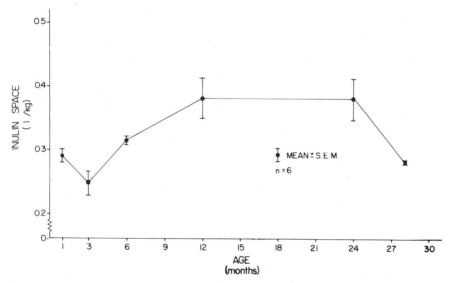

Figure 1. Water content and distribution in rat left atria as a function of age. *a*) Total tissue water, determined in atria freshly excised from rats at the ages indicated, and calculated as the difference between wet and dry weight (expressed as percent wet weight). n = 6 at 1 month, 13 at 3, 10 at 6, 18 at 12 months, 12 at 24 and 10 at 28 months.

b) Inulin space, determined on atria excised from rats at ages indicated and incubated in ^{14}C-inulin containing modified Krebs-Henseleit solution at 37 C for 2 hours stimulated at 60 Hz, calculated as counts taken up in 2 hours. n = 5 at 1 and 12 months, 6 at 3 and 6 months, and 3 at 28 months.

excitable membranes. For developing mammalian heart and skeletal muscle, the literature contains reports of observed alterations in electrical properties (4, 7) and water and ionic content (8, 9). Evidence that aging muscles continue to undergo alterations was provided by a study of the electrical properties of atrial muscle membranes from rats of 1 month to 28 months of age (2).

In view of the foregoing observations, a study was instituted to examine rat cardiac tissue with respect to ionic content and movement throughout the life cycle of the animal, so that the effects of both maturation and aging could be observed.

METHODS

Atria from rats aged 1, 3, 6, 12, 24 and 28 mo were isolated and analyzed for the following: total water content; total sodium (Na) and potassium (K) contents; extracellular space; and influx and efflux of Na and K. Ion content was determined by flame photometry. Extracellular space was determined as the ^{14}C-inulin space after 2 hours of incubation. Ionic fluxes were determined by the methods of Page et al. (6, 13) and of Holland et al. (10, 11) in atria stimulated at 60 Hz.

Influx and efflux rate constants for radioactive sodium (^{22}Na) and potassium (^{42}K) were calculated by fitting a linear regression line to the data from individual experiments. In the ^{22}Na efflux studies, multicompartmental analysis was performed using the method of Riggs (14). Intracellular concentrations of ions were calculated from the experimentally determined values for total ion content, total water content, and inulin space. It should be pointed out that statistical significance was determined by analysis of variance followed by Student's two-tail t test.

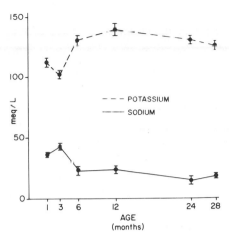

Figure 2. Intracellular Na and K concentrations in rat left atria as a function of age. $(Na)_i$ (solid line) and $(K)_i$, (dashed line) calculated at ages indicated by method described in text.

RESULTS

The total tissue water was highest in the 3 and 24 mo animals, and in both cases was significantly greater than in the 1 mo group (Fig. 1). The extracellular volume as measured by the inulin space did not decrease significantly between 1 and 3 mo, and increased significantly between 3 and 6 mo (Fig. 1). There was no apparent change in extracellular space thereafter including the 28 mo group which was not significantly different than the 24 mo group.

The increase in intracellular Na observed during the maturation stage, that is, between 1 and 3 mo, proved to be of significance (Fig. 2). However, intracellular Na decreased significantly between 3 and 6 mo, and thereafter remained relatively constant. Intracellular K concentration at 6 mo differed significantly from that at 1 and 3 mo; after 6 mo, the K concentration did not change appreciably (Fig. 2).

The Na influx rate constant exhibited a significant upward trend as a function of age with the exception of the 24 mo group (Fig. 3). The 24-month-old animals had a significantly lower rate constant than the 3-, 6-, 12- and 28-month-old animals. The K influx rate constant did not undergo any significant change as a function of age (Fig. 3).

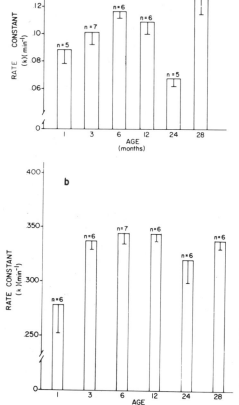

Figure 3. Sodium and potassium influx in rat left atria as a function of age. Influx rates of ^{22}Na (*a*) and ^{42}K (*b*) in atria excised at ages indicated were determined as accumulation rates by methods described in text.

The efflux of Na from the myocardium was found to be multiexponential. At least two rate components were obtained in ^{22}Na efflux studies (k_1, k_2). Figure 4 shows that k_1 decreased significantly between 6 and 12 mo, and remained relatively constant until 28 mo. The rate constant k_2 exhibited changes with age which did not prove to be significant. Potassium efflux experiments revealed one rate constant; efflux rate of ^{42}K was significantly greater at 1 and 3 mo than at the other ages (Fig. 5).

DISCUSSION

Our results indicate that ionic concentrations and ionic movements in myocardial tissue undergo changes during the life cycle of the rat. With respect to K, the increase in intracellular concentration between the ages of 1 and 6 mo may be accounted for by the decreased efflux of the ion during this period of life or by the increased extracellular space. Thereafter, efflux appeared to remain constant, thus accounting for the stabilized intracellular K concentration between the ages of 6 mo through 28 mo. These findings are consistent with the observations of Cavoto et al. (2) on the age-correlated changes of electrical properties of rat atria. These authors found that both the duration of the plateau and the time to 95% repolarization of the action potential increased with age up to 12 mo.

With Na, we have observed an age-correlated decrease in the intracellular concentration of this ion despite a concomitant small increase in influx and hardly any change in the k_2 rate constant of efflux. However, it should be kept in mind that the resting Na exchange, which is thought to contribute significantly to the total Na exchange, has not as

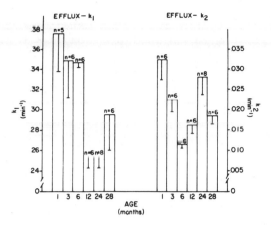

Figure 4. Sodium efflux in rat left atria as a function of age. Atria from rats at ages indicated were loaded with ^{22}Na and efflux was followed as rate of ^{22}Na disappearance by methods described in text.

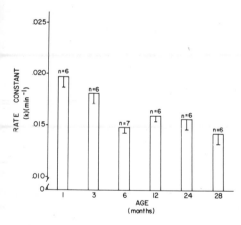

Figure 5. Potassium efflux in rat left atria as a function of age. Atria from rats at ages indicated were loaded with ^{42}K and efflux was followed as rate of ^{42}K disappearance by methods described in text.

yet been determined in these age-dependent studies. It is suggested that in view of the large increase of the inulin space after 3 mo, the sodium most likely redistributes with the water to the outside of the cell. Al-ternatively, the calculated decrease of $(Na)_i$ could occur if the inulin space were an overestimation of the extracellular space in older animals.

Both our studies and those of Cavoto et al. (2) demonstrate age-related changes at the level of the excitable membranes of the myocardium. Such changes may very well, therefore, be responsible for the observed overall functional alterations of the heart as it ages. Furthermore, the reactivity of the heart to pharmacological agents used in cardiovascular therapy would be expected to be influenced by such age-related physiological changes. Our experiments are now being extended to include the study of the effects of age on the reactivity of the heart to therapeutic agents.

REFERENCES

1. BERG, B. N. J. Gerontol. 10: 420 423, 1955.
2. CAVOTO, F., G. KELLIHER AND J. ROBERTS. Am. J. Physiol. 226: 1293–1297, 1974.
3. CHERASKIN, E., AND W. M. RINGSDORF, JR. J. Am. Geriat. Soc. 19: 271–275, 1971.
4. COUCH, J. R., T. C. WEST AND H. E. HOFF. Circulation Res. 24: 19–31, 1969.

5. EVERITT, A. V. *Gerontologia* 2: 204–212, 1958.
0. GOERKE, J., AND E. PAGE. *J. Gen. Physiol.* 48: 933–948, 1965.
7. HARRIS, J. B., AND A. R. LUFF. *Comp. Biochem. Physiol.* 33: 923–931, 1970.
8. HAZELWOOD, C. F. *Johns Hopkins Med. J.* 127: 136–145, 1970.
9. HAZELWOOD, C. F., AND B. L. NICHOLS. *Johns Hopkins Med. J.* 125: 119–133, 1969.
10. HOLLAND, W. C., AND R. L. KLEIN. *Circulation Res.* 6: 516–521, 1958.
11. KLEIN, R. L., AND W. C. HOLLAND. *Am. J. Physiol.* 193: 239–243, 1958.
12. MORI, K., AND J. P. DURUISSEAU. *Can. J. Biochem. Biophys.* 38: 919–928, 1960.
13. PAGE, E., AND A. K. SOLOMON. *J. Gen. Physiol.* 44: 327–344, 1960.
14. RIGGS, D. S. In: *The Mathematical Approach of Physiological Problems.* Cambridge, Mass.: The MIT Press, 1970, p. 120.
15. SHAH, G. B., S. R. SHAH AND H. C. MERCHANT. *Indian Heart J.* 7: 278–288, 1968.
16. WILLEMS, J. L., J. ROELANDT, H. DE-GEEST, H. KESTELOOT AND J. V. JOOSSENS. *Circulation* 42: 37–42, 1970.

Enzymatic studies on the skeletal myosin A and actomyosin of aging rats[1,2]

G. KALDOR AND B. K. MIN

Department of Physiology and Biophysics
The Medical College of Pennsylvania
Philadelphia, Pennsylvania 19129

ABSTRACT

Myosin A and actomyosin were isolated from the skeletal muscle of old and young rats. The velocity of the Ca^{2+} activated myosin A ATPase was increased in the case of the older animals. On the other hand the velocity of the Mg^{2+} activated actomyosin ATPase was decreased in the skeletal muscle of the aging rats. At 5×10^{-5}M EGTA concentration the inhibition of the Mg^{2+} activated myosin B ATPase of the 1-month-old rats was two- to threefold smaller than that of the older animals. It was shown that the myosin A component of the actomyosin was responsible for the decreased troponin inhibition in the case of the 1-month-old rats. Between the ages of 1 month and 29 months the number of free myosin A SH groups decreases by 50%. The lipid peroxidation in the muscle tissue of the 29-month-old rats was threefold greater than that in the muscle of the 1-month-old animals.
—KALDOR, G., AND B. K. MIN. Enzymatic studies on the skeletal myosin A and actomyosin of aging rats. *Federation Proc.* 34: 191–194, 1975.

It is well known that muscular strength decreases with age. The cause of this decline is not understood. For this reason it appeared to be important to obtain information about the enzymatic and molecular characteristics of the contractile proteins of aging animals. The objective of this study was to compare some molecular and enzymatic properties of myosin A and actomyosin molecules obtained from young adult and old rats.

[1] From Session VI, *Development and Aging at the Molecular Level*, of the FASEB Conference on *Biology of Development and Aging*, presented at the 58th Annual Meeting of the Federation of American Societies for Experimental Biology, Atlantic City, N.J., April 11, 1974.

[2] Supported by National Institutes of Health Grants HD 06267 and NB 06517.

Abbreviations: K_m = Michaelis constant; V_m = maximal velocity; E_{act} = Energy of activation; SDS = Sodium dodecyl sulfate; EGTA = Ethylene glycol-bis-(β-aminoethylether)-N, N-tetra acetic acid; P_i = inorganic phosphate; μmole P_i mg prot^{-1} min^{-1} = μmole inorganic phosphate liberated by 1 mg enzyme protein in 1 minute.

MATERIALS AND METHODS

Myosin A and Myosin B were prepared essentially as described by
Mommaerts (9). Myosin A was further
purified by centrifugation at 30,000
rpm in the presence of 10 mM ATP
and Mg^{2+}. The myosin A used for gel
electrophoresis was further purified
by ammonium sulfate fractionation
(12). Natural tropomyosin (tropomyosin + troponin) was prepared
according to the method of Ebashi
and Ebashi (4). Troponin-free actin
was obtained as described by Bailin
and Barany (1). Subfragment 1 was
prepared according to the method of
Lowey et al. (8). These proteins were
purified from the skeletal muscle of
CD Fischer rats. The yields were the
same from the tissues of old and
young animals.

In previous publications we have
described the methods used for the
determination of molecular weight
(6), helical content (5), protein side
chains (6), K_m, V_m and E_{act} (13),
steady-state ATPase (13) and pre-

steady-state ATPase activities (7, 11).
Starch gel electrophoresis was performed in a 10% polyacrylamide gel
containing 0.1% SDS (10). Peroxidation of lipids in the muscle tissue
was measured by the method of Bernheim et al. (3).

RESULTS

It may be seen from Fig. 1 that the
Ca^{2+} activated myosin A ATPase
doubled between 1 month and 3
months of age and that the Mg^{2+}
activated actomyosin ATPase decreased between 6 months and 29
months of age. The results compiled
in Table 1 show that the V_m of the
rat myosin A enzyme increased significantly between 1 month and 29
months of age. The E_{act} of the rat
myosin A ATPase decreased slightly
while the K_m of the same enzyme
increased but not significantly, between 1 month and 29 months of
age.

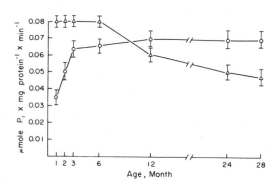

Figure 1. The Ca^{2+} activated myosin A ATPase
and the Mg^{2+} activated actomyosin ATPase of
rat skeletal muscle between 1 month and 24
months of age. ○ Each tube contained 1 mg/ml
myosin A, 5 μmole ATP, 5 μmole Ca^{2+}, 50
μmole KCl, and 25 μmole, pH 7.5 Tris buffer
in 1 ml total volume. △ Each tube contained
1 mg myosin B, 5 μmole ATP, 5 μmole

Mg^{2+}, 0.1 μmole Ca^{2+}, 50 μmole KCl, and
25 μmole, pH 7.5 Tris buffer, in 1 ml total
volume. An average of 4–6 experiments was
used to determine the individual points represented on the graphs. The verticle bars indicate the standard deviations. The incubations
were performed at 37 C.

TABLE 1. Some kinetic constants of rat myosins

| Age, mo | K_m, mole/l | | Steady-state ATPase | | | | | | P_i burst,[b] μmole P_i M^{-1} | | No. of expt. |
| | | | V_m [a] | | E_{act} | | | | | | |
	$\bar{x}$	SD	$\bar{x}$	SD	$\bar{x}$	SD	No. of expt.		$\bar{x}$	SD	
1	2×10^{-5}	0.8×10^{-5}	0.055	0.004	13,500	1,500	4		0.8	0.2	5
3	5×10^{-5}	1.0×10^{-5}	0.100	0.006	11,000	1,400	3				
6	4×10^{-5}	1.2×10^{-5}	0.120	0.006	11,000	1,500	3				
12	5×10^{-5}	1.0×10^{-5}	0.130	0.008	10,000	1,300	3				
24	5×10^{-5}	0.7×10^{-5}	0.140	0.006	9,500	1,300	3		1.5	0.4	3
29	6×10^{-5}	1.0×10^{-5}	0.130	0.006	9,600	1,000	3		1.8	0.4	4

[a] V_m, μmole P_i mg^{-1} min^{-1}. [b] P_i burst = Presteady-state phosphate burst.

TABLE 2. Some molecular parameters of rat myosins

| Age, mo | MW | No. of expt | Helical content, % | No. of expt | His | | Tyr | | Try | | No. of expt | SH | | No. of expt |
					$\bar{x}$	SD	$\bar{x}$	SD	$\bar{x}$	SD		$\bar{x}$	SD	
1	510,000	1	68	1	16	1.6	18	0.5	5	0.3	3	9.6	0.4	6
6	—	—	69	1	17	1.6	19	0.7	4	0.3	3	6.0	0.3	4
12	—	—	67	1	18	1.7	18	0.6	4	0.3	3	6.3	0.3	4
24	500,000	1	69	1	16	1.6	17	0.6	5	0.3	3	4.2	0.3	5

The results shown in Table 1 and Fig. 2 demonstrate that the myosin A enzyme of the 1-month-old rat produced 0.8 mole P_i per mole of myosin and the same enzyme obtained from the 24-month-old animal cleaved 1.8 mole P_i per mole of protein in the presteady state. On the other hand the presteady-state phosphate bursts of the actomyosins obtained from 1-month-old and 24-month-old rats were 7.8 mole per 600,000 g protein and 6.0 mole per 600,000 g protein respectively.

These kinetic studies indicated an alteration on the active site or sites of the myosin A molecule during the development and aging of the rat. We therefore investigated the molecular characteristics of rat myosins obtained from young and old animals in some detail.

Polyacrylamide gel electrophoresis of highly purified myosin A and subfragment 1 obtained from 1-month-, 12-month- and 24-month-old animals failed to disclose any qualitative or

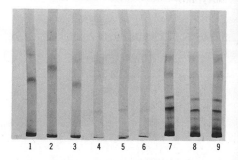

Figure 3. Electrophoresis of rat myosin A and subfragment 1 on SDS-polyacrylamide gel. *1)* Myosin A, 1 mo, loading 5 µg, electrophoresis time 4 hours; *2)* myosin A, 12 mo, loading 5 µg, electrophoresis time 5 hours; *3)* myosin A, 24 mo, loading 5 µg, electrophoresis time 4 hours; *4)* subfragment 1, 1 mo, loading 1 µg, electrophoresis time 4 hours; *5)* subfragment 1, 12 mo, loading 2 µg, electrophoresis time 4 hours; *6)* subfragment 1, 24 mo, loading 1 µg, electrophoresis time 4 hours; *7)* trypsinized myosin A, 1 mo, loading 7 µg, electrophoresis time 4 hours; *8)* trypsinized myosin A, 12 mo, loading 7µg, electrophoresis time 4 hours; and *9)* trypsinized myosin A, 24 mo, loading 7 µg, electrophoresis time 4 hours.

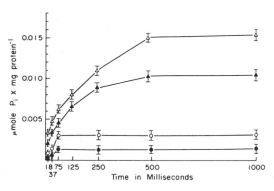

Figure 2. The presteady-stage ATPase activity of myosin A and myosin B obtained from 1-month-old and 24-month old rats. Each tube contained 0.5 µmole/ml ATP, 2 µmole/ml Mg^{2+}, 0.1 µmole/ml Ca^{2+}, 50 µmole/ml KCl, and 25 µmole/ml, pH 7.5 Tris buffer, to which the following were added: △ myosin B, 1 mo, ▲ myosin B, 24 mo, ○ myosin A, 1 month, ● myosin A, 24 month. An average of 6 experiments was used to determine the individual points represented on the graphs.

The vertical bars indicate the standard deviations. Radioactive ATP was used for the assay in 4 experiments with myosin A and in 2 experiments with myosin B. In these experiments the protein concentration was 1 mg/ml in the mixtures. In 2 experiments with myosin A and in 4 experiments with myosin B, a colorimetric method was used to determine ATPase activity. In these experiments the protein concentration was 5 mg/ml. The assays were performed at 37 C.

quantitative differences. (Fig. 3, gels 1–6). A brief treatment of these myosin A proteins by trypsin produced a number of split products that migrated into the gel. The qualitative and quantitative distribution of these split products after the trypsin treatment was the same for all myosins obtained from 1-month-, 12-month- and 24-month-old rats. (Fig. 3, gels 7–9). The experimental results compiled in Table 2 show that the molecular weight, helical content and number of histidine, tyrosine and tryptophan sidechains were similar for the myosin A enzymes obtained from the muscle of old and young rats. On the other hand one mole of myosin A obtained from the 1-month-old rat contained 9.6 mole of SH groups while the myosin A of the 24-month-old rat contained only 4.2 moles of SH groups per mole of protein.

Peroxidation has been implicated as a possible cause of damage in aging tissues (2). Our experimental results (Table 3) show that peroxidation in the muscle tissue of the 24-month-old

rat was three to four times higher than that of the 2-month-old animal. This was true whether or not the peroxidation was enhanced by the addition of $FeCl_3$ and ADP.

To explore further the physiological implications of the observed enzymatic and molecular alterations of the developing and aging myosin A molecule we investigated the effect of EGTA on the ATPase activity of myosin B obtained from young and old rats. Figure 4 demonstrates that the ATPase activity of the myosin B enzymes obtained from the 3-month-, 6-month- and 12-month-old rats decreased by 75% if 5×10^{-5}M EGTA was added to the mixtures. Under similar experimental conditions the ATPase activity of myosin B of the 1-month-old rat decreased only by 25% and that of the 24-month-old rat by 60%.

It was of interest to determine which protein component of myosin B was responsible for the decreased EGTA sensitivity observed in the enzyme obtained from the 1-month-old rat. Therefore, the various com-

TABLE 3. Peroxidation of muscle tissue[a]

Age, mo	Time of incubation, min	No addition		μmoles malonyl dialdehyde, 30μM FeCl$_3$ + 3μM ADP added		No. of expt
		$\bar{x}$	SD	$\bar{x}$	SD	
2	30	0.28	0.05	0.47	0.17	5
	60	0.56	0.12	0.94	0.15	5
12	30	0.80	0.15	1.73	0.30	3
	60	1.25	0.28	2.56	0.38	3
24	30	1.15	0.15	2.50	0.36	5
	60	1.68	0.28	2.98	0.50	5
28	30	1.20	0.20	2.41	0.30	4
	60	1.72	0.32	3.27	0.50	4

[a] A 10% suspension of muscle homogenate 27 mg prot/ml was incubated for 30 or 60 min at pH 7.5 and at 37 C. In the presence or absence of 30μMFeCl$_3$ + 3μM ADP malonyl dialdehyde formation was assayed as described in the text.

ponents of myosin B were purified from 1-month-old and 24-month-old rats. Figure 5 shows the inhibitory effect of natural tropomyosin on the Mg²⁺ activated ATPase activity of various synthetic actomyosins in the presence of 1×10^{-4} M EGTA. It may be seen that both "old" and young natural tropomyosin had a greater inhibitory effect on the ATPase activity of those synthetic actomyosins that contained a myosin A component prepared from the muscle of 24-month-old rats. This was true in the

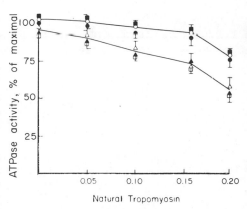

Natural Tropomyosin

Figure 5. The effect of natural tropomyosin on the ATPase activity of synthetic actomyosins assembled from 1-month-old and 24-month-old rats. Each tube contained 5 μmole ATP, 5μmole Mg²⁺, 0.1 μmole EGTA, 50 μmole KCl, and 25 μmole, pH 7.5 Tris buffer with the following additions: ■ 1 mg myosin A, 1 mo + 0.5 mg actin, 24 mo + natural tropomyosin, 24 mo; ○ 1 mg myosin A, 1 mo + 0.5 mg actin, 24 mo + natural tropomyosin, 1 mo; ● 1 mg myosin A, 1 mo + 0.5 mg actin, 1 mo + natural tropomyosin, 24 mo; △ 1 mg myosin A, 24 mo + 0.5 mg actin, 1 mo + natural tropomyosin, 1 mo; ▲ 1 mg myosin A, 24 mo + 0.5 mg actin, 24 mo + natural tropomyosin, 24 mo; and □ 1 mg myosin A, 24 mo + 0.5 mg actin 1 mo + natural tropomyosin, 24 mo. The total volume of the mixtures was 1 ml. The experiments were performed at 37 C. The average of 3–4 experiments was used to determine the individual points represented on the graph. The vertical bars indicate the standard deviations.

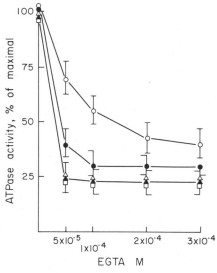

EGTA   M

Figure 4. The effect of EGTA on the Mg²⁺ activated ATPase activity of myosin B obtained from rats between 1 month and 24 months of age. Each tube contained 5 μmole ATP, 5 μmole Mg²⁺, 50 μmole KCl, and 25 μmole, pH 7.5 Tris buffer to which the following were added: ○ 1 mg myosin B, 1 mo, △ 1 mg myosin B, 3 mo, ▲ 1 mg myosin B, 6 mo, □ 1 mg myosin B, 12 mo, and ● 1 mg myosin B, 24 mo. The total volume of the mixtures was 1 ml. The incubations were performed at 37 C. An average of 4–6 experiments was used to determine the individual points represented on the graph. The vertical bars indicate the standard deviations.

presence of the actin that was obtained from the 1-month-old rat and also in the presence of the actin prepared from the 24-month-old animal. Conversely both natural tropomyosins inhibited the ATPase activity of the synthetic actomyosins to a lesser extent if these molecules contained myosin A obtained from the skeletal muscle tissue of 1-month-old rats whether the actin component of the mixture was obtained from young or old rat muscle.

DISCUSSION

The enzymatic studies performed on the myosin A and actomyosin of young, adult and old rats clearly showed that the maximal velocity of these enzymes was changing during the aging process (Fig. 1, Fig. 2 and Table 1). The presteady-state phosphate burst measurements suggested that in the absence of actin only one of the two myosin A heads were active in the myosin A enzyme of the 1-month-old rat. On the other hand both myosin A heads seemed to be active in the case of proteins obtained from the 24-month-old rats (Fig. 2).

We have compared several important molecular parameters of the myosin A molecules of young, adult and old rats (Table 2). It was found that there was a gradual decrease in the free SH group content of this protein during the aging process (Table 2). Furthermore the peroxidation was significantly higher in the muscle homogenates of old rats than in those of young rats. Increased cellular peroxidation may explain the decreased SH content of the myosin A molecule of the aging rats. The decreased SH content of these proteins may be related to an altered physiological function or stability in the case of the aging animals. We offer this "mechanism" as one possible explanation for our experimental results. It has to be realized that in this case the causal correlation between peroxidation, protein SH,

and function remains to be proven.

It was also shown that the actomyosin ATPase activity of adult and old rats was more sensitive to Ca^{2+} than that of the young rats (Fig. 4). The experiments performed with purified myosin A, actin, and natural tropomyosin have shown conclusively that the decreased Ca^{2+} sensitivity of the young actomyosin molecule was due solely to its myosin A component.

REFERENCES

1. BAILIN, G., AND M. BARANY. *J. Mechanochem. Cell Motility* 1: 189, 1972.
2. BARBER, A. A., AND F. BERNHEIM. *Advan. Gerontol. Res.* 2: 355, 1967.
3. BERNHEIM, F., M. L. C. BERNHEIM AND K. M. WILBUR. *J. Biol. Chem.* 171: 257, 1948.
4. EBASHI, S., AND F. EBASHI. *J. Biochem, Tokyo* 55: 604, 1964.
5. KALDOR, G. *Arch. Biochem. Biophys.* 127: 22, 1968.
6. KALDOR, G., J. GITLIN, F. WESTLEY AND B. W. VOLK *Biochemistry* 3: 1137, 1964.
7. KALDOR, G., AND Q. S. HSU. *Physiol. Chem. Phys.* 6: 67, 1974.
8. LOWEY, S., H. S. SLAYTER, A. G. WEEDS AND H. BAKER. *J. Mol. Biol.* 42: 1, 1969.
9. MOMMAERTS, W. F. H. M., *Methods Med. Res.* 7: 1, 1958.
10. PATERSON, B., AND R. C. STROHMAN. *Biochemistry* 9: 4094, 1970.
11. SCHLIESELFELD, L. H., AND G. KALDOR. *Biochim. Biophys. Acta.* 328: 481, 1973.
12. TSAO, T. C., *Biochim. Biophys. Acta* 11: 368, 1953.
13. WACHSBERGER, P., AND G. KALDOR. *Arch. Biochem. Biophys.* 143: 127, 1971.

Index